Parsley

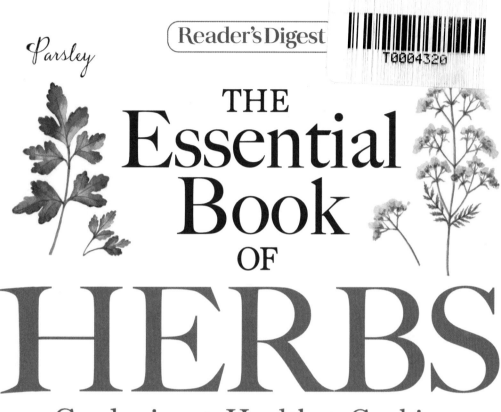

THE
Essential
Book
OF
HERBS

Gardening * Health * Cooking

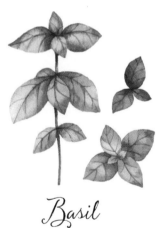

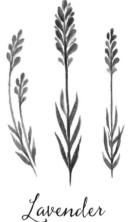

Basil *Lavender* *Oregano*

New York / Montreal

A READER'S DIGEST BOOK

ISBN 978-1-62145-548-6 (pbk)
ISBN 978-1-62145-549-3 (epub)

Library of Congress catalogued the previous edition of this book as follows:
Library of Congress Cataloging-in-Publication Data

The complete illustrated book of herbs : growing, health & beauty, cooking, crafts.
      p. cm.
      Includes index.
1. Herbs. 2. Herb gardening. 3. Herbs--Therapeutic use. 4. Cookery (Herbs)
I. Reader's Digest Association.
      SB351.H5C65 2009
      635'.7--dc22
                  2008046082

We are committed to both the quality of our products and the service we provide
to our customers. We value your comments, so please feel free to contact us.

    Reader's Digest Adult Trade Publishing
    44 South Broadway
    White Plains, NY 10601

For more Reader's Digest products and information, visit our website:
    www.rd.com (in the United States)
    www.readersdigest.ca (in Canada)

Printed in China

1 3 5 7 9 10 8 6 4 2

IMPORTANT NOTE FOR OUR READERS

Growing herbs: Some herbs can become invasive and may be toxic to livestock. This information
has been given where possible, but regulations do change from time to time. Readers are
advised to consult local plant services if they have any concerns.

Herbal medicine: While the creators of this book have made every effort to be as accurate and
up to date as possible, medical and pharmacological knowledge is constantly changing. Readers
are advised to consult a qualified medical specialist for individual advice. Moreover, even though
they are natural, herbs contain chemical substances that can sometimes have marked side
effects. If used unwisely, they can be toxic. The writers, researchers, editors, and publishers
of this book cannot be held liable for any errors, omissions, or actions that may be taken as a
consequence of information contained in this book.

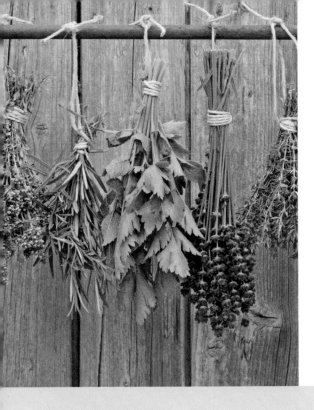

Contents

Herb directory   4

An A-to-Z guide to more than 100 herbs
and the various ways to use them

Gardening   138

Tips on growing herbs
successfully, from seed or plant

Herbal medicine   156

Herbal remedies to boost general
health and well-being and treat
common ailments

Index   214

Introduction

Herbs have been used for thousands
of years to flavor and preserve food,
treat ailments, ward off pests and
diseases, freshen the air, and decorate
and enhance our lives. Over the centuries
they have also become associated with
fascinating myths, legends, and folklore.

In general terms, an herb is a plant
that is valued for its flavor, aroma, or
medicinal properties, and different parts
of an herb — such as the stalks, flowers,
fruits, seeds, roots, or leaves — may
have important applications. From small
herbs growing beside our highways
to bushy shrubs in mountain areas to
tall trees in lush tropical rain forests,
there are literally thousands of plants
all over the world that belong to the
herb family.

In *The Essential Book of Herbs* we have
combined traditional knowledge and
herbal wisdom with up-to-date advice
from herbalists, natural therapists,
gardening experts, and cooks to show
you how to grow herbs successfully and
make the best use of them in your daily
life. The comprehensive information
on more than 100 herbs in the A-to-Z
directory, together with the chapters
on how to use them, will enable you to
improve your health, save money, and
use fewer chemicals in your home.

With herbal remedies, gardening
know-how, safe and delicious recipes,
this practical reference guide to herbs is
packed with information and illustrated
with beautiful photographs. We hope you
will find it a source of inspiration.

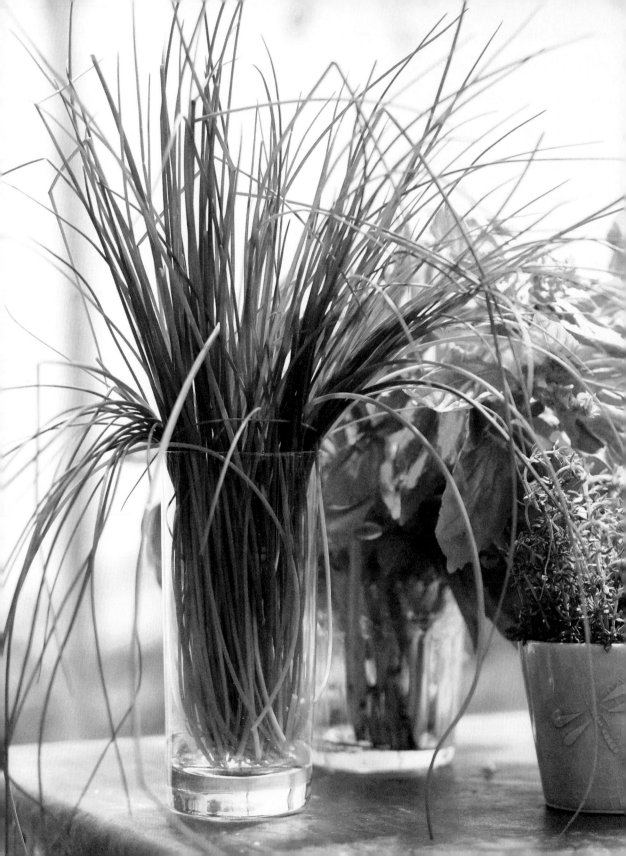

Herb directory

The history of herbs, their uses, and methods of cultivation are fascinating, rewarding topics. This practical guide to more than 100 herbs, most of which can be grown in a home garden, tells you how to cultivate, use and store herbs.

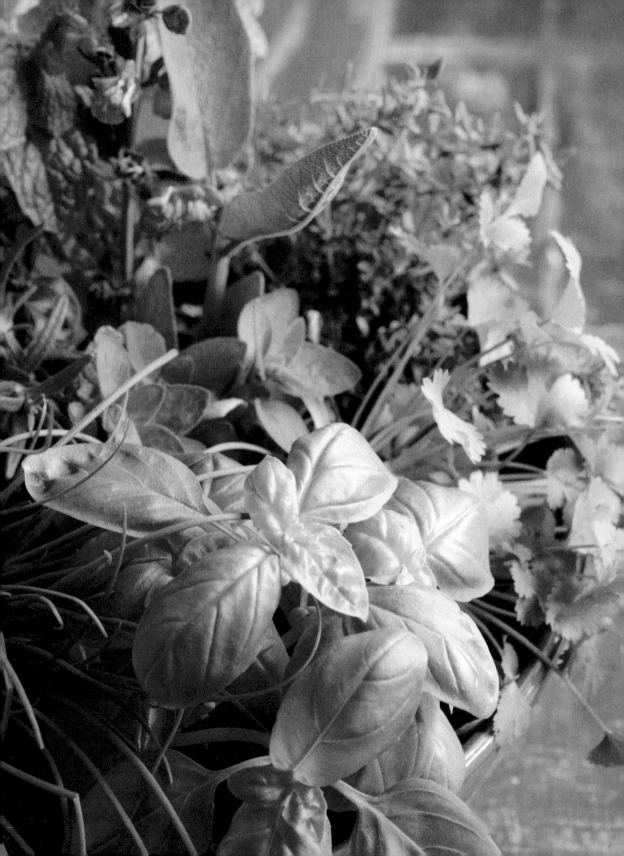

Herb directory

Aloe vera	8	
Angelica	9	
Anise	10	
Anise hyssop	11	
Arnica	12	
Artemisia	13	
Basil	14	
Bay	17	
Bergamot	20	
Borage	21	
Brahmi	22	
Burdock	23	
Calendula	24	
Caraway	25	
Catnip	26	
Celery	27	
Chamomile	28	
Chervil	29	
Chili	30	
Clove pinks	34	
Comfrey	35	
Coriander	36	
Curry plant	37	
Dandelion	38	
Dill	39	
Echinacea	40	
Elder	41	
Eucalyptus	42	
Evening primrose	44	
Eyebright	45	
Fennel	46	
Feverfew	47	
Flax	48	
Galangal	49	
Garlic & onions	50	
Ginger	54	
Ginkgo	55	
Ginseng	56	
Gotu kola	57	
Heartsease	58	
Hops	59	
Horseradish & wasabi	60	
Horsetail	61	
Hyssop	62	
Iris	63	
Jasmine	64	
Lavender	66	
Lemon balm	69	
Lemon grass	70	
Lemon verbena	71	
Licorice	72	
Lime	73	
Lovage	74	
Mallow & hollyhock	75	
Marjoram & oregano	76	
Meadowsweet	78	
Mint	79	
Nettle	81	
Parsley	82	
Passionflower	84	
Peony	86	
Perilla	87	
Plantain	88	
Poppy	89	
Primrose & cowslip	91	
Purslane	92	
Red clover	93	
Rocket or arugula	94	
Rose	96	
Rosemary	100	
St. John's wort	104	
Sage	105	
Salad burnet	108	
Savory	109	
Scented geranium	110	
Sorrel	112	
Sweet cicely	113	
Sweet myrtle	114	
Sweet violet	115	
Sweet woodruff	117	
Tansy	118	
Tarragon	119	
Tea	120	
Tea tree	122	
Thyme	123	
Turmeric	125	
Valerian	126	
Vervain	127	
Viburnum	128	
Watercress & nasturtium	129	
White horehound	130	
Yarrow	131	
Spices	132	
Berries	134	
Trees	136	

Aloe vera

Latin Name *Aloe vera* syn. *A. barbadensis, A. vulgaris* Aloeaceae
Other common names **Barbados aloe, bitter aloe, Curacao aloe**
Part used **Leaves**

The ancient Egyptians called it the "plant of immortality," and Cleopatra used its juices to help preserve her beauty. The clear gel from the cut leaves has soothing and healing properties. Aloe vera is suitable for large pots and rockeries and as an indoor plant.

Gardening

Aloe vera is a succulent plant with very fleshy light green leaves that create a fan from the stemless base. In warm climates it produces narrow tubular yellow flowers. Cape aloe (*A. ferox*) is a tall single-stemmed species that has long, grayish, spiny succulent leaves and tall, handsome spikes of tawny orange flowers.

Position ▶ Aloe requires a sunny position and a very well-drained soil.

Propagation ▶ Aloe vera can be raised from seed, but it rarely sets seed in other than warm climates. Propagate it from offsets that form at the base of the plant. Allow these plantlets to dry for two days before planting them into small pots filled with a gritty free-draining potting mix. Once they are well established, transfer them to their permanent position.

Maintenance ▶ Aloe is affected by even light frosts, and in areas where winter temperatures fall below 40°F (5°C), it is best grown in pots and brought indoors in cool weather. It makes an excellent indoor plant in good light.

Pests and diseases ▶ Mealybug may prove a problem for plants grown indoors, although it rarely occurs on those grown in the garden. Spray with insecticidal soap, which is nontoxic to animals and leaves no residue. Apply it late in the afternoon, because it can burn sensitive plants in full sun or at high temperatures.

Harvesting and storing ▶ Harvest leaves as needed, using only as much of the leaf as required. Cut the used end back to undamaged tissue, then wrap in plastic wrap and store in the refrigerator for further use.

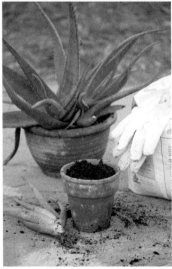

Plant the dried-out plantlets into small pots filled with gritty free-draining potting mix.

Aloe vera

Herbal medicine

Aloe sp., including *Aloe vera syn. A. barbadensis and A. ferox.* Part used: leaves. The clear mucilaginous gel from the center of the aloe vera leaf has anti-inflammatory and healing properties. Probably best known for its ability to encourage the healing of burns, aloe vera gel can also be applied to wounds, abrasions, eczema, psoriasis, and ulcers.

The exudate from the cut aloe vera leaf acts as an extremely cathartic laxative, and consequently, homemade preparations of aloe vera should not be consumed. Commercial preparations (without the laxative constituents) are available, and preliminary research indicates that they may be beneficial in a range of conditions, including non-insulin-dependent diabetes mellitus and high blood lipid levels.

For the safe and appropriate use of aloe vera, see First aid, *page 194*. Note: Do not take aloe vera internally if you are pregnant or breastfeeding. Topical application is considered safe during these times.

Natural beauty

Ultra-soothing and nourishing for even the most parched and dehydrated skin, aloe vera is also a mild exfoliant, gently removing dead skin cells and stimulating cell regeneration, helping to prevent scarring and diminish wrinkles.

Angelica

Latin Name **Angelica archangelica** Apiaceae
Other common name **Archangel**
Parts used **Leaves, stems, seeds, roots**

A showy, aromatic herb, angelica has both medicinal and culinary uses. Angelica's name honors the archangel Raphael, who is said to have revealed to a monk that the plant could cure the plague.

Gardening

Native to northern Europe, *Angelica archangelica* grows to 4 ft. (1.2 m) and has ribbed hollow stems, compound leaves and a flowering stem that can reach 6 ft. (1.8 m), although it often does not appear until the third year.

Ornamental angelica (*A. pachycarpa*) grows to about 3.5 ft. (1 m) high and has shiny dark green leaves. It is mostly grown for its ornamental value. Purple-stem angelica (*A. atropurpurea*) has similar uses to *A. archangelica*. It grows to about 6 ft. (1.8 m), has stems suffused with purple, and pale green to white flowers. The most striking species is the beautiful *A. gigas*, which grows to 6 ft. (1.8 m), with deep garnet buds opening to large wine red to rich purple flowers.

Position ▶ Angelica requires a shady position in well-drained but moist and slightly acidic soil that has been enriched with compost. Allow a distance of 3.5 ft. (1 m) between plants.

Propagation ▶ Plant angelica seed soon after collection. Mix the seed with damp, but not wet, vermiculite and place the mixture in a sealed plastic bag (see also *page 40*). Store in the crisper section of the refrigerator for six to eight weeks before planting into seed trays. Barely cover the seed, and keep the soil moist. Transplant seedlings when around 4 in. (10 cm) high or when the fifth and sixth leaves emerge.

Maintenance ▶ Plants die once the seed has matured, but you can delay this by removing the emerging flower stem. First-year plants will die back in winter but will grow readily in spring. Water regularly.

Pests and diseases ▶ This plant is virtually pest- and disease-free. The flowers are attractive to many beneficial insects, including parasitoid wasps and lacewings.

Harvesting and storing ▶ Harvest the leaves and flowering stalks in the second year. Dig the roots at the end of the second year, then wash and dry them. Gather the seed when brown and dry.

Herbal medicine

Angelica archangelica. Part used: roots. Angelica is an important digestive tonic in European herbal medicine. It stimulates the production of gastric juices and can relieve symptoms of poor appetite, dyspepsia and nausea. Angelica can also reduce the discomfort of flatulence, stomach cramps and bloating. It is a warming herb and suited to individuals who suffer from the effects of cold weather.

For the safe and appropriate use of angelica, consult your healthcare professional. Do not use angelica in greater than culinary quantities.

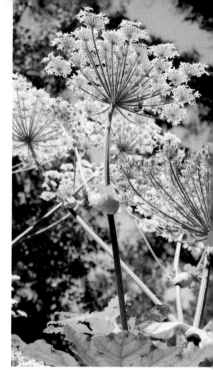

Angelica (*Angelica archangelica*)

Cooking

Angelica is a popular boiled or steamed vegetable dish in some Scandinavian countries; it has a musky, bittersweet taste. The dried seeds and stems are used (in maceration or via the essential oil) in vermouth and liqueurs such as Chartreuse and Benedictine. Crystallized leaves and young stems are a popular decoration for cakes and sweets.

Blanch young shoots for use in salads. Use leaves and stalks in marinades and in poaching liquids for seafood. Add leaves to recipes for tart fruits, such as rhubarb. They cut the acidity, and their sweetness allows you to reduce the amount of sugar.

Anise

Latin Name *Pimpinella anisum* Apiaceae
Other common names **Aniseed, common anise**
Parts used **Roots (anise only), leaves, seeds, dried fruits (star anise only)**

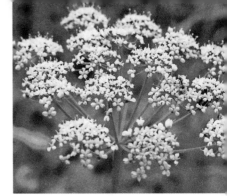

Anise (*Pimpinella anisum*)

Anise is responsible for much of the "licorice" flavoring in baked goods, liqueurs, teas, and chewing gum. Chinese star anise and aniseed myrtle, although unrelated to anise, have a similar flavor.

Gardening

Anise is an aromatic annual with stalked, toothed leaves. The slender flowering stems bear clusters of white flowers followed by ridged gray seeds.

Chinese star anise (*Illicium verum*, Family Illiciaceae), an evergreen tree, bears fruits that open to an eight-pointed star. Do not confuse it with the neurotoxic Japanese star anise (*Illicium anisatum*) or the inedible Florida anise (*I. floridanum*).

Position ▶ Anise prefers an enriched, light, well-drained and fairly neutral soil.

Propagation ▶ Sow anise seed directly in spring. Propagate Chinese star anise by semi-ripe cuttings; they will grow in well-drained but moist, acidic soil in light shade. Propagate aniseed myrtle from semi-hardwood cuttings. It is quite hardy, will grow in full sunlight, and prefers a deep, rich, moist acidic soil.

Maintenance ▶ Keep anise free of weeds.

Pests and diseases ▶ Anise repels aphids and attracts beneficial insects, such as parasitoid wasps.

Harvesting and storing ▶ Cut anise when the seeds are fully developed. Tie bunches inside paper bags and hang them upside down to dry and catch the seed. Harvest leaves as required. Dig up roots in autumn. Harvest star anise fruits just before ripening, and harvest firm leaves of aniseed myrtle anytime.

Herbal medicine

Pimpinella anisum, Illicium verum. Part used: dried ripe fruits. Anise and its Chinese equivalent, star anise, are used medicinally for similar purposes. Despite belonging to different plant families, the essential oils derived from the seeds of each plant both contain a high percentage of a compound called anethole, which imparts the licorice-like flavor. They both possess calming and antispasmodic properties, making them ideal remedies for alleviating flatulence, intestinal colic, and bloating. Do not give star anise to infants and young children, as it has produced serious side effects. For the safe and appropriate use of anise and star anise, see Indigestion, *page 178*, and Wind, bloating & flatulence, *page 180*. For aniseed myrtle consult your healthcare professional. Do not use these herbs in greater than culinary quantities if you are pregnant or breastfeeding.

Cooking

Anise seeds and oil are used throughout Europe in drinks such as the French pastis, the Greek ouzo, and Turkish raki. Use the seeds whole or crushed, but for the best flavor grind them as you need them.

Use them in bakery goods, confectionery, tomato-based dishes, vegetable and seafood dishes, curries, pickles, soups, and stews. Add the young leaves sparingly to green salads, fish dishes, fruit salads, and cooked vegetables.

The leaves of aniseed myrtle are a major Australian bush-food spice. Use dried or fresh to flavor desserts, preserves, sweet or savory sauces, and marinades.

A culinary star

Star anise is an essential ingredient in many Asian cuisines. In Vietnamese cooking it is used to flavor the noodle soup known as pho. Along with Sichuan pepper, cloves, cassia and fennel seeds, it is a component in Chinese five-spice mix (ingredients pictured below) and in Indian garam masala.

You can use star anise whole, broken, or ground. Add it to pork, chicken, or duck stews. Insert a whole star anise into the cavity of a chicken or duck before roasting.

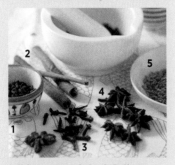

1. Sichuan pepper 2. Cassia 3. Cloves
4. Star anise 5. Fennel seeds

Anise hyssop

Latin Name *Agastache foeniculum* syn. *A. anethiodora* Lamiaceae
Other common names **Anise mint, giant blue hyssop, licorice mint**
Parts used **Leaves, flowers**

Many agastaches have fragrant foliage, their scents ranging from anise to mint and citrus. The leaves are used to make herbal tea, for flavoring, and in medicines, while the ornamental flower spikes, which attract beneficial insects, make a pretty addition to salads.

Gardening

Anise hyssop (*A. foeniculum*) is a hardy perennial with a sweet anise scent. Both balsamic and peppermint pennyroyal–scented forms are available.

Varieties ▶ Two varieties are 'Golden Jubilee', with its golden foliage, and white-flowered 'Alabaster', while fragrant varieties and hybrids include 'Heather Queen' and 'Just Peachy'.

Korean mint (*A. rugosa*), similar to anise hyssop, is a short-lived perennial, slightly more frost-tender, with a flower that ranges in color from rose to violet.

Licorice mint (*A. rupestris*) is a perennial with small licorice-scented

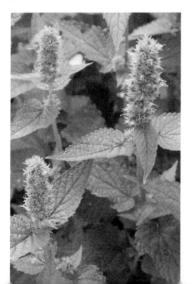

leaves and spikes of nectar-rich apricot flowers.

Hummingbird mint (*A. cana*) is a spectacular perennial species growing to 3 ft. (90 cm) with long, dense spikes of large rosy pink flowers and aromatic foliage.

Position ▶ *A. foeniculum, A. rugosa,* and *A. urticifolia* prefer light shade and a slightly acid to neutral soil. Most other species are from areas with a dry climate, are water-thrifty, prefer a light well-drained soil and sunny position, and are well suited to pot culture.

Propagation ▶ Sow agastache seed in spring; just cover the seed with soil. It takes 6 to 8 weeks to germinate. Plant in pots when large enough. Established plants produce many basal shoots in spring. Propagate these as softwood cuttings and plant outside in summer, or multiply plants by root division.

Maintenance ▶ Agastaches are generally hardy. In cool-climate areas keep plants in a greenhouse and transfer to the garden in their second spring; in warm-climate areas do so in the first summer.

Pests and diseases ▶ Leaf-chewing insects can be a minor problem.

Harvesting and storing ▶ Use the leaves and flowers freshly picked, or dry them by hanging them upside down in small bunches away from direct sunlight. They will retain their color and scent.

◀ Korean mint (*A. rugosa*), with its lavender blue flowers, is also known as wrinkled giant hyssop.

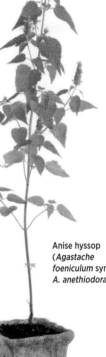

Anise hyssop (*Agastache foeniculum* syn. *A. anethiodora*)

Cooking

The flowers of anise hyssop yield large quantities of nectar, which was popular with North American beekeepers in the 19th century for producing a faintly aniseed-flavored honey. Native American Indians used it as a tea and a sweetener.

Infuse the dried leaves to make a hot or cold drink. Also, use them to season lamb, chicken or salmon. Add the seeds to cakes and muffins. Use the flowers or fresh leaves of anise hyssop or Korean mint in salads. Korean mint has a peppermint and aniseed flavor and aroma and is a good substitute for mint.

Arnica

Latin Name *Arnica montana* Asteraceae
Other common names **Leopard's bane, mountain tobacco**
Part used **Flowers**

There are about 30 species of Arnica, and all of them are perennials that spread by rhizomes. With its cheerful golden flowers, arnica has long been used for sprains and bruises as well as homeopathic treatments.

Gardening

Arnica montana is an aromatic hardy perennial that forms a basal rosette of leaves. From late spring to late summer, it produces flowering stems up to 2 ft. (60 cm) high, and each terminates in a single, golden daisy flower.

Varieties ▶ Most varieties are native to subalpine areas. European arnica (*A. montana*) is also known as mountain tobacco and leopard's bane (not to be confused with the ornamental perennial leopard's bane, *Doronicum orientale*, which is also poisonous, from the family Asteraceae). Native to the northern Iberian peninsula northward to Scandinavia, its natural habitat is low, ferte meadows to an altitude of about 1,000 ft. (3,000 m). *Arnica montana* is becoming rare, due to over-collection and the inroads of agriculture, and wild collection is being curtailed.

Consequently, the American species *A. chamissonis* is sometimes used in its place in herbal treatment.

Position ▶ Arnica requires a cool climate and full sun as well as slightly acid to slightly alkaline free-draining soil. In areas with wet winters, grow it in raised beds to prevent fungal attack.

Propagation ▶ You can raise arnica from seed but you'll need a period of moist cold. In climates with cold winters, sow the seed outside in autumn. In milder winter areas, stratify the seed by mixing it with a little damp vermiculite or sterile sand. Seal it in a plastic bag, and place it in the crisper tray of the refrigerator for about 12 weeks before sowing. Propagate mature plants by division in spring.

Maintenance ▶ Arnica is a slow grower and resents competition from pasture weeds such as white clover. Mulch well and weed regularly, or grow plants in weed mat.

Pests and diseases ▶ Fungal rots occur in wet winters.

Harvesting and storing ▶ Gather the flowers when fully open and dry them.

Herbal medicine

Arnica montana, A. chamissonis. Part used: flowers. Arnica flowers have significant anti-inflammatory and mild analgesic properties. They are applied topically in the form of infused oils, ointments and creams to bruises, sprains and strains to encourage healing and to reduce the discomfort of pain and swelling. The pain-relieving effects of arnica

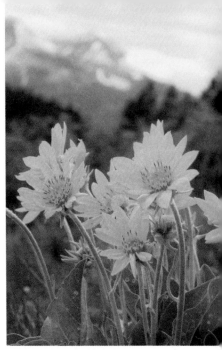

Arnica (*Arnica montana*) is toxic in all but the tiniest doses. In some countries, it is restricted to external use only.

also make this a suitable topical remedy for the treatment of sore and aching muscles and rheumatic joint problems.

Internally, *Arnica montana* is taken as a homeopathic remedy, in a very dilute preparation of the herb. It may help with the emotional effects of trauma as well as shock resulting from injury. It may also help to alleviate the physical complaints described above.

Arnica has been ruled unsafe in some countries. For the safe and appropriate use of arnica, see First aid, *page 194*. Do not use arnica if you are pregnant or breastfeeding.

The name "arnica" most likely derives from the Greek "arnakis," meaning "lamb's skin," due to the soft texture of the leaves.

Artemisia

Latin Name *Artemisia* sp. Asteraceae

Other common names *Artemisia absinthium*: wormwood, old woman.
  A. pontica: Roman wormwood, old warrior. *A. abrotanum*: southernwood,
  lad's love, maiden's ruin, old man. *A. afra*: wilde als

Parts used **Aerial parts, roots**

Named for the Greek goddess Artemis, *Artemisia* is a genus containing about 300 species. A number of species inhibit other plants, sometimes to the point of death.

Gardening

Wormwood (*A. absinthium*) forms a woody shrub to about 2.5 ft. (74 cm) with a bittersweet smell. Its deeply incised gray-green leaves are densely covered in fine hairs.

Tree wormwood (*A. arborescens*) resembles wormwood but grows upright to about 5 ft. to 6 ft. (1.5 m to 1.8 m), with narrower leaf segments; it smells less strongly.

Roman wormwood (*A. pontica*) is a low-growing plant to about 1.5 ft. (40 cm), with finely cut, scented leaves. It spreads by rhizomes.

White sage or native wormwood (*A. ludoviciana*) has silvered foliage. An aromatic upright subshrub to 4 ft. (1.2 m) that that is used as an ornamental ('Silver King' is popular).

Mugwort (*A. vulgaris*) is a perennial that spreads via rhizomes. It grows to about 3 ft. (90 cm), with deeply incised leaves that are deep green above and grayish white below.

Southernwood (*A. abrotanum*) forms an upward-growing bush to about 3 ft. (90 cm) with threadlike, finely divided leaves with a "lemon and camphor" smell.

Wilde als (*A. afra*) is indigenous to Africa, from the Western Cape up to Ethiopia. A popular garden plant, it forms clumpy bushes from 1.5 ft. to 6.5 ft. (0.5 to 2 m).

Varieties ▶ Some excellent ornamental forms of *A. absinthium* include 'Lambrook Silver' and aromatic 'Powis Castle,' a hybrid.

Position ▶ Most species prefer full sun, good drainage and almost neutral soil, (although mugwort tolerates partial shade). As it is strongly insecticidal, use it as a companion plant in the edge of gardens.

Propagation ▶ Propagate all perennial artemisias by semi-hardwood cuttings taken from midsummer to autumn, or raise from seed. Propagate rhizomatous species by root division in autumn. Directly sow the annual species *A. annua* into the garden in spring, or raise as seedlings and transplant at 6 weeks.

Maintenance ▶ Lightly prune and shape perennial bushy artemisias in spring. Prune southernwood heavily in spring. Artemisias are a drought-tolerant group once they are established, and perennial forms have good frost tolerance.

Pests and diseases ▶
Wormwoods are very rarely troubled by pests and diseases.

Harvesting and storing ▶
Harvest the leaves as required to use fresh or dried.

Herbal medicine

A. absinthium. Parts used: aerial parts. Wormwood is used to treat symptoms associated with poor digestion, including wind. In many cultures it is regarded as a valuable remedy for worm infestations and

Tree wormwood
(*Artemisia aborescens*)

other parasitic infections of the gut. It is also used as a nerve tonic and to treat fever and menstrual complaints.

A. vulgaris. Parts used: aerial parts. Mugwort is used as a digestive stimulant and nerve tonic, and is also used to treat menstrual problems.

A. annua. Parts used: aerial parts. According to traditional Chinese medicine, Chinese wormwood (qing hao) is a cold remedy and is used for treating fevers, rashes and nosebleeds. It is the subject of intense scientific research.

A. afra. Parts used: leaves, stems, roots. Wilde als is used as a traditional medicine by many African cultures, and like wormwood and mugwort, is sometimes taken as a digestive tonic. Other traditional applications include respiratory problems, such as colds, flu, sore throats and nasal congestion, for which it is sometimes applied topically.

For the safe and appropriate use of these herbs, consult your healthcare professional. Do not use these herbs if you are pregnant or breastfeeding.

Basil

Latin Name *Ocimum* sp. Lamiaceae
Parts used **Leaves, flower spikes**

Sweet basil, with its savory clove fragrance, is the quintessential Italian culinary herb and is available in an amazing range of forms and fragrances — from lemon, lime, anise, spice, cinnamon and thyme to incense and sweet camphor.

Gardening

There are 64 basil species, all native to the subtropics and tropics, but generally speaking, they are annuals, or evergreen perennials and shrubs, with simple aromatic leaves and spikes of lipped flowers arranged in whorls.

Varieties ▶ Many varieties of sweet basil (*O. basilicum*) have been developed, particularly in the Mediterranean region.

Compact small-leafed forms of sweet basil are popular in Greece and for pot and windowsill culture.

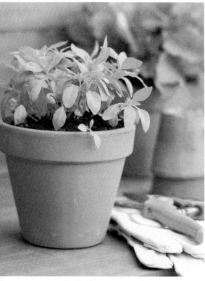

Lemon basil (*Ocimum americanum*) has a fresh lemon scent with sweet basil undertones.

They include 'Greek Bush' and 'Green Globe.'

Large-leafed sweet basils include 'Lettuce Leaf' and 'Mammoth' (both have leaves that are large enough to use as food wraps); the very ornamental 'Magical Michael'; and 'Medinette,' a large-leafed dwarf form suitable for pot culture.

Colored-leaf forms are widely used as modern ornamental plantings, as well as for culinary purposes. They include 'Red Rubin' and the frilly leafed 'Purple Ruffles.' The variety 'Ararat' is green, deeply suffused with purple, and has a licorice-and-clove fragrance.

Citrus-flavored varieties include lemon basil (*O. americanum*). Hybrid varieties (*O. x citriodorum*) include 'Sweet Dani' and 'Mrs Burn's Lemon,' which are richly lemon-scented and ideal for culinary use. The variety 'Lesbos' or 'Greek Column' contains heady spice, floral and citrus notes. A similar variety, known as 'Greek' or 'Aussie Sweetie' in Australia, is a separate introduction from Greece. 'Lime' basil (*O. americanum*) has a fresh lime and sweet basil scent.

Strongly spice-scented varieties of *O. basilicum* include 'Oriental Breeze,' a purple-flowered form much used for ornamental and culinary purposes; 'Cinnamon'; 'Spice' (often incorrectly sold as 'Holy Basil'), with its heady, almost incenselike fragrance; and 'Blue Spice,' which contains additional vanilla notes.

'Peruvian Basil' (*O. campechianum* syn. *O. micranthum*) is a spice-

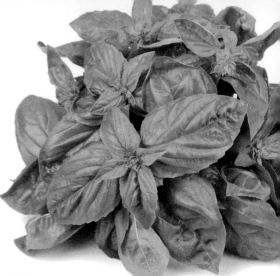

Sweet basil (*Ocimum basilicum*)

"A man taking basil from a woman will love her always."

Sir Thomas More
Tudor statesman and philosopher, 1478–1535

scented species. 'Sacred Basil' or 'Holy Basil' (*O. tenuiflorum* syn. *O. sanctum*), which is available in both green- and purple-leafed strains, has a mild spice scent and is widely planted in India around temples and in gardens.

'Anise Basil' (*O. basilicum*), also sold as 'Licorice Basil,' has a sweet anise scent and purple-suffused leaves. The basil encountered in the cooking of Thailand and Vietnam, 'Thai Basil' (*O. basilicum*), has a light, sweet anise scent, glossy green foliage and ornamental lavender flowers. Several selections have been made, including the very aromatic 'Queenette' and 'Siam Queen,' with a spicy anise fragrance.

Some handsome perennial basils are the result of hybridization between *O. basilicum* and

O. kilimandscharicum, the camphor-scented perennial species. They have a spicy clove fragrance, with a hint of balsam. They include white-flowered, green-leafed 'All Year' basil, and the beautiful purple-suffused 'African Blue.'

Tree basil, or East Indian basil (*O. gratissimum*), is native to tropical Africa but widely grown in India and South America. The plant is pleasantly thyme- and clove-scented and makes a substantial bush to about 1.5 m. Another strain of this species, sold as 'Mosquito Plant' or 'Fever Plant,' has a strong thyme scent.

Position ▶ Basils require a protected, warm, sunny site with a well-drained soil.

Propagation ▶ With the exception of the perennial basils mentioned above, basils are generally treated as annuals and propagated from seed. Do not plant seeds directly in the garden until the soil warms. For an early start, plant into seed trays kept in a warm and protected

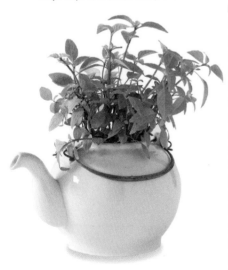

Thai Basil, another variety of *O. basilicum*, has a sweet aroma that combines anise and licorice.

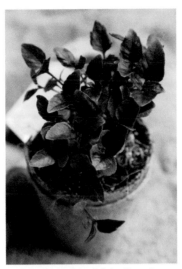

'Dark Opal,' a variety of *O. basilicum*, bears long cerise flowers and has a delicate scent.

environment. Grow seedlings of smaller varieties in pots or spaced about 1 ft. (30 cm) apart, larger bush types about 1.5 ft. (45 cm) apart. Basils cross very readily between varieties, so seeds saved in a mixed planting will not grow true to type in the following year unless you prevent cross-pollination by bees. You can also take cuttings from side shoots.

Maintenance ▶ Water regularly. Being a tropical plant, basil grows rapidly at temperatures in excess of 60°F (16°C), and is frost-sensitive. Pinch out flower heads to promote bushy plant growth and to prolong the plant's productive life.

Pests and diseases ▶ A fungal disease called fusarium wilt can attack plants, causing sudden wilting. Remove and destroy affected plants (do not compost them), and do not replant basil in the contaminated soil. Consider planting basils among other plants, rather than en masse. They make a fashionable addition to the ornamental garden.

Harvesting and storing ▶ Harvest mature leaves and flower spikes for fresh use at any time.

To dry the leaves, cut bushes at the base and hang out of direct light, then store in an airtight container in a cool place.

Herbal medicine

Ocimum basilicum. Part used: leaves. Sweet basil is known more for its pleasant taste than for its medicinal effects. Due to its mild sedative properties, herbalists traditionally prescribed basil as a tea for easing nervous irritability.

Ocimum tenuiflorum syn. *O. sanctum*. Part used: leaves. Holy basil, an important herb in Ayurvedic medicine, is used for a range of complaints. Scientific research supports its role in the management of diabetes (due to a hypoglycaemic effect) and as a supportive herb during times of stress. It may also improve concentration and memory and, due to an antiallergic effect, may be beneficial in treating hay fever and asthma.

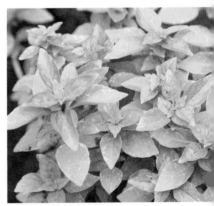

In Greece, Greek basil (*Ocimum minimum* 'Greek') is placed on tables to deter flies.

For the safe and appropriate use of basils, consult a professionally trained medical herbalist. Do not use these herbs in greater than culinary quantities if you are pregnant or breastfeeding.

Basil *Continued*

Around the home

Basil is a natural disinfectant. Use the essential oil in combination with other antiseptic herbal oils to make disinfectant sprays for cleaning household surfaces. Plant basil in a pot close to the back door to deter flies. Cut a bunch of basil as an aromatic table centerpiece when you eat outdoors. The dried flower heads add a sweet and spicy note to a potpourri.

Cooking

Basil is one of the great culinary herbs; different varieties are used extensively in both European and Asian cooking. If a recipe specifies simply "basil," sweet or common basil (*Ocimum basilicum*) is the type generally meant. Fresh sweet basil is highly aromatic, with a distinctive scent and flavor reminiscent of aniseed, and tends to be either loved or loathed. Dried basil tastes more of curry, and is a poor substitute for the fresh herb and should be avoided.

Using a knife to cut basil can bruise and darken the leaves. For salads and pasta sauces where appearance matters, shred the leaves with your fingers. Young leaves have the best flavor, while old ones have a coarser, stronger taste.

In cooked dishes, basil quickly loses its aroma and the leaves tend to darken, so add it to give depth of flavor during cooking and then, for fragrance and visual appeal, stir in a little more just before serving.

Tomato dishes, chicken, egg and rice dishes, spaghetti sauces, fish and vegetables — especially beans, capsicum and eggplants — all go well with basil. Basil is a good addition to stuffings. The most famous use of basil is in pesto (or pistou in French). Citrus-scented and spice-flavored varieties of basil work well in a range of Asian recipes.

Classicaly Italian

Insalata Caprese ("salad in the style of Capri"), in the colors of the Italian flag, is a light, summery salad that showcases the flavor of basil and ripe tomatoes. Arrange tomato slices on a plate. Intersperse with slices of fresh bocconcini (baby mozzarella). Season well. Add a dash of olive oil and a scattering of fresh basil leaves. ▶

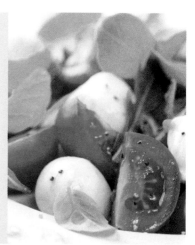

Aromatic basil oil

◀ Preserve basil the Italian way. Layer the leaves in a jar and sprinkle each layer with salt. Then at the top add a good-quality olive oil. Seal the jar securely and store in the refrigerator, allowing several days for the oil to be infused with the flavor of the basil. Use the leaves and the oil for making pesto. (Drizzle a little oil over pizzas or salads. Also, try adding a dash to a marinade.

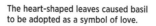

The heart-shaped leaves caused basil to be adopted as a symbol of love.

Bay

Latin Name *Laurus nobilis* Lauraceae
Other common names **Bay laurel, Grecian bay, sweet bay**
Parts used **Leaves, flower buds, fruits, bark, roots**

The bay is a long-lived and slow-growing, pyramid-shaped evergreen tree. According to folklore, a bay tree in the garden or at the front door keeps away evil as well as thunder and lightning.

Gardening

While a bay tree can reach about 50 ft. (15 m) over a long period, its slow, dense upright growth habit makes it an ideal specimen for a large pot, whether it is allowed to grow into its natural form or is shaped into an ornamental topiary or standard. In this form, a small garden can accommodate a bay without concern; its growth is even slower when cultivated in a pot. Bay generally flowers only in warm climates, and the small, very fragrant flower buds open to tiny cream flowers, after which come blue-black berries.

Varieties ▶ There are two species of bay, *L. nobilis* and *L. azorica*; the latter is used ornamentally. There is a gold-leafed form of *L. nobilis* called 'Aurea,' as well as a willow-leaf form, 'Angustifolia.'

Several other species are known as bay or laurel, and some are also classified as herbs or spices. The northern bayberry (*Myrica pensylvanica*), which is the source of bayberry candles; the bay rum tree (*Pimenta racemosa*), used in men's colognes; and Indonesian bay (*Eugenia polyantha*) have all been used for cooking.

The ornamental plants cherry laurel (*Prunus laurocerasus*) and mountain laurel (*Kalmia latifolia*) are easily confused with sweet bay due to a similar leaf shape. However, the leaves of these species are very poisonous if ingested, and even the honey harvested by bees can be toxic.

Position ▶ Bay trees prefer a deep soil, so if you are growing one in a pot, plant it in one of generous depth, in a compost-enriched potting mix. Provide full sun and good air circulation. Bay prefers a moist, rich, well-drained soil.

Propagation ▶ Seed may take 6 months to germinate. Cuttings, best made from semi-ripe wood, may take 3 or more months to form roots, and must never be allowed to dry out.

Maintenance ▶ In areas with cold winters, sweet bay is best grown in pots and brought inside during the

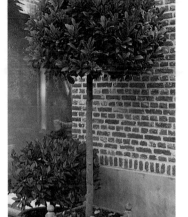

Bay tree (*Laurus nobilis*)

History and myth

The bay tree was considered sacred to the sun god Apollo and later to his son Asclepius, the Greek god of medicine. According to myth, Apollo fell in love with Daphne, a beautiful nymph who, rather than returning his affection, appealed to the gods to rescue her from him. She was duly changed into a bay tree, the perfect disguise. Apollo declared the tree sacred and thereafter wore a bay laurel wreath in Daphne's honor.

Bay is considered an herb of strong magic, able to attract good fortune and wealth and keep away evil. The death of bay trees was considered a portent of evil times; when the city of Rome fell to invasion from the north in the 4th century, all the bay trees allegedly died.

During outbreaks of the plague, Roman citizens burned bay leaves in the public squares, and the herb was still used for this purpose into the 16th century.

The leaves are mildly narcotic in quantity; it is said that the Oracle of Delphi in Greece chewed bay leaves before she entered a prophetic trance. The temple at Delphi was roofed with protective branches of bay.

Bay (*Laurus nobilis*)

Bay Continued

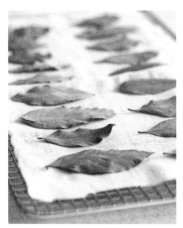

A cake rack covered with kitchen paper is ideal for drying individual leaves, or you could stretch mesh over a frame.

winter months or if the temperature is likely to drop below 5°F (−20°C). Check plants regularly for both scale and fungal infestations. Re-pot potted specimens into larger containers with fresh additional soil as required; when transplanting, disturb the root system as little as possible.

Pests and diseases ▶ Bay is generally trouble-free but can suffer from scale insects, which may infest the underneath of leaves and stems. To remove these, blend 2 cloves of garlic with a cup of water, filter, and add a little liquid soap. Apply to the insects with cotton buds. Alternatively, apply horticultural oil in the same manner. Plants grown without adequate ventilation and light can develop disfiguring gray mildew, which should be treated with sulphur while the plant is wet with morning dew.

Harvesting and storing ▶ Pick green leaves for use at any time. Dry leaves out of direct sunshine and store in an airtight bottle. Also see Harvesting, preserving & storing, *page 152.*

Around the home

To deter weevils in your pantry, add a few bay leaves to containers of flour and rice. Bay leaves placed between the pages of a book may also help to repel silverfish. As the leaves will lose their pungency, they need to be regularly replaced.

Cooking

Sweet bay is indispensable in French and other Mediterranean cookery. The tough leaves withstand long cooking, so use them in soups and stews. Apart from meat and fish, they go well in dishes that contain lentils or beans. Two leaves are sufficient in a dish that serves six people.

Bay is essential in a bouquet garni, which is made with fresh herbs or dried herbs wrapped in muslin. Bay is also used in pickling spice and garam masala.

Fresh leaves tend to be bitter, but the taste will diminish if they are left to wilt for a few days. Fresh sprigs stripped of a few leaves make aromatic skewers for meat or fish cooked on the barbecue.

Dried leaves retain their flavor for about a year. Remove dried leaves from dishes before serving.

Crowning glory

Bay's botanical name, *Laurus*, stems from the Latin word *laus*, or "praise," in reference to the crown of bay leaves worn by the ancient Romans to celebrate victory. Other herbs were often incorporated into wreaths. The Roman emperor Tiberius always wore a wreath of bay laurel when thunderstorms were raging, because he believed that it would provide protection from the gods of thunder and lightning.

Vanilla bay custard

Bay complements fish, meat and poultry dishes; sauces such as béarnaise and, surprisingly; perhaps, sweet custards such as this, where it imparts a slightly spicy taste.

Place 5 fl. oz. (150 ml) milk, 5 fl. oz. (150 ml) thick cream, 1 split vanilla pod and 1 bay leaf in a saucepan. Bring to a simmer, remove from heat, and leave to infuse for 15 minutes. Remove pod and leaf. Beat 3 egg yolks and 1 tablespoon soft brown sugar in a bowl. Add infused milk, mixing thoroughly. Return mixture to a clean saucepan. Cook over a low heat, stirring, until custard thickens; do not let it boil. Serve warm with hot fruit pies and steamed puddings.

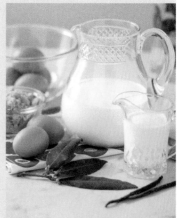

Opposite page: Bouquet garni, a bundle of classic herbs, usually includes bay, thyme, parsley, and peppercorns.

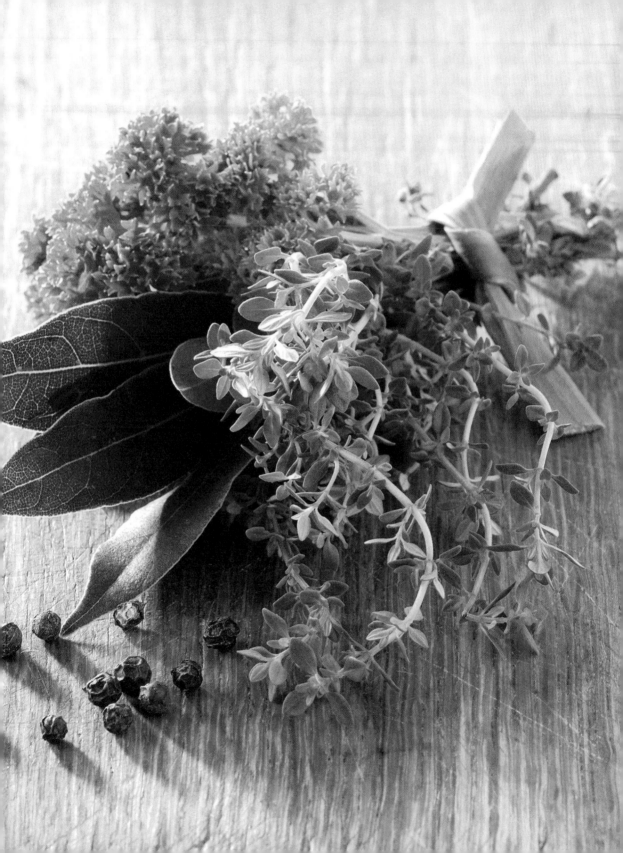

Bergamot

Latin Name *Monarda* sp. Laminaceae

Other common names **Bee balm, Monarda, Oswego tea**

Part used **Leaves**

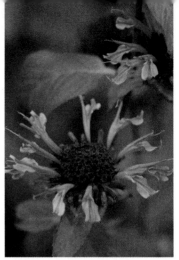

Wild bergamot (*Monarda fistulosa*)

Native Americans used *Monarda* to make medicinal tisanes. After the Boston Tea Party, in 1773, when American colonists dumped tea shipped by the British East India Company in protest against British rule, the bergamot tea of the Oswego Indians became a popular substitute.

Gardening

Monarda obtained its common name in Europe because the scent of its foliage resembled that of bergamot orange (*Citrus bergamia* syn. *C. aurantium* var. *bergamia*), a small tree that resembles Seville orange (*C. aurantium*). Bergamot's leaf fragrances range from oregano to lemon. This herb's spectacular flowers attract bees and birds.

Oswego tea (*M. didyma*) is a perennial growing to 4 ft. (1.2 m), with several stems terminating in heads surrounded by dense whorls of long-tubed, scarlet flowers. The leaves have a very pleasant citrus scent.

Wild bergamot (*M. fistulosa*) is found on well-drained hillsides and in light woodland. Two botanical varieties to 4 ft. (1.2 m) are grown, both with lance-shaped leaves. *M. fistulosa* usually has whorled heads of lavender flowers (occasionally pink), and different strains have thyme- or rose geranium-scented leaves.

The cold-hardy *M. menthifolia*, known as oregano de la Sierra, has a true oregano scent and flavor. Spectacular spotted bergamot (*M. punctata*) has densely whorled heads of cream flowers speckled purple and showy lavender bracts. Lemon bergamot (*M. citriodora*) is a tall annual species with heads of large, lipped, pink or lavender flowers.

Varieties ▶ Most garden bergamots are hybrids (*M. x media*) and include varieties such as 'Blue Stocking' and 'Mohawk.'

Position ▶ With the exception of *M. fistulosa*, which is drought-resistant, bergamots prefer a sunny position and an enriched, moist but well-drained soil.

Propagation ▶ Propagate by seed, or by dividing perennials in early spring. You can also take stem cuttings in summer.

Maintenance ▶ Clear dead material from plants in winter. Divide plants every 3 years.

Pests and diseases ▶ Some of the garden varieties are susceptible to powdery mildew, which, although it is disfiguring, does not appear to cause any permanent damage.

Harvesting and storing ▶ Harvest the edible flowers as required. Collect leaves in late spring and dry them.

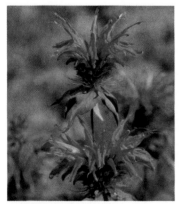

Oswego tea's nectar-rich blossoms attract bees and honey-seeking birds.

Herbal medicine

Monarda didyma, M. fistulosa. Part used: leaves. *M. didyma* has been used medicinally to ease flatulence and colic and reduce fevers. It is reputed to contain thymol, an essential oil compound that is also found in thyme and marjoram, and may explain the calming effect that the plant has on the digestive system.

Do not confuse this herb with bergamot essential oil. For the safe and appropriate use of *M. didyma* and *C. bergamia*, consult your healthcare professional. Do not use these herbs if you are pregnant or breastfeeding.

Bergamot orange

The aromatic yellow peel of the bergamot orange (*Citrus bergamia* syn. *C. aurantium* var. *bergamia*) is used to flavor Earl Gray tea and also yields bergamot essential oil, which is used for aromatherapy purposes. It can be beneficial for a range of skin conditions, including an oily complexion and acne, but take care when applying skin creams and oils containing the essential oil: One of its compounds, bergapten, has a known photosensitizing effect.

Borage

Latin Name *Borago officinalis* Boraginaceae
Other common name **Starflower**
Parts used **Leaves, flowers**

Borage
(*Borago officinalis*)

Considered a cure for "melancholia" in ancient times, borage is a hardy annual herb and an excellent companion plant, helping to deter tomato hornworm and Japanese beetles, and stimulating the growth of strawberries.

Gardening

Borage forms a rosette of large ovate leaves before sending up hollow flowering stems to 3 ft. (90 cm). The whole plant has a cucumber scent, is coarsely hairy and can irritate sensitive skin. The flower is five-petaled with a white ring in the center and a cone of black stamens.

Varieties ▶ There are three species of borage, but only *B. officinalis* is used as an herb. There are three color variants. The common form has intense blue flowers, but some plants have flowers suffused with pink. There is also a rare white form.

Position ▶ Borage requires a sunny, well-drained position and prefers a well-dug and composted oil.

Propagation ▶ Sow plants directly into the ground in spring and in autumn. You can sow them in pots, but you should transplant them while they are young, because they develop a large taproot. Borage germinates readily, in 3 to 5 days. Thin the plants to a spacing of 1.5 ft. (45 cm).

Maintenance ▶ Keep the soil moist, and fertilize in spring.

Pests and diseases ▶
Generally pest- and disease-free.

Harvesting and storing ▶
Harvest borage year-round as required. Dry the leaves in a very cool oven or in a well-aired place, out of direct sunlight.

Herbal medicine

Borago officinalis. Part used: seed oil. Borage seed oil is a rich source of gamma-linolenic acid (GLA), an omega-6 fatty acid that is also found in evening primrose oil. GLA exhibits anti-inflammatory activity; some research suggests that it may be of therapeutic value in the treatment of dry and itching skin conditions, including eczema and psoriasis. The latest evidence suggests that better therapeutic results may be achieved when GLA and other omega-6 oils are taken in combination with omega-3 essential fatty acids, such as those found in flax seed and fish.

The leaves are used as a poultice for sprains, bruises and inflammation, and in facial steams for dry skin.

For the safe and appropriate use of borage seed oil, consult your healthcare professional. Do not use borage seed oil if you are pregnant or breastfeeding.

Cooking

Remove the sepals from flowers and use them in salads, or crystallize for use as cake decorations.

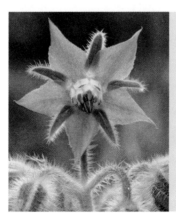

The age of chivalry

During the Crusades, borage was infused in stirrup cups and offered to Crusaders about to depart for the Holy Land, in the belief that it would grant them courage. Ladies traditionally embroidered its star-like flowers onto scarves, which they gave to their chosen knights before they went into combat.

Brahmi

Latin Name *Bacopa monnieri* Scrophulaceae
Other common names Bacopa, thyme-leafed gratiola, water hyssop
Parts used Whole plant above ground

This tropical herb is reputed to improve both brain function and memory, and the dried plant is used in many traditional Ayurvedic formulations. Brahmi makes an attractive hanging basket. You can also grow it in an ornamental pond.

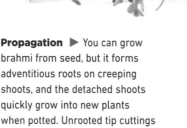

Brahmi (*Bacopa monnieri*)

Gardening

Bright green brahmi is a modest ground-hugging perennial plant that grows in wetland environments. The leaves are simple, oval, arranged in opposite pairs, smooth-edged and bitter-tasting. It is slightly succulent and bears small five-petaled flowers that are white, which faintly turn blue on the petal backs, over many months. The fruits are small, flat capsules.

Position ▶ Brahmi requires a moist soil and preferably light shade. It grows well in a pot, preferably with a diameter of 1 ft. (30 cm) or more, and makes an attractive hanging basket if grown in the shade. It is frost tender, so grow brahmi under protection in winter.

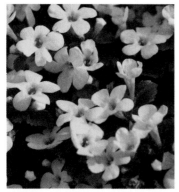

Brahmi is an aquatic herb, ideal for growing in damp places in the garden or even in a pond.

Propagation ▶ You can grow brahmi from seed, but it forms adventitious roots on creeping shoots, and the detached shoots quickly grow into new plants when potted. Unrooted tip cuttings also strike quickly.

Maintenance ▶ As brahmi has very shallow roots, water it regularly, especially if exposed to direct hot sunshine. Promote rapid growth with liquid seaweed fertilizer diluted to the recommended strength.

Pests and diseases ▶ None of note.

Harvesting and storing ▶ Harvest stems and leaves when plant is 5 months old, leaving 2-in. (5-cm) stems so that plant can regenerate for further harvesting. Dry leaves in the shade at room temperature and store in airtight containers.

Herbal medicine

Bacopa monnieri. Parts used: whole herb. In Ayurvedic medicine, brahmi is prescribed by herbalists to improve memory, learning and concentration. Scientific research has provided encouraging evidence for some of these effects, but suggests improvements take around 3 months to occur. Brahmi is also renowned as an exceptional nerve tonic, so it is notable that a reduction in anxiety levels was also observed in some clinical studies, supporting its use during times of anxiety and nervous exhaustion.

For the safe and appropriate use of brahmi, see Memory & concentration, *page 187*. Do not use brahmi if you are pregnant or breastfeeding.

Food for the brain

Keeping our brains healthy is as important as keeping our bodies in shape. Brahmi has been used as a "brain workout" herb in the Ayurvedic tradition of medicine for about 500 years. Researchers hypothesize that it may help by improving the way the nervous system transmits messages in the brain. Gotu kola (*Centella asiatica* syn. *Hydrocotyle asiatica*) is also sometimes confusingly referred to by the common name brahmi and is a "brain" herb in its own right. However, the two plants are easily distinguished by their different leaf shapes (see Gotu kola, *page 57*).

Burdock

Latin Name **Arctium lappa** Asteraceae
Other common names **Beggar's buttons, great burdock**
Parts used **Leaves, roots, seeds**

Burdock is enjoying a resurgence in popularity, both as a vegetable and as a traditional medicinal plant. It is regarded as a weed in the Northern Hemisphere, where it grows well on rough ground in a sunny position.

Gardening

Burdock is a strong-growing biennial. The fairly bitter but tender young foliage of spring regrowth is used as a green vegetable. The leaves are large and oval, and the numerous purple thistlelike flowers are quite remarkable in their perfect symmetry. Burdock can grow as high as 8 ft. (2.4 m).

Varieties ▶ Some named varieties are grown as a vegetable for their slender, crisp, textured taproots, which can grow as long as 4.5 ft. (1.3 m). These include two Japanese varieties — 'Takinogawa Long' and 'Watanabe Early'. Both have a flavor between that of parsnip and Jerusalem artichoke. *Arctium minus* is a very bitter weedy species that is found all over North America.

Position ▶ Burdock requires a moist humus-rich soil and full sun, although it will tolerate some light shade. It is also fully cold-hardy, and dies down in winter.

Propagation ▶ Propagate from seed in spring or late autumn. Although the seed usually germinates easily, soak the seed overnight in warm water before sowing, then lightly cover it with soil and firm down. Thin seedlings to about 6 in. (15 cm) apart. To produce high-quality, long, straight roots, dig the soil to a depth of 2 ft. (60 cm)

and incorporate well-rotted compost before sowing.

Maintenance ▶ Keep the soil moist and weed the crop regularly, particularly when the plants are young. Remove the flowers and burrs to promote root growth.

Pests and diseases ▶ Burdock is rarely affected by pests and diseases.

Harvesting and storing ▶ For cooking, collect young shoots and leaves in spring. Lift the roots in autumn, about 100 days after planting, when they are at least 1 ft. (30 cm) long. For medicinal purposes, dry the grayish brown roots, which are white on the inside.

Herbal medicine

Arctium lappa. Part used: roots. In Western herbal medicine, burdock root is used as an alterative or blood purifier. These terms describe its gentle detoxifying effect on the body and stimulation of the body's eliminatory channels, namely the lymphatic, digestive and urinary systems. It is commonly prescribed for chronic inflammatory skin and joint conditions, which traditional herbalists regard as the result of

a buildup of unwanted toxins in the body. When used over a long period of time, burdock root can be particularly effective in clearing dry, scaly skin complaints, such as eczema and psoriasis, and improving rheumatic joint conditions.

For the safe and appropriate use of burdock, consult your healthcare professional. Do not use burdock if you are pregnant or breastfeeding.

Cooking

Burdock is not an important edible plant, although the cultivated Japanese form, gobo, is used as a vegetable and also in various pickles and a miso-based condiment. It is also eaten as a vegetable in Korea. Scrape the young leaf stalks and cook them as you would celery. Use the roots raw as a salad vegetable, or cooked in stir-fries like carrots.

Burdock (*Arctium lappa*)

Making it stick

The evenly distributed hooks on the burdock burrs, which kept sticking to his clothes on walks in the countryside, inspired George de Mestral to invent Velcro in 1945. The name comes from the French words *velour,* meaning "velvet" and *crochet* or "hook." The invention has been applied to a wide range of items, from fasteners on clothes, bags and shoes to stainless-steel hook and loop fasteners that are used to attach car parts.

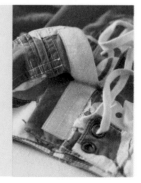

Calendula

Latin Name *Calendula officinalis* Asteraceae
Other common names **Golds, marigold, pot marigold, ruddles**
Part used **Petals**

Calendula has large daisylike flowers in golden yellow or orange. In ancient Rome, the herb was used to make a broth that was said to uplift the spirits. In India, the bright flowers decorated the altars in Hindu temples.

Gardening

Native to the Mediterranean, calendula forms a dense clump of simple lance-shaped aromatic leaves. The flowers resemble large daisies.

Varieties ▶ The original calendula of the herb garden was the single form; however, in the 20th century, double-flowered forms were extensively bred, yielding much larger harvests of petals. Two notable choices are 'Pacific Beauty' and the dwarf 'Fiesta Gitana.' 'Erfurter Orangefarbigen' from Germany is used for commercial medicinal flower production in Europe. A remarkable heirloom single variety from the Elizabethan period, *C. officinalis* 'Prolifera,' is still grown. This is the quaint 'Hen and Chickens,' which has a central flower encircled by a number of miniature flowers.

Position ▶ Plants need full sun but will tolerate partial light shade. They prefer a moderately fertile, well-drained soil.

Propagation ▶ Calendula is an annual that is very easy to grow from seed.

Maintenance ▶ In hot summers, calendulas usually cease flowering.

Regular deadheading will help to prolong flowering.

Pests and diseases ▶ Plants are prone to mildew in autumn. The variety 'Orange King' has good resistance. Spider mite can be a problem in midsummer, although reducing water stress lessens the severity of attack.

Harvesting and storing ▶ Gather petals after the dew has dried, and spread them very thinly over paper on racks, out of direct sunlight, in a well-ventilated place. When they are dried, store them in airtight containers.

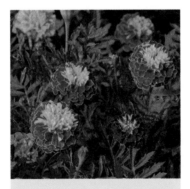

Globetrotting

Pot marigold should not be confused with the Mexican genus *Tagetes*, which includes the so-called African and French marigolds above as well as the coriander-tasting Andean herb huacatay or Peruvian black mint *Tagetes terniflora*, and the closely related *T. minuta*.

Calendula
(*Calendula officinalis*)

Herbal medicine

Calendula officinalis. Part used: flowers. Brightly colored calendula flowers possess significant wound-healing and local anti-inflammatory properties. To aid the healing of wounds, cuts and burns, apply them topically in the form of an ointment, cream or infused oil.

Calendula's slight astringency may help to staunch bleeding, while its antimicrobial effects help to keep the site of injury free from infection. Use a calendula tincture as an effective mouthwash against gum infections and mouth ulcers and also as a topical antifungal agent for some skin conditions.

Traditionally, calendula flowers are taken internally for infections and inflammation of the gut, including stomach and duodenal ulcers, and also as a lymphatic remedy for the treatment of swollen lymph nodes.

For the safe and appropriate external use of calendula, see First aid, *page 194*. For internal use, consult your healthcare professional. Do not take calendula internally if you are pregnant or breastfeeding. Topical application is considered safe at these times.

Caraway

Latin Name *Carum carvi* Apiaceae

Other common name **Persian cumin**

Parts used **Leaves, roots, dried ripe fruits (known as seeds) and their essential oil**

Caraway was a popular Middle Eastern herb before being introduced into Western Europe in the 12th century. Its seeds are used as an anise-scented spice in cooking. The herb also has medicinal and cosmetic uses.

Gardening

Caraway is a biennial with divided fernlike leaves and a parsley–dill fragrance. It has a spindle-shaped taproot, which can be cooked as a root vegetable, like carrot. The flowering stem, about 2 ft. (60 cm) tall, bears tiny white flowers touched with pink that are followed by crescent-shaped ridged 'seeds.' *C. roxburghianum*, known as ajmud, is a popular Indian spice.

Varieties ▶ 'Sprinter' is high-yielding and the seeds don't shatter, making it easier to save the seeds.

Position ▶ Caraway requires a well-drained fertile soil and a warm sunny position. Thin plants to 6 in. (15 cm) apart.

Propagation ▶ Sow caraway seed directly into the soil in either spring or autumn (the latter crop will seed the following summer).

Maintenance ▶ Regularly weed and water the crop, because the seed is often slow to germinate.

Pests and diseases ▶ Caraway is rarely troubled by pests. To prevent fungal diseases of foliage, water in the morning; do not water from above.

Harvesting and storing ▶ Gather leaves at any time. Lift roots after harvesting seed. Cut flowering stems when the seeds begin to darken and ripen. Secure stems in small bunches to allow air movement, and hang the bunches upside down until dry. Then shake bunches over sheets. The seeds often contain insects, such as weevils, so freeze to kill the eggs before storage.

Herbal medicine

Carum carvi. Part used: dried ripe fruits. Caraway's ability to dispel wind and exert a calming, antispasmodic effect on the gastrointestinal tract makes it

Caraway
(*Carum carvi*)

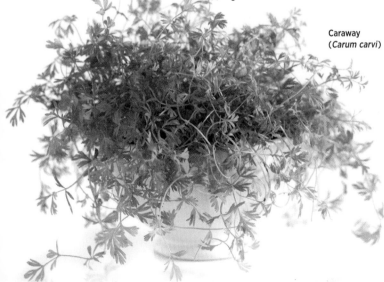

a reliable remedy in cases of flatulence, intestinal colic and bloating. As a result of its slightly drying nature, it is also prescribed with other appropriate herbs to assist in the relief of diarrhea.

For the safe and appropriate use of caraway, see Wind, bloating & flatulence, *page 180*. Do not use caraway in greater than culinary quantities if you are pregnant or breastfeeding.

Cooking

Caraway seeds are used to flavor rye bread, sausages, cabbage dishes, cheeses, soups, pork dishes, goulash and cooked apples, as well as liqueurs and spirits such as schnapps. A digestive known as "sugar plums" is made from sugar-coated seeds. Use the feathery caraway leaves in salads and soups. Their taste resembles a mixture of parsley and dill.

Caraway crackers

Roll out ready-made pizza dough or puff pastry on a lightly floured work surface. Whisk 1 egg yolk with 2 tablespoons water until combined and brush lightly over dough. Cut dough into squares. Combine 2 tablespoons each of poppy seeds, caraway seeds, sunflower seeds and chopped almonds. Sprinkle over squares. Cook in preheated 400°F oven for 10–15 minutes, or until pastry is golden. Serve warm. Makes 36.

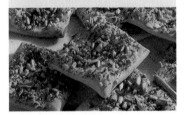

Catnip

Latin Name *Nepeta cataria* Lamiaceae
Part used **Leaves**

Many cats that encounter this velvety, curiously scented perennial react by rolling in it, rubbing against it and generally behaving as though the aroma is irresistible. Catnip is used to relieve fevers, colic and teething pain in young children.

Gardening

Catnip is a short-lived perennial native to Europe that resembles its relative, mint. It has soft, hairy, aromatic gray-green leaves and small, white, lipped flowers. The chemicals responsible for the amazing response of many cats are nepetalactones. A lemon-scented variety, *N. cataria* var. *citriodora*, has a similar effect. Not all cats exhibit such reactions: young kittens and older cats show almost no response.

Varieties ▶ There are some 250 species of *Nepeta*, many of which contain nepetalactones and attract cats. These include two common garden perennials that are both called catmints, namely *N. mussinii* and *N. x faassenii*.

Position ▶ Catnip needs a well-drained soil, and preferably full sun.

Propagation ▶ Grow catnip from seed, if possible in seed trays; seeds germinate best between 68°F and 86°F (20°C and 30°C). You can also propagate it easily by tip cuttings, and by root division in early spring.

Maintenance ▶ Cover young transplants in wire netting to protect them from felines. Plants grow rapidly in summer to form quite large, floppy bushes, so you'll need to stake them. Water regularly.

Pests and diseases ▶ In warm humid climates, septoria leaf spot may cause spotting, followed by yellowing of mature leaves. The nepetalactones effectively repel insect pests.

Harvesting and storing ▶ Once the bush is well grown, harvest catnip at any time after the dew has dried. Secure small bunches of stems with string and hang them upside down in a well-aired place. When perfectly dry, strip the foliage and store it in an airtight container.

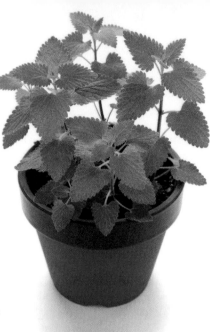

Catnip (*Nepeta cataria*)

Herbal medicine

Nepeta cataria. Parts used: leaves, flowers. An excellent remedy for children, catnip helps to resolve feverish conditions, and its antispasmodic properties alleviate flatulence and colic. It is a mild sedative and can reduce sensitivity to the pain of teething and improve irritability.

Catnip can also be used to treat the symptoms of colds, flu, digestive bloating, nausea and cramping in adults, and it is particularly effective when stress is a contributing factor.

For the safe and appropriate use of catnip, consult a healthcare professional. Do not use catnip if you are pregnant or breastfeeding.

Around the home

Catnip is a useful herb to have on hand in the home. Nepetalactones are a very powerful mosquito repellent, and cockroaches don't like them much, either.

Catnip cat toy

Trace a fish outline onto some thin cardboard and cut out a template. Place two fabric 5 x 6 ½ in. rectangles right sides together. Trace the fish onto the wrong side of one rectangle, remembering to add ¼-in. seam allowance all around.

Stitch the two shapes together, leaving a small opening for turning. Trim seam, clip curves and turn right side out. Fill with dried catnip and stitch opening closed. Stitch a small bell to the head of the fish.

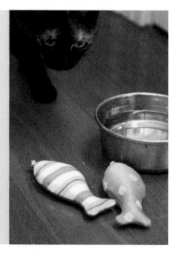

Celery

Latin Name **Apium graveolens** Apiaceae
Other common names **Cutting leaf celery, smallage**
Parts used **Leaves, seeds, roots**

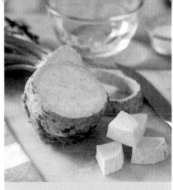

Rich in vitamins and minerals, wild celery has been used as a food and flavoring since ancient Egyptian times. The Greeks crowned the victors in the Nemean Games with garlands of its leaves, and also made funeral wreaths from them.

Gardening

The deep green leaves of wild celery may reach 2.5 ft. (74 cm), while the flowering stem bears compound umbels of inconspicuous white-tinged green flowers. The whole plant, including the tiny brown seeds, is very aromatic. Chinese celery or kin tsai (*A. graveolens*) is strongly flavored, with thin stalks that can be dark green to white in color. *A. prostratum* is a creeping, shiny-leaved, somewhat succulent Australian coastal plant with a strong celery flavor. It is now used as a flavoring in commercial bush foods.

Varieties ▶ Excellent selections include 'French Dinant' and the Dutch 'Soup Celery d'Amsterdam.'

Position ▶ Celery prefers a well-drained soil enriched with rotted compost and a sunny but protected position, and is tolerant of saline soils.

Propagation ▶ Grow wild celery from seed in spring. Space plants about 1.5 ft. (45 cm) apart.

Maintenance ▶ Keep the soil moist with regular watering.

Pests and diseases ▶ Celery has good disease tolerance, although septoria leaf spot can occur.

Harvesting and storing ▶ Harvest leaves from midsummer to autumn, as required. Pick ripe seeds, then dry, deep-freeze for several days to kill any insect eggs, and store in an airtight container.

Herbal medicine

Apium graveolens. Part used: dried ripe fruits (seeds). Celery seed has a strong diuretic effect and enhances elimination of uric acid and other toxins from the body via the urinary system. This action may help to explain its use as a specific remedy for the treatment of painful joint conditions, such as gout and arthritis, in which an accumulation of toxins in the joint area may be partly responsible for the characteristic symptoms of pain and swelling.

As a result of its diuretic properties, celery seed can also be used to treat fluid retention. Due to its slightly antiseptic nature, it can be of assistance in treating urinary tract infections.

For the safe and appropriate use of celery seed, see Arthritis & gout, *page 198*. Do not use celery seed in greater than culinary quantities if you are pregnant or breastfeeding.

Celeriac

Celeriac is a selected form of *Apium graveolens* with a very large taproot, which is grown as a root vegetable. Slice off the rough, tough outer skin rather than peel it, then use it raw or cooked in soups and baked dishes. The root and hollow stems have a celery flavor; slice the stems and use them as straws for drinking Bloody Marys.

Cooking

Celery's tiny edible seeds are aromatic and slightly bitter, tasting of celery. The whole seeds retain their flavor well; crush as needed and use to complement fish and seafood dishes, pickles and relishes, soups, stews, egg dishes, salad dressings, breads and savory biscuits.

Celery
(*Apium graveolens*)

Chamomile

Latin Name *Chamaemelum nobile* syn. *Anthemis nobilis*
and *Matricaria recutita* Asteraceae

Parts used Flowers, leaves

Roman or perennial chamomile or manzanilla (*C. nobile*), the annual German chamomile (*M. recutita*) and dyer's chamomile (*Anthemis tinctoria*) share the same common name. The flowers of both Roman and German chamomile are used medicinally, while the flowers of dyer's chamomile yield a golden brown dye.

Gardening

Roman chamomile is a densely carpeting and low-growing, cold-hardy plant. Its feathery green leaves have a ripe apple scent, and the flowers of the species are single white daisies. It is often confused with German chamomile, an upright growing annual with fine ferny leaves and white daisy flowers. Another annual species, pineapple weed (*Matricaria matricarioides*), has greenish yellow flowers and foliage with a pineapple scent.

Roman chamomile (*Chamaemelum nobile*), foreground; German chamomile (*Matricaria recutita*), background

Varieties ▶ A non-flowering variety, *C. nobile* 'Treneague,' is popular for lawns. An attractive fully double variety, *C. nobile* 'Flore Plena,' is grown commercially for its essential oil in many countries. Varieties of dyer's chamomile include the golden-flowered 'Kelwayi.'

Position ▶ All these chamomiles require a sunny position and well-drained soil.

Propagation ▶ Raise each species from seed in spring. Propagate perennial varieties by cuttings or root division.

Maintenance ▶ Weed regularly, especially if you are establishing a chamomile lawn.

Pests and diseases ▶ There are no significant problems.

Harvesting and storing ▶ Gather the flowers when fully open. German chamomile will reflower if harvested in summer. Dry the flowers and store them in an airtight container.

A multipurpose herb

For a relaxing sleep, try combining the essential oils of both chamomile and lavender in an oil burner. Chamomile is also antifungal and antibacterial. Next time you make chamomile tea, brew a second cup that's extra strong and use the liquid to wipe down the kitchen sink and table, or to wipe out a cabinet to rid it of a musty smell. Also, spray it onto plants and vegetables to deter fungal diseases such as mildew in the yard.

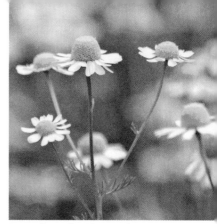

Roman chamomile (*Chamaemelum nobile*)

Herbal medicine

Matricaria recutita. Part used: flowers. Chamomile has a mild sedative effect on the nervous system. Chamomile's relaxing effects extend to the gut, helping to ease colic, and also to the female reproductive system, alleviating the pain of menstrual cramps. Chamomile's bitter-tasting compounds can help to stimulate the digestion and relieve the discomfort of nausea. Chamomile is a gently acting herb, suitable for children.

Topically, the soothing and anti-inflammatory effects of chamomile are excellent for treating itchy and inflamed skin conditions; it has also been shown to promote wound healing.

Chamaemelum nobile syn. *Anthemis nobilis*. Part used: flowers. Roman chamomile is commonly used in essential oil form, and the dried flowers can be hard to obtain. Some herbalists suggest that the Roman variety has a more pronounced relaxing effect on the gut and uterus, and can be used in a similar way to German.

For the safe and appropriate use of these herbs, see Nausea, page 179. Do not use these herbs in greater than culinary quantities if you are pregnant or breastfeeding.

Chervil

Latin Name *Anthriscus cerefolium* Apiaceae
Other common name **Garden chervil**
Parts used **Leaves, stems**

This delicious culinary herb, used since Roman times, has a delicate flavor between tarragon and parsley that is indispensable in French cuisine. Either use it raw or add it at the last minute, after the dish has been taken off the heat and is ready to serve.

Gardening

Apicius, the renowned gourmet of 1st-century Rome, set his seal of approval on chervil, which is an annual plant with delicate and lacy, fernlike foliage that forms a low-growing rosette. The tiny white

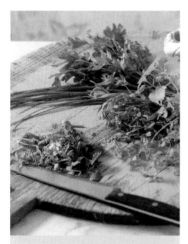

Fines herbes

Chervil is especially popular in French cooking, and essential (along with parsley, chives and tarragon) in the classic herb blend called fines herbes, which is used fresh with poached fish, shellfish and chicken and in green salads and egg dishes such as omelettes.

Grow chervil to lure slugs away from nearby vegetable crops.

flowers, borne in umbels on slender stems, are followed by thin black seeds.

Varieties ▶ There are flat-leafed and lightly curled forms as well as a strain called 'Brussels Winter,' which is tolerant of colder conditions.

Position ▶ Chervil requires good drainage and a moist soil that is close to neutral, preferably enriched with compost. Grow chervil in a lightly shaded position, because excessive sun exposure will cause the leaves to burn and turn rose pink. In warm climates, grow chervil in spring, autumn and even winter, as it has some cold tolerance and will withstand light frosts.

Propagation ▶ Scatter seed over the soil, press down lightly and water regularly. Seedlings usually emerge in about 10 to 14 days. Plants are ready for harvesting about 8 to 10 weeks after planting. Chervil has a long taproot and bare-rooted seedlings do not easily transplant. It will not germinate in soil that is too warm. In cool-climate areas with mild summers, grow chervil for a continuous supply during the growing season, although light shade promotes lush growth, and the

Chervil (*Anthriscus cerefolium*)

season can be further extended with the use of protective covers.

Maintenance ▶ Water regularly to promote lush growth.

Pests and diseases ▶ There are no significant problems.

Harvesting and storing ▶ Harvest leaves from the outside, preferably with scissors, because the plant is delicate. Leaves can also be deep frozen in sealed plastic bags.

Cooking

Chervil flowers, leaves and roots are all edible, although it is the faintly anise-flavored leaves that are most frequently used. There are various types, including curly leafed varieties that make a pretty garnish. Use fresh chervil in cooking, because its delicate flavor is destroyed by heat or drying. It goes well with glazed carrots and in butter sauces and cream-based soups. Chervil frozen into ice cubes adds a refreshing taste to summery fruit drinks.

Chervil butter makes a delicious spread for savory biscuits or bread. Also, use it as a flavorsome topping for barbecued fish, meat or poultry.

Chili

Latin Name *Capsicum* sp. Solanaceae
Part used **Fruits**

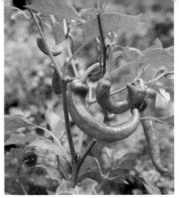

'New Mexico,' a variety of *C. annuum*, has a sweet flavor and can be either green or red.

Part of the South American diet for at least 7,000 years, chili varieties are the world's most frequently used culinary spice. The heat is mostly concentrated in the seeds and the white pith, so remove either or both for a milder hit.

Gardening

All *Capsicum* species are indigenous to South America. The most commonly grown is *C. annuum*, which contains many chili varieties as well as the bell peppers, pimentos and other sweet capsicum varieties, such as 'Banana' and 'Cubanelle.' Chilies and bell peppers differ from each other by a single gene that produces the fiery-flavored compound capsaicin.

C. baccatum, a species less known outside South America, requires a long growing season.

The rocoto pepper (*C. pubescens*), from the Andes and upland Mexico, forms a perennial bush that is tolerant of cooler weather and that produces purple flowers and thick-

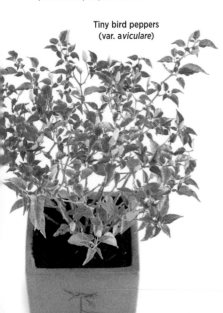

Tiny bird peppers (var. *aviculare*)

walled, fruity-flavored hot fruits with black seeds.

Varieties ▶ There are possibly hundreds of named varieties of *C. annuum*, and these have been selected worldwide for climate tolerance, color, size, shape, degree of heat and flavor, which may vary from citrus and prune to smoky, coffee, raisin, almond and tobacco. They are all divided into groups by shape: cherry-shaped (Cerasiform), cone-shaped (Coniodes), clustered elongated cones (Fasciculatum), sweet peppers (Grossum) and long hot peppers (Longum).

Among the best-known varieties of *C. baccatum* are 'Anaheim,' with large, long, tapering, mildly pungent fruit; 'Poblano,' which has large, medium-hot, heart-shaped fruits (and is known as 'Ancho' in its dried form); 'Pasilla,' a large raisin-flavored tapering variety; 'Jalapeño,' a thick-walled variety that is used in salsas or smoked (when it is known as chipotle); 'Guajillo,' a leathery, dark reddish brown variety that is moderately hot; and 'Mirasol,' a reselection of a pre-Columbian Mexican variety.

Some — such as 'Purple Tiger,' 'Filius Blue,' Variegata syn. 'Bellingrath Gardens' — are very ornamental and widely grown for landscape purposes. They are all edible.

The tiny bird peppers — including the wild pepper of New Mexico, the 'Chiltepin' or 'Tepin' — all belong to *C. annuum* var. *aviculare*. 'Tabasco' is the most widely known variety of the species *C. frutescens*.

The species *C. chinense* contains some of the hottest chili varieties,

including the 'Habañero' and its variants, the 'Scotch Bonnet' or 'Jamaican Hot,' and the somewhat milder Puerto Rican 'Rocatillo.' All three types are excellent for culinary use and widely grown in the Caribbean. The best-known variety, 'Aji Amarillo' or 'Kellu-Uchu,' is widely used in the cuisine of Peru.

Position ▶ All chili varieties require good drainage, full sunshine and an enriched soil. Do not grow chilies where related species of the family Solanaceae, such as tomatoes and eggplants, have recently been grown.

Propagation ▶ Even the fastest-maturing chili varieties of *C. annuum* require a minimum growing season of 3 months. In cooler areas, grow seedlings under protection before planting them out after the last frost. Although the flowers are self-pollinating, they also readily cross-pollinate, so carefully isolate plants intended for seed saving with fine netting.

Maintenance ▶ You may need to protect your plants from birds. Control aphids to prevent the spread of viral diseases; destroy any plants that have mottled or distorted leaves.

Pests and diseases ▶ Plant rotation will minimize verticillium wilt and other soil-borne diseases. Vegetable bugs may damage leaves.

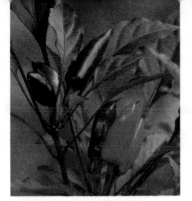

The dark purple fruits of Thai chili (*C. annuum* var. *fasciculatum*) turn red when ripe.

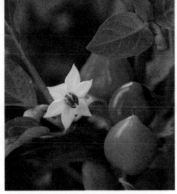

Chili 'Ebony Fire' is one of many chili varieties whose name indicates the intensity of its heat.

Harvesting and storing ▶ Pick peppers at any time. They reach peak heat when they turn red.

Cooking

Some cuisines — Indian, West Indian, African and Asian cuisines in general — are almost unthinkable without chilies, yet they were unknown in those regions until after 1492, when Columbus introduced them from the New World.

Chilies are always green when unripe; when ripe, they may be red, yellow, purple or almost black. Their heat level varies from negligible to incendiary. Generally, the smaller the

chili, the hotter it will be.

Varieties lacking the capsaicin gene produce sweet fruits that taste more like capsicum (to which they are related) and have a fruity flavor but little or no heat. The heat level may vary considerably even among chilies of the same variety, so the stated quantity in a recipe should always be adjusted to taste.

To check the heat level of your chilies, cut the end off one and give it the tiniest, tentative lick. A remedy for chili burn on the palate is dairy foods, such as milk or yogurt.

To minimize irritation from the fumes when grinding chilies, use a

Too hot to handle!

Most of the capsaicin that's responsible for the heat in peppers is stored in the seeds and the white septae within the fruit. To reduce the heat in a dish, you need to remove these before cooking. Capsaicin is not water-soluble, and neither water nor beer will neutralize the heat. It is, however, fat-soluble, and a glass of milk or yogurt, or the Indian yogurt-based drink lassi, are effective.

Wear protective gloves when chopping quantities of chili peppers, because they can numb your fingertips for many hours. Also, avoid touching your face, eyes or genitals after preparing them. Do not feed pets food containing chili, because it is fatal for some breeds.

Chili heat is commonly measured in Scoville Heat Units (SHU), with the 'Habañero' equating to between 200,000 and 300,000 SHU. Until recently, the world's hottest chili was an infamous variety of *C. chinense* known as the 'Red Savina Habañero,' which measured 577,000 SHU. Far less lethal for the tastebuds, 'Tabasco' is a mere 30,000 to 50,000. In 2007, a new record was established by a variety from Assam in India known as 'Bhut Jolokia,' which reached a very dangerous 1,000,000 SHU.

High-pressure liquid chromatography (HPLC) is now used to measure SHU. A relative heat scale, based on a simple 0 to 10 rating, has also been developed, with bell peppers rating 0 and 'Habañero' 10.

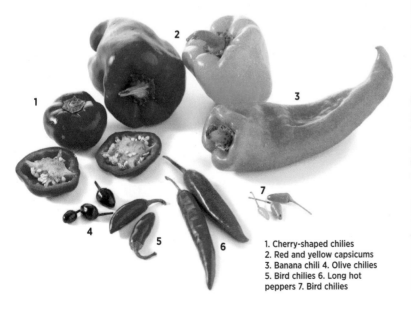

1. Cherry-shaped chilies
2. Red and yellow capsicums
3. Banana chili 4. Olive chilies
5. Bird chilies 6. Long hot peppers 7. Bird chilies

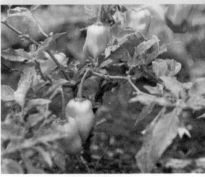

Habañero, a *C. chinese* variety, is among the hottest chilies in common use.

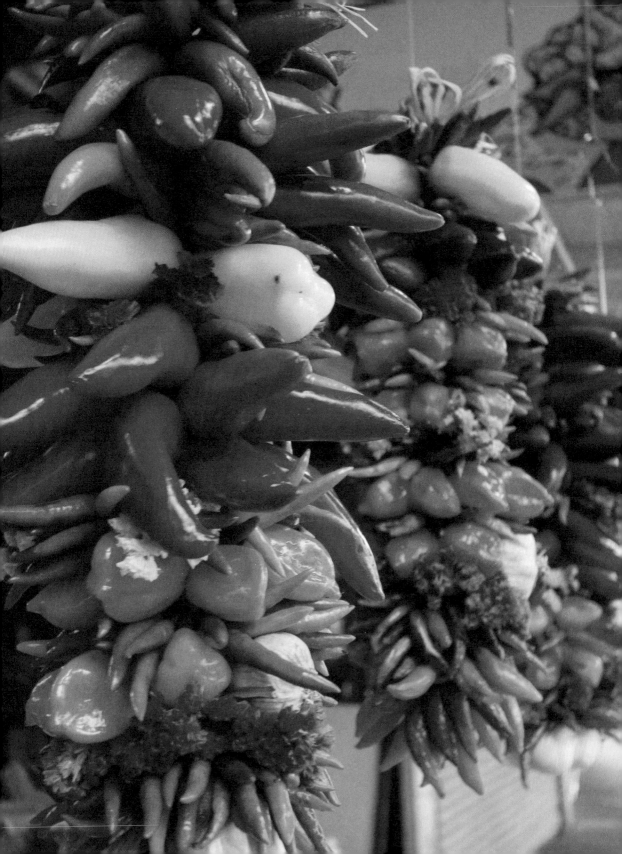

Chili *Continued*

spice grinder rather than a mortar and pestle.

Choose firm, shiny fresh chilies; avoid those that are wrinkled. Green chilies are always used fresh; red chilies can be used fresh or dried. Dried chilies differ in flavor to fresh, being fruitier and sweeter, although still retaining their heat. Buy dried chilies whole, crushed or powdered, and fresh chilies whole, or chopped and preserved in vinegar in jars; these are a good substitute for fresh.

In one of those transatlantic differences in spelling, "chilli" — together with the less often used "chilie" — are both used in the UK, while the Spanish-originated 'chile' is commonly used in the United States and Mexico. The term "chili" is reserved for a regional hot and spicy stew, originally from Mexico, which the United States subsequently made its own.

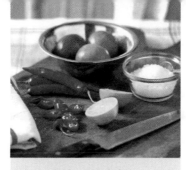

Chili and lime sauce

This Caribbean sauce recipe is delicious with barbecued or baked fish or vegetables. Baste the food with it, or serve it separately.

2 fresh red chilies
1 tablespoon sea salt
1 cup (250 ml) fresh lime juice

Remove the seeds and white pith from the chilies if you do not want too much heat. Slice chilies finely and pack into a jar. Dissolve the salt in the juice and pour over the chilies. Seal and store in a cool place to let the flavors develop. It is ready for use after 4 days and keeps for up to 4 weeks.

Chili condiments

There is a range of chili condiments to choose from.

- **Paprika** is a mildly hot, sweet, bright red chili powder that is produced by drying and grinding suitable varieties. Spain and Hungary are the world's largest producers. Suitable varieties, which must be intensely red when fully ripened, include 'Hungarian,' 'Paprika Supreme' and 'NuMex Conquistador.'

- **Cayenne** is a spice powder that is derived from dried hot red chilies. 'Cayenne' is a pre-Columbian variety from French Guiana. A number of cayenne-type varieties have been developed from it, including 'Hot Portugal,' 'Long Red,' 'Ring of Fire' and 'Hades Hot.' Dried chilies and chili flakes are also used.

Cayenne pepper

- **Tabasco**, the most famous chili sauce, is made in Louisiana, according to a 3-year process invented in 1868 by Edmund McIlhenny.

- **Peri Peri** is a sauce developed by the Portuguese from the tiny but powerfully hot Southern African variety 'Peri Peri'; it includes lemons, spices and herbs.

- **Mole poblano** — compounded of chili (such as pasilla), chocolate, spices and seeds or peanuts — is a popular sauce in Mexico, and increasingly abroad.

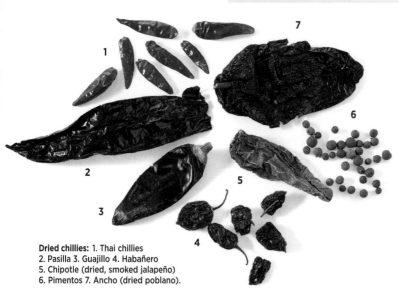

Dried chillies: 1. Thai chillies
2. Pasilla 3. Guajillo 4. Habañero
5. Chipotle (dried, smoked jalapeño)
6. Pimentos 7. Ancho (dried poblano).

Opposite page: These colorful strings of chilies include only a fraction of the varieties available.

Clove pinks

Latin Name *Dianthus caryophyllus* and *D. plumarius* Caryophyllaceae
Other common name **Gillyflower**
Parts used **Petals, whole flowers**

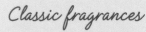

With an intoxicating spicy fragrance, the pretty flowers of clove pinks resemble small carnations. The fresh petals are edible and are used in mulled wines, cordial nerve tonics, salads and desserts, while the essential oil is used in perfumery.

Gardening

Clove pinks were bred from the grass pink or cottage pink (*D. plumarius*) and *D. caryophyllus* (which also gave rise to the carnation). They form a dense, low, spreading cushion of grasslike foliage, from which emerge many flower stems in early summer. All are perennial.

Varieties ▶ A remarkable number have survived the centuries, including 'Sops in Wine,' used in Elizabethan times to flavor mulled wines. 'Bridal Veil,' 'Queen of Sheba,' 'Ursula le Grove' and 'Pheasant's Eye' date from the 17th century. Eighteenth-century heirlooms include the Paisley Pinks, such as 'Dad's Favorite' and 'Paisley Gem,' which were bred to resemble intricate Paisley fabric patterning, as well as 'Inchmery' and 'Cockenzie.' Nineteenth-century large double-flowered forms include 'Mrs Sinkins,' 'Earl of Essex,' 'Rose de Mai' and 'Mrs Gullen.' 'Napoléon III' is a historic variety that involves a cross with sweet william (*D. barbatus*). The Carthusian pink (*D. carthusianorum*) was used in medicinal liqueurs by the Carthusian monks.

The famed Allwoodii 20th-century pinks include 'Arthur,' 'Kestor,' 'Doris' and 'Fusilier.' Other very fragrant modern pinks include 'Kim Brown,' 'Tuscan Lace,' 'Highland Fraser,' 'Pretty,' 'Tudor Manor,' 'Jean d'Arc,' 'May Queen,' 'Falstaff' and 'Gloire Lyonnaise.'

Position ▶ These plants require a well-drained, sunny position. They grow well in pots, and are both drought- and cold-tolerant once established. Pinks thrive in alkaline soil; if gardening on acid soil, add dolomite or garden lime. Alternatively, tuck small pieces of concrete rubble under the plant. These will leak lime into the soil during watering.

Propagation ▶ Mixed seed of perennial pinks are available. Named varieties must be propagated by cuttings.

Maintenance ▶ Clove pinks are hardy and easily grown. Do not let these plants be overshadowed.

Pests and diseases ▶ There are no significant problems.

Harvesting and storing ▶ Harvest flowers as required. To use fresh, remove the bitter white heels of the petals.

Classic fragrances

Like the spice clove, the flowers of clove pinks and carnations are rich in eugenol, and the perfume absolute is used in many high-quality perfumes, including Floris's Malmaison, Nina Ricci's L'Air du Temps, Guerlain's Samsara and L'Heure Bleu, Worth's Je Reviens, Hermès's Bel Ami, Estée Lauder's White Linen and Bvlgari's Bvlgari for Men. It takes 1,100 lb. (500 kg) of flowers to produce 3.5 fl. oz. (100 ml) of the essential oil, so synthetics such as eugenol and isoeugenol are often used in modern perfumery.

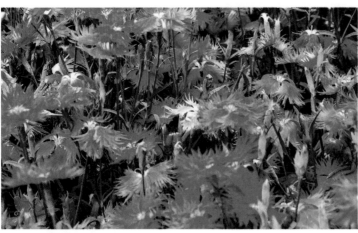

Clove pinks (*Dianthus caryophyllus*)

Comfrey

Latin Name *Symphytum officinale* Boraginaceae
Other common name **Knitbone**
Parts used **Leaves, roots (high in toxic alkaloids)**

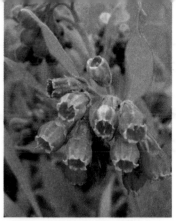

Comfrey comes in many color variations, including pink, lavender, or white.

Comfrey's other common name, knitbone, is a clue to its traditional use in poultices to encourage the healing of broken bones. Comfrey is also a fabric dye and dynamic compost accelerator.

Gardening

Common comfrey is a vigorous perennial, with mauve bell-shaped flowers, that grows to about 30 in. (80 cm). Varieties are not commonly available. Comfrey is also an "accumulator," a deep-rooted plant that taps into minerals in the subsoil. A "soup" made from rotting comfrey leaves in water makes a great organic liquid feed for crops. Other species are the ornamental cream-flowered groundcover *S. grandiflorum*, and *S. asperum*, which has bright blue flowers.

Position ▶ Comfrey grows readily from segments of root and, once established, is difficult to remove.

Propagation ▶ Dig the site deeply, incorporating ample compost or rotted manure. Space plants 3.5 ft. (1 m) apart. Lay out segments of root horizontally and cover with about 2 in. (5 cm) of soil.

Maintenance ▶ Comfrey requires ample nitrogen; an annual top dressing of rotted manure is recommended. Water regularly in the first season.

Pests and diseases ▶ Comfrey is generally trouble-free. Some strains are prone to rust, usually when the plants are water-stressed.

Harvesting and storing ▶
Harvest mature plants up to 5 times a year. Cut with shears and wear gloves, because the hairs on the leaves are an irritant. Leaves can be dried. Do not harvest in the first year or after early autumn.

Herbal medicine

Symphytum officinale. Parts used: leaves, roots. Traditionally, comfrey has been used as a topical application for bruises, fractures and wounds. It has a remarkable reputation for hastening the repair and renewal of damaged tissue as well as reducing inflammation. One of the compounds found in comfrey, called allantoin and thought to be responsible for many of the healing effects of this herb, has been shown to have a regenerative action on connective tissue.

While traditionally comfrey was also prescribed for internal use, these days such practice is strongly discouraged. Comfrey contains pyrrolizidine alkaloids that have been shown to have toxic effects.

For the safe and appropriate topical use of comfrey, refer to Sports injuries, sprains & strains, *page 196*. Do not use comfrey if you are pregnant or breastfeeding.

Dyes from herbs and plants

For centuries, dyes have been made from herbs and other plants. Comfrey leaves produce a golden yellow dye, while dandelion roots create a reddish one. Until indigo from the Far East was traded with Europe, woad (*Isatis tinctoria*) was used to produce a blue dye, and the characteristic war paint of the ancient Britons and Celts was made from it. In today's commercial world, synthetic dyes are favored over natural ones because they are resistant to fading from exposure to light. To make your own herbal dyes, consult the Internet or craft books.

Comfrey (*Symphytum officinale*)

Coriander

Latin Name **Coriandrum sativum** Apiaceae
Other common names **Chinese parsley, cilantro**
Parts used **Leaves, seeds, roots**

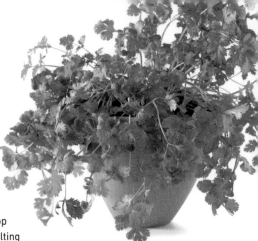

For more than three millennia, coriander has been cultivated for its aromatic foliage, roots and seeds, all found in the tombs of the pharaohs.

Gardening

Coriander resembles flat-leaf parsley, although it is more tender in texture, forming rosettes of long, thinly stalked leaves arising from a crown. The leaves are dissected into wedge-shaped segments, developing a fernlike appearance. Vietnamese coriander or rau ram (*Polygonum odoratum*) is a leafy perennial used in tropical areas. The leaves of Mexican coriander or cilantro (*Eryngium foetidum*) are strongly aromatic.

Varieties ▶ 'Spice' is popular for its seeds, while 'Santo' is a variety in which premature flowering is delayed and profuse deep green foliage develops.

Position ▶ Good air circulation, a sunny position and adequate fertilizing will minimize disease problems.

Propagation ▶ Sow this annual directly in the garden in spring after the last frost. Assist germination by rubbing the seed, separating it into halves and then presoaking the halved seeds for 48 hours.

Maintenance ▶ Weed the crop regularly. To stop premature bolting of varieties grown for foliage, protect the plants from water stress. Apply seaweed liquid fertilizer to promote leaf growth over flowering.

Pests and diseases ▶ Late crops may be susceptible to mildew and fungal leaf spot.

Harvesting and storing ▶ Harvest the seed crop when half the seeds on the plant have turned brown. Tie harvested stems into bunches and then hang them upside down inside paper bags to trap the falling seed. Once the plant is full-size, harvest foliage to use fresh at any time.

Herbal medicine

Coriandrum sativum. Part used: dried ripe fruits (seeds). Seeds have antispasmodic properties and a stimulating effect on the appetite. Coriander is often used in conjunction with caraway, fennel, cardamom and anise to ease symptoms of indigestion, including spasm, flatulence, and abdominal distension.

For the safe and appropriate medicinal use of coriander, consult your healthcare professional. Do not use coriander in greater than culinary quantities if you are pregnant or breastfeeding.

Cooking

The pungent leaves and stalks are popular in Southeast Asian, Middle Eastern, South American and Mexican cooking, in salads, soups, legume dishes, curries and stir-fries. In India, the leaf is used in types of fresh chutneys. Long cooking destroys the flavor of the leaves, so add them just before serving.

Roast the seeds to enhance their flavor. Used whole or ground, their mild, slightly sweet taste works well in sweet and savory dishes and in sauces such as harissa. The fiber in ground seeds absorbs liquid and helps to thicken curries and stews.

The root has a more intense flavor than leaves. It is used in Thai cooking, especially pounded into curry pastes.

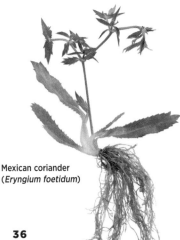

Mexican coriander
(*Eryngium foetidum*)

Coriander (*Coriandrum sativum*)

Coriander and figs

Palathai, or fig cakes, date from Roman times. They are popular in Egypt and Turkey. Remove stalks from ¾ lb. (400 g) dried figs (select soft ones). Process figs to a paste in food processor. Shape into an oval cake with your hands. Combine 1 teaspoon freshly ground coriander seeds and 1 teaspoon flour. Dust cake with mixture. Serve wedges for dessert.

Curry plant

Latin Name **Helichrysum italicum** syn. *H. angustifolium* Asteraceae
Other common names **Strawflower Italian everlasting**
Parts used **Leaves, flowers**

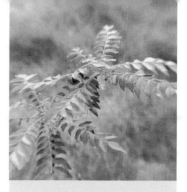

The intensely silvered needlelike foliage of this plant releases a mouthwatering fragrance of curry. The flowers can be dried and included in floral arrangements or used in craft work, while the essential oil is used in perfumery.

Gardening

The common form of curry plant found in herb gardens is *H. italicum* subsp. *italicum*, a form widely sold in the nursery trade as *H. angustifolium*. It is an upright but eventually semi-sprawling shrub to about 2 ft. (60 cm), with densely arrayed, needle-shaped leaves covered in very fine hairs, which give the plant a silvered appearance.

Varieties ▶ Other forms that are less commonly grown include the dwarf curry plant (*H. italicum* subsp. *microphyllum*), which is popular for edging herb gardens. *H. stoechas* is also used as a source of essential oil for the fragrance industry. The oil of both species is known as 'immortelle' or 'helichrysum.'

Position ▶ Curry plant requires an open sunny position and a very well-drained soil. Plants may suffer temporary dieback after light frosts. In areas where the temperature can drop below 23°F (–5°C), grow plants under protection in winter.

Propagation ▶ Take tip cuttings in spring and autumn.

Maintenance ▶ Curry plants respond well to a light pruning and shaping.

Pests and diseases ▶ Pests are rarely a problem but curry plant is affected by prolonged rain, often developing fungus on the foliage. To avoid this, mulch around the plant with gravel and ensure that the plant has excellent air circulation.

Harvesting and storing ▶ As an herb, curry plant is only used fresh. Pick sprigs as required.

Cooking

The entire plant is strongly aromatic of curry, particularly after rain. Add sprigs to egg, rice and vegetable dishes to impart a mild curry flavor, but cook only briefly.

To enhance fruit flavors, the oil and the extract are used commercially in food and beverage processing.

Curry tree

Curry plant is sometimes confused with the curry tree (*Murraya koenigii*), which is used in Ayurvedic medicine. This small tree with pinnate leaves is also intensely curry-scented and may eventually reach 10 ft. to 13 ft. (3 m to 4 m). Use fresh leaves in Indian dishes, adding them just before serving. The curry tree makes an attractive container plant, preferring a warm climate in full sun to partial shade.

Curry plant responds well to trimming, so consider using it in a low-growing, aromatic hedge.

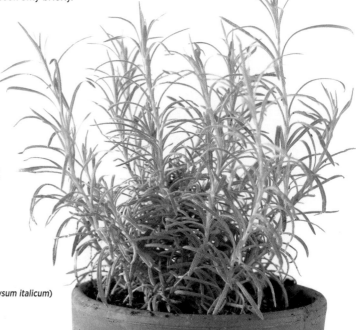

Curry plant (*Helichrysum italicum*)

Dandelion

Latin Name *Taraxacum officinale* Asteraceae
Other common names **Clocks and watches, fairy clocks**
Parts used **Leaves, roots, flowers**

Dandelion
(*Taraxacum officinale*)

Dandelion flowers make a delicious wine. The vitamin-rich, slightly bitter young leaves are used in cooking and the roots are used to make herbal coffee.

Gardening

Dandelion is a perennial with a thick, fleshy, deep taproot and a rosette of coarsely toothed leaves. From the leaves emerge many unbranched flower stalks, each terminating in a double golden-yellow flower. The flowers are followed by spherical balls of seed, or 'clocks,' which are dispersed by the wind.

Varieties ▶ Improved forms were developed in France in the 19th century. 'Thick Leaved' has tender, broad, thick leaves. 'Improved Full Heart' has profuse foliage that is easily blanched.

Position ▶ Despite its weedy reputation, dandelion crops will thrive if you dig the soil deeply and enrich it with rotted compost. It requires a sunny situation and prefers a neutral to slightly alkaline soil.

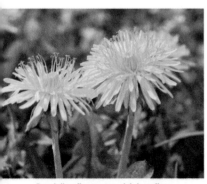

Dandelion flowers are rich in pollen and nectar, attracting beneficial insects such as bees.

Propagation ▶ Sow the seed directly into the soil in spring. The plants die down in winter.

Maintenance ▶ Cut spent flowers to prevent reseeding.

Pests and diseases ▶ The leaves are prone to mildew, particularly late in the season. Root rot can occur in poorly drained soil.

Harvesting and storing ▶ Blanch the leaves for culinary purposes by covering them from the light for 2 to 3 weeks before harvesting in late spring and before flowering occurs. Lift roots at the end of the second season. Both leaves and roots can be dried for herbal use.

Herbal medicine

Taraxacum officinale. Parts used: leaves, roots. Dandelion is well known for its therapeutic effects on both the kidneys and liver, hence its traditional reputation as a cleansing cure in the spring months. The leaf exerts a powerful diuretic action on the urinary system and may reduce fluid retention and assist the removal of toxins from the body. It also contains high levels of potassium and helps to replenish potassium that would otherwise be lost as a result of increased urination.

The root, which has a bitter taste, is utilized when a stimulating action on the digestive system is required. It promotes bile secretion and is a valuable remedy for many liver and gallbladder conditions. Dandelion root can improve a sluggish digestion and provide a laxative effect.

For the safe and appropriate use of dandelion, see Liver & gallbladder support, *page 182*. Do not use dandelion in greater than culinary quantities if you are pregnant or breastfeeding.

Cooking

The variety 'Thick Leaved' has leaves that can be used fresh in salads, or cooked in a similar way to spinach.

Dandelion and burdock is a traditional British, naturally fizzy soft drink made from fermented dandelion and burdock roots — in much the same way as root beer and sarsaparilla.

Clock flower

Dandelion has acquired a number of names, including *piss-en-lit* (French for 'wet the bed'), a reference to its diuretic effect. Other names include fairy clocks, and clocks and watches, derived from a game played by children in which they believe time can be revealed based on the number of puffs needed to blow the filamentous achenes, or the downy white seed head of a dandelion after flowering.

Dill

Latin Name *Anethum graveolens* Apiaceae
Other common name **Dillweed**
Parts used **Leaves, seeds**

Traditionally, if you suffered from hiccups, insomnia or indigestion, dill was an ideal remedy. Its name comes from the old Norse word *"dylla,"* meaning to soothe or lull. With its slight caraway taste, dill has a long history of use in Indian cooking and medicine.

Gardening

Dill is an annual plant with feathery, aromatic, blue-green foliage and attractive flat-headed compound umbels of yellow flowers, which are followed by small elliptical flat seeds.

Varieties ▶ Dill varieties suited to dillweed harvesting that are also slow to bolt include 'Hercules,' 'Tetra Leaf' and 'Dukat,' which is strongly flavored. Dwarf varieties suited to pot culture include 'Fernleaf' and 'Bouquet.' If you are growing dill for seed, 'Long Island Mammoth' is a good dual-purpose heirloom variety.

Position ▶ Dill requires full sun and a well-drained, moist soil.

Propagation ▶ Sow seeds directly into the soil in spring after the last frost, lightly cover them with soil and keep them moist until they germinate, or plant seedlings with the potting soil attached. In frost-free areas, plant it in late autumn.

Maintenance ▶ You may need to stake some tall varieties. Thin plants to about 1.5 ft. (45 cm) apart.

Pests and diseases ▶ Dill has no noteworthy pests or diseases.

Harvesting and storing ▶ Harvest leaves as required. Spread them thinly on paper, then microwave them to retain good color and fragrance. Store in an airtight container in a cool, dry place. Store fresh leaves in a plastic bag in the refrigerator, or chop them finely, put into ice-cube trays, top with water and freeze. Harvest the seeds after the heads have dried on the plant.

Herbal medicine

Anethum graveolens. Part used: dried ripe fruits (seeds). The essential oil found in dill seed is a key ingredient in the preparation of dill water, a popular treatment for flatulence and intestinal colic in infants and children. Dill seeds have been used to improve the flow of breast milk in breastfeeding mothers. Used in this way, even culinary quantities of dill seeds can allow the herb's medicinal properties to be passed on to the child.

Dill seeds can be used in adults for gastrointestinal conditions characterized by wind, bloating and cramping as a result of its antispasmodic effects.

For the safe and effective medicinal use of dill, see Wind, bloating & flatulence, *page 180*. Do not use dill in greater than culinary quantities if you are pregnant or breastfeeding except under professional supervision.

Cooking

With a taste reminiscent of anise and parsley, the fresh leaves complement soft cheeses, white sauces, egg dishes, seafood and chicken, salads, soups and vegetables dishes, especially potatoes. Dill is often used in salmon dishes. Add fresh dill to hot dishes just before serving, because cooking diminishes its flavor.

Dill seeds are used in pickling spice mixtures, in breads (especially rye bread), and in commercial seasonings for meat.

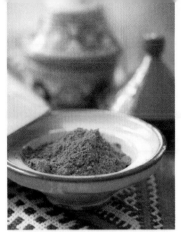

Dill seed is used in the spice mix, ras el hanout.

Dill (*Anethum graveolens*)

Echinacea

Latin Name **Echinacea** sp. Asteraceae
Other common name **Coneflower**
Parts used **Roots, leaves, flowers, seed**

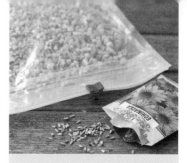

Echinaceas are not only strikingly beautiful, butterfly-attracting plants, they are also among the most significant medicinal herbs, widely used as an immune-system stimulant, with antiviral, fungicidal, bactericidal, anti-inflammatory and detoxifying properties.

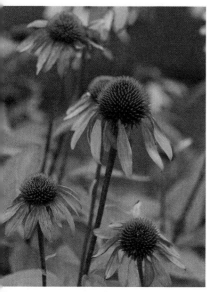

Echinacea (*Echinacea* sp.)

Gardening

There are nine species of echinacea, all North American, of which three are commonly used medicinally. *Echinacea purpurea* syn. *Rudbeckia purpurea* is the best known and the most widely grown species. Its roots are the most potent part of the plant, but the leaves and seeds are also used in herbal medicine.

Varieties ▶ A number of varieties are valued as ornamentals and as cut flowers while retaining their herbal potency. They include 'Magnus,'

with rose-purple flowers; 'White Swan,' which is believed to have a similar potency to the pink forms; and the large-flowered 'Primadonna' series, available in deep rose and pure white. The extraordinary 'Doppelganger' has a crownlike second tier of petals emerging from the top of the cone. 'Fancy Frills' resembles a fragrant pink sunflower.

Narrowleaf echinacea (*E. angustifolia*) and pale purple echinacea (*E. pallida*) are more potent medicinally than *E. purpurea*. Yellow echinacea or yellow coneflower (*E. paradoxa*) is a handsome species that has large flowers with narrow yellow petals and a chocolate center. Its roots have similar properties to those of *E. pallida*.

Position ▶ Echinaceas require a well-drained, sunny position. The plants are deep-rooted and, if grown in areas with shallow soil, should be planted into raised beds. They are drought resistant once they are established.

Propagation ▶ Echinaceas are perennials, and can be divided in autumn and spring or propagated by root cuttings. However, most propagation is by seed, which will germinate more readily after stratification (see box above right).

Maintenance ▶ Plants require little except watering and weeding.

Pests and diseases ▶ No serious pests or diseases are likely to occur.

Harvesting and storing ▶ Dig up the roots of mature plants in autumn, then clean and dry them. Gather flowers and foliage from mature plants as required.

Stratifying seed

To speed germination, stratify your seeds. Mix seed with moist sterile sand or vermiculite and place in a sealed plastic bag in the crisper section of the refrigerator for 4 weeks. Plant treated seed in pots. Transplant into the ground once the roots have filled the pots.

Herbal medicine

Echinacea angustifolia, E. purpurea, E. pallida. Parts used: roots, aerial parts. Echinacea's reputation as an effective treatment for the common cold, flu and acute upper respiratory infections has been the focus of extensive scientific research. The results of many clinical trials indicate that echinacea can indeed reduce the symptoms and duration of such conditions.

Traditionally, echinacea has been used as a popular and valuable herbal remedy for the treatment of many contagious illnesses and skin infections. It has a significant immune-stimulating effect, enhancing the body's ability to fight off bacteria, viruses and other disease-causing microorganisms.

Consequently, individuals who have weakened immune systems due to prolonged ill health or drug therapy may also benefit from using echinacea.

For the safe and appropriate use of echinacea, see Immune support, *page 176*. Do not use echinacea if you are pregnant or breastfeeding.

Elder

Latin Name *Sambucus nigra* Caprifoliaceae
Other common names **Bore tree, devil's wood, Frau Holle, Judas tree, pipe tree**
Parts used **Flowers, ripe berries, leaves (insecticidal only)**

There is a continuing belief in the mystical and magical powers of the elder, so many people ask the tree's permission before harvesting its flowers or berries. The flowers are used to brew elderflower champagne and to flavor desserts, while the berries are the nutritional equal of grapes.

Gardening

The European elder is a multi-stemmed shrub tree with deep green compound leaves that repel flies, mosquitoes and midgets. The large lacy inflorescences bear tiny, creamy white, fragrant flowers. The leaves, bark, green berries and roots are poisonous if consumed.

Varieties ▶ Ornamental varieties of elder include 'Black Lace' syn. 'Eva,' with finely cut purple-black foliage and pink flowers; 'Black Beauty' syn. 'Gerda,' with similar coloring; and the bronze-purple semi-dwarf 'Guincho Purple' syn. 'Purpurea.' European red elder (*S. racemosa*), which has large bunches of red berries, is also used herbally, while the 'Sutherland Gold' and 'Plumosa Aurea' varieties both have golden foliage.

Position ▶ These cold-hardy plants prefer a moist but well-drained, humus-rich soil and full sun to partial shade.

Propagation ▶ Collect fresh seed in autumn or stratify older seed for 4 weeks (see *page 40*). Alternatively, propagate by suckers, by semi-ripe wood cuttings taken in late summer or by cuttings of ripe wood in autumn.

Pests and diseases ▶ Elder is resistant to honey fungus. To repel aphids, mites, leafhoppers, whitefly and cabbage loopers from the garden, make a strong infusion of the leaves.

Harvesting and storing ▶
Harvest the berries when they are black. Pick flowers early on a dewless morning, spread the heads on clean kitchen paper and leave in a warm, dark, dry place for several days.

Herbal medicine

Sambucus nigra. Parts used: flowers, berries. Elder flowers and berries have a long history of

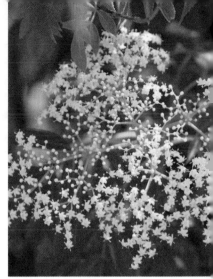

Elder (*Sambucus nigra*)

use for alleviating the symptoms of colds and flu, in particular fever and congestion of the nose and sinuses. Elder flowers have also been used to reduce mucus production in hay fever, sinusitis and middle-ear infections.

Recently, clinical trials found that a commercial elderberry syrup reduced both the symptoms and duration of flu in sufferers. Laboratory studies suggest that constituents in the berries may activate certain immune cells and act directly on viruses to reduce their infectivity.

For the safe and appropriate use of elder, see Sore throats, colds and flu, *page 174*. Do not use elder if you are pregnant or breastfeeding.

Cooking

Use the fresh flowers to make elderflower wine or cordial or an herbal infusion; such processing results in a pleasant floral-tasting beverage. High in vitamins A and C, the berry juice is fermented to produce elderberry wine. Freeze the berries for later use, but cook them for a few minutes first and use them in baked goods.

Ripe elderberries are the nutritional equal of grapes.

Eucalyptus

Latin Name *Eucalyptus* sp., *Corymbia* sp. Myrtaceae
Other common name **Gum tree**
Parts used **Leaves, gum (kino)**

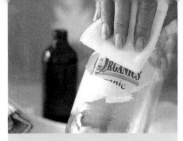

Largely indigenous to Australia, the eucalypts are rich in essential oils that are valued for both their medicinal applications and their fragrance, which ranges from lemon to peppermint and turpentine.

Gardening

The genus *Eucalyptus* has undergone taxonomic revision and a number of botanical names have been changed, although older names still prevail in much of the literature. Kino, a gum produced as a response to wounding of the tree, is gathered commercially from species such as scribbly gum, also known as white gum kino (*E. haemostoma*), and the red blood-wood (*E. gummifera*). Some eucalyptus species have shown weedy tendencies in parts of the world, such as South Africa, so consult local plant services before growing them.

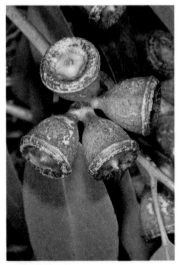

Eucalyptus seeds or "gum nuts"
(*Eucalyptus* sp.)

Varieties ▶ Many species are steam-distilled for their essential oil. These include the lemon-scented gum (*Corymbia citriodora* syn. *Eucalyptus citriodora*) and lemon ironbark (*E. staigeriana*), which has a fragrance of lemon and rosemary, and *E. globulus*, the most significant species. Narrow-leafed peppermint (*E. radiata*) yields a sweet, fruity essential oil with some camphor. The commercial chemotype of broad-leafed peppermint (*E. dives*) produces a pepperminty essential oil with sweet balsamic notes; it is used in toiletries and aromatherapy. Gully gum (*E. smithii*) essential oil is used in aromatherapy.

Position ▶ Most species require a sunny position and do not tolerate low temperatures. In general, eucalypts require a well-drained soil and are quite drought-tolerant once established. When mature, they are able to regenerate after fire.

Propagation ▶ Raise from seed.

Maintenance ▶ Water regularly during the establishment phase. Plantation-grown crops are usually coppiced for ease of harvesting and to improve yields.

Pests and diseases ▶ The oils in eucalypt leaves render them distasteful to most insects; they are not susceptible to fungal diseases of the leaves. Heavy beetle infestation, particularly during droughts, will cause dieback and eventually the death of the whole tree.

Harvesting and storing ▶ The foliage of mature or regenerated coppiced trees is harvested for steam distillation.

Stain remover

Eucalyptus oil is invaluable for removing stains — particularly grease and perspiration — from clothing and other fabric. (Moisten a clean rag with a little oil and dab the stain from the edge to the middle, then launder as usual.)
You can also use it to remove scuff marks, sticky spills from all types of hard flooring and stubborn jar labels.

Herbal medicine

Eucalyptus globulus. Part used: leaves. The essential oil from eucalyptus leaves possesses significant antibacterial and antiviral effects.

Eucalyptus essential oil is used today as a popular remedy for upper respiratory tract infections, predominantly as a decongestant for catarrhal conditions. It is commonly used as an external preparation in the form of a chest rub or as an inhalant with a few drops added to a vaporizer or put on a handkerchief. Internal use of the essential oil is not recommended except in commercial preparations, such as cough lozenges and cough mixes, in which the oil is present in a diluted form.

The oil can also be used topically, especially as a cold sore treatment. It is also common in a number of ointments used to relieve muscle aches and joint pain.

For the safe and appropriate use of eucalyptus, consult your healthcare professional. Do not use eucalyptus if you are pregnant or breastfeeding.

Opposite page: Eucalyptus

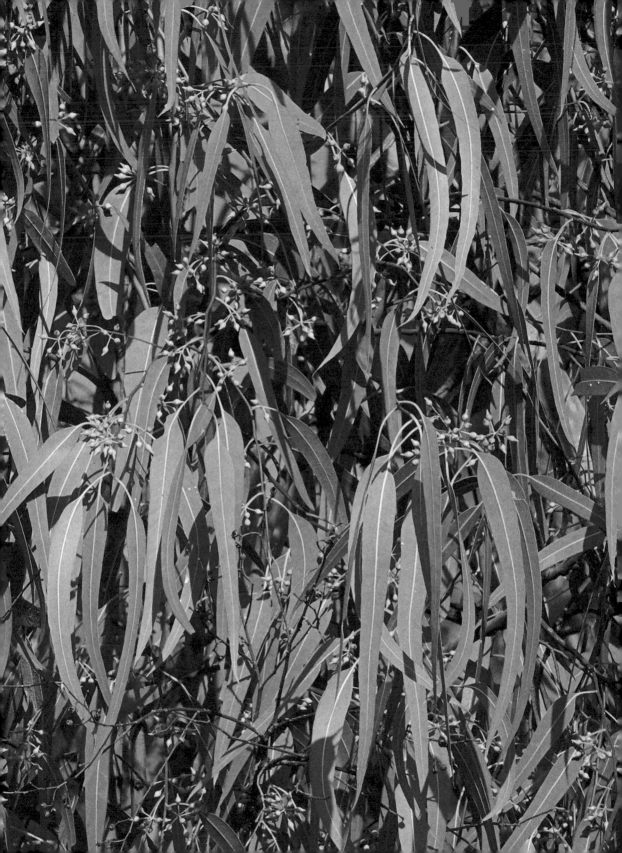

Evening primrose

Latin Name *Oenothera* sp. Onagraceae
Other common names **Suncups, sundrops**
Parts used **Seeds, roots, leaves**

The beautiful evening primroses gain their name from the many species that are pollinated by moths, opening their flowers at night and pouring forth exquisite fragrance. Evening primrose oil has applications in the beauty and health industries.

Gardening

The principal species cultivated for evening primrose oil extraction is *O. biennis*, a biennial forming a basal rosette of leaves from which emerges a central flowering stalk. This terminates in a cluster of buds that open during successive nights. The large, circular, faintly phosphorescent lemon-colored flowers mimic the moon and, together with their sweet lemon and tuberose fragrance, draw the attention of moths, which are their chief pollinators. By the following morning, the flowers begin to wither and turn reddish orange, later developing slender pods, which are filled with tiny seed.

Taming the beast

Theophrastus (371–c. 287 BCE) wrote two influential botanical volumes, *On the Causes of Plants* and *Enquiry into Plants*; this led to him being regarded by some as the Father of Taxonomy.

He named evening primrose *Oenothera*, possibly from the Greek words *oinos*, meaning wine, and *thera*, meaning hunt. It is thought that Theophrastus recommended using evening primrose for taming wild beasts.

Varieties ▶ Other *Oenothera* species used as sources of evening primrose oil include *O. lamarckiana* (sometimes considered a synonym of *O. glazioviana*) and *O. parviflora*.

Position ▶ Wild *Oenothera* species require a sunny position. They are, however, very tolerant of freely draining, poorer, sandy loam soils and are also fairly drought-tolerant and frost hardy.

Propagation ▶ Propagate plants by seed sown in spring to early summer. Extreme heat in summer reduces the gamma-linolenic content.

Maintenance ▶ Keep free of weeds. *O. lamarckiana* is a much better competitor than the other species mentioned above.

Pests and diseases ▶ Where plants are overcrowded, powdery mildew may affect the foliage. In inadequately drained soils, root rot may also occur.

Harvesting and storing ▶ Gather the fresh young leaves as required. Lift roots at the end of the second season and use them as a vegetable. Gather the seed when ripe; shattering can be a problem.

Herbal medicine

Oenothera biennis. Part used: seed oil. Evening primrose oil (EPO) contains significant levels of omega-6 essential fatty acids, especially gamma-linolenic acid (GLA), thought to be involved in many of the oil's therapeutic effects. GLA has notable anti-inflammatory activity, and several clinical studies suggest that this effect may be of benefit in alleviating the symptoms

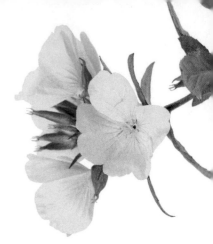

Evening primrose (*Oenothera biennis*)

of rheumatoid arthritis, diabetic neuropathy, eczema and dermatitis.

Further research also indicates that EPO supplementation may help to reduce high blood pressure and improve some of the symptoms of PMS. However, results of other trials have been negative. The latest research suggests that a greater therapeutic effect may be achieved if EPO or GLA supplements are taken in combination with omega-3 essential fatty acids, found in flax seeds and fish.

For the safe and effective use of EPO, consult your healthcare professional. Do not use EPO if you are pregnant or breastfeeding.

Natural beauty

Evening primrose oil is widely used in cosmetics. To make your own skincare treatment.

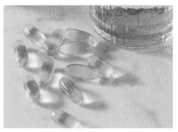

Evening primrose oil tends to be taken in high doses, so capsules are the most convenient.

Eyebright

Latin Name *Euphrasia officinalis*
Orobanchaceae
Parts used **Whole plant**

Eyebright is a European alpine wildflower that takes its common name from its use in various eye ailments, including conjunctivitis, styes and the inflammation and congestion caused by hay fever and colds.

Gardening

The use of eyebright dates back to the Middle Ages when it was cultivated in Northern European monastic herb gardens. All *Euphrasia* species are semi-parasitic on the roots of host plants, namely grasses, plantain (*Plantago* sp.) and clover (*Trifolium* sp.). The genus is widely distributed around the world.

Varieties ▶ The principal species used herbally as eyebright are *E. officinalis*, *E. brevipila* and *E. rostkoviana*, all annual herbs with small, toothed, rounded leaves and yellow-throated white flowers, striped or spotted with purple. The lower flower lip is three-lobed, and each lobe is incised.

Position ▶ These particular species, which will not thrive under hot summer conditions, require a moist soil. Eyebright's native habitat is meadowland with alkaline soil and a cool climate.

Propagation ▶ If you have these conditions in your garden, you can establish these three species by scattering seed around host grasses during spring. Alternatively, grow seedlings in pots, but add generous amounts of dolomite or lime to the soil and also some established soft meadow grasses.

Maintenance ▶ Ensure that the soil remains moist.

Pests and diseases ▶ No problems of significance has been noted.

Harvesting and storing ▶ Harvest the whole plant when in flower, and dry it for use in herbal preparations.

Herbal medicine

Euphrasia officinalis. Parts used: leaves, flowers. Eyebright, as noted above, has traditionally been used as a specific remedy for irritated or inflamed conditions of the eye. The combined astringent and anti-inflammatory effects of eyebright

also make it well suited to the treatment of catarrhal conditions of the upper respiratory tract. It can also help to clear up postnasal drip, middle-ear infections and sinus congestion.

Eyebright is regarded as an effective hay fever remedy and can ease many of the symptoms experienced by hay fever sufferers, including itchy, weeping eyes, watery secretions of the nose and also sinus headaches.

For the safe and appropriate use of eyebright, see Hay fever & sinusitis, *page 177*. Do not use eyebright if you are pregnant or breastfeeding.

Natural beauty

The pretty flowers of this plant have a toning, cooling and mildly astringent effect on the eye. Eyebright may be used as a compress or topical lotion to relieve common eye disorders and infections.

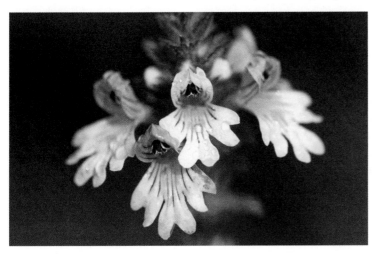

Eyebright (*Euphrasia officinalis*)

Fennel

Latin Name *Foeniculum vulgare* Apiaceae
Parts used **Leaves, flowers, seeds, stems, roots**

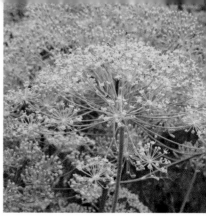

Fennel (*Foeniculum vulgare*)

Some varieties of fennel have a particular sweetness and some ornamental qualities, while others are eaten as a vegetable or used to flavor pickles and baked goods.

Gardening

Fennel plants are annual or perennial and can reach 5 ft. (1.5 m) or more, with one to several erect, hollow stems coming from the base and bearing fine, glossy aromatic pinnate foliage. The tiny yellow flowers, borne in umbels, are used in pickling and the small seeds are very aromatic.

Varieties ▶ There are two subspecies: a large group classified under *F. vulgare* subsp. *vulgare*, with the second, *F. vulgare* subsp. *piperitum*, containing only the pepper or Italian fennel. *F. vulgare* subsp. *vulgare* is further divided into three botanical varieties: var. *vulgare*, which contains perennial fennel; var. *azoricum*, which contains the annual Florence fennel, with its enlarged bulbous leaf bases grown as a

vegetable; and var. *dulce*, known as sweet or Roman fennel. Many superb Italian regional varieties of Florence fennel include 'Romanesco' and 'Fennel di Firenze.'

Position ▶ It prefers a light, well-drained, slightly alkaline soil in a sunny position but is adaptable and tolerates the cold well.

Propagation ▶ Raise all fennel varieties by seed sown in spring. Propagate perennial forms by division in spring.

Maintenance ▶ Cut down and remove old stems.

Pests and diseases ▶ Fennel rarely has any problems.

Harvesting and storing ▶ Harvest foliage and flowers as required. Harvest seeds when ripe, then dry and freeze for a few days to kill any insects. Lift roots in autumn and dry them.

Herbal medicine

Foeniculum vulgare. Part used: dried ripe fruits (seeds). Fennel has calming effects on the digestive system, relieving flatulence, bloating and abdominal discomfort, and its pleasant taste and gentle action make it popular for such conditions in children. Fennel has also been taken by breastfeeding mothers as a remedy for improving breast milk flow; used in this way, the therapeutic effects of fennel can be passed on to young infants experiencing colic and griping.

Fennel has long been used to treat respiratory complaints with catarrh and coughing, and is suitable for treating these conditions in adults and children.

For the safe and appropriate medicinal use of fennel, consult your healthcare professional. Do not use fennel in greater than culinary doses if you are pregnant or breastfeeding except on the advice of a healthcare professional.

Around the home

Fennel is a natural flea repellent. Crush a handful of fresh fronds and rub them all over your dog or cat. Put handfuls of fennel fronds under your pet's bedding.

Cooking

Slice the raw bulb thinly and add to salads, or cut in half and roast as a vegetable to bring out its sweetness. Use fresh fennel leaves in salads, salad dressings and vinegars, with fish, pork and seafood dishes, or as a garnish. The dried seeds are used in cakes and breads, Italian sausages, salads, pickles, curries and pasta and tomato dishes.

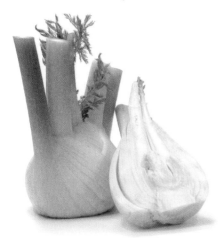

The bulbous leaf bases of Florence fennel are delicious sliced raw in salads or roasted.

Field of Marathon

The ancient Greek name for fennel, *marathon*, was also the name of the battlefield to the north of Athens where, in 490 BCE, a Greek army defeated the invading Persian force.

Feverfew

Latin Name *Tanacetum parthenium* syn. *Chrysanthemum parthenium*, *Matricaria parthenium* Asteraceae

Part used **Leaves**

With a long history in European herbal medicine, the name feverfew is derived from "febrifuge," because it was said to dispel fevers. Its excellent ornamental flower is as fresh-looking as checked gingham. Feverfew is used as an insect repellent and a companion plant.

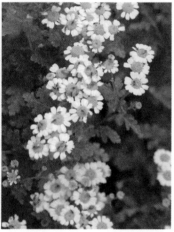

Daisy-like feverfew. Varieties can be confused with pyrethrum (*Tanacetum cinerariifolium*).

Gardening

Feverfew is a perennial, forming a clump of deeply incised compound leaves to about 1.5 ft. (45 cm). The tall branched inflorescence contains many small, white-petaled, yellow-centered daisy flowers.

Varieties ▶ In addition to the species, several varieties are commonly grown. 'Golden Feather' has golden yellow foliage, and there is also a compact form called 'Golden Ball' and a dwarf form, 'Golden Moss.' Double-flowered forms include 'Flore Pleno' and the ivory-flowered 'Snowball,' 'White Bonnet' and 'Tom Thumb.'

Position ▶ It is a very easygoing plant, which responds to a sunny position, good soil, regular watering in summer and good drainage. The plants remain evergreen in winter and are frost-hardy.

Propagation ▶ Feverfew self-seeds readily, but you can also grow it from seed, by cuttings or by root division.

Maintenance ▶ After flowering is finished, cut back the tall flowering stalks.

Pests and diseases ▶ The leaves of feverfew are bitter and highly aromatic, and act as an insect repellent. No fungal diseases are of significance.

Harvesting and storing ▶ Harvest the fresh leaves at any time. (Take note that handling plants can cause dermatitis in some sensitive individuals.)

Herbal medicine

Tanacetum parthenium. Part used: leaves. Feverfew is used as a valuable remedy for the treatment and prevention of migraine headaches. Clinical trials have shown that the herb can reduce the severity of symptoms, including visual disturbances and nausea. Laboratory studies suggest that the therapeutic effects of feverfew are a result of its anti-inflammatory and pain-relieving properties as well as a muscle relaxant action.

Fresh leaves of feverfew are sometimes chewed for medicinal purposes. However, feverfew

is more likely to cause adverse effects if taken this way, so the use of commercially produced feverfew extracts may be preferable.

For the safe and appropriate use of feverfew, see Headache & migraine, *page 189*. Do not use feverfew if you are pregnant or breastfeeding.

Around the home

Feverfew is noted for its moth-repellent qualities.

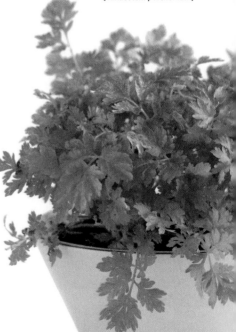

Feverfew
(*Tanacetum parthenium*)

Flax

Latin Name *Linum usitatissimum* Linaceae
Parts used **Whole plant, seeds, stems**

Beautiful blue-flowered flax is one of the oldest-known crop plants. It produces a fiber that's used to make linen, and flaxseed oil, also known as linseed oil, which is a source of linolenic acid (omega-3). Seeds, whole or cold-milled, are used in cooking.

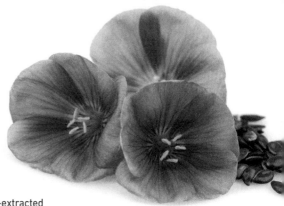

Flax (*Linum usitatissimum*)

Gardening

Linum usitatissimum is a crop species developed by humans that has been cultivated for at least six millenia. The species has been developed as two distinct types: the taller forms known generically as long-stalked flax (for fiber); the shorter, more floriferous types known as crown flax (for seed production). The plants are slender, erect, narrow-leafed annuals, with multiple stems from the base. In summer, they bear single, upward-facing, sky-blue flowers, followed by round capsules, about 0.4 in. (1 cm) in diameter, filled with glossy, flattened oval seeds. The seed is milled and extracted for flaxseed oil, also known as linseed oil. The industrial-grade oil is used in a range of products, from printing inks, paints and varnishes to linoleum; the residual linseed cake is used as feed for cattle. The cold-extracted oil is used for quality human nutritional supplements.

Linola is a new crop specifically bred for the production of a cooking oil that is comparable to that of sunflower and corn oil. Flaxseed is also used in bakery and cereal products.

Position ▶ It requires a sunny position and a well-drained, open soil.

Propagation ▶ Sow the seed directly into prepared ground in spring.

Maintenance ▶ Keep flax weeded so it does not compete against weeds.

Pests and diseases ▶ A 3-year crop rotation is recommended. Flax may be vulnerable to fungal problems.

Harvesting and storing ▶ When mature, cut plants for fiber. Harvest the seed when ripe. Store the seed whole in the refrigerator, or preserve in oil.

Herbal medicine

Linum usitatissimum. Parts used: seeds, oil. Taken whole or crushed with a little water, the seeds of flax have a gentle laxative effect and are a popular remedy for constipation. The mucilage content of the seed produces a soothing effect on many irritable and inflamed conditions of the gut.

The seed oil is the most concentrated plant source of the omega-3 essential fatty acid, alpha-linolenic acid (ALA), which is often deficient in the Western diet, especially for vegetarians.

Supplementing the diet with flaxseed oil or alpha-linolenic acid may have numerous health benefits. Human studies indicate that ALA has positive effects on cholesterol levels and a potential role in the treatment of other cardiovascular diseases. The anti-inflammatory omega-3 oils can also be useful for treating inflammatory skin conditions such as eczema and psoriasis.

For the safe and appropriate use of flaxseed, see Eczema & psoriasis, *page 191.* Do not use flaxseed if you are pregnant or breastfeeding.

New Zealand flax

Native to New Zealand, *Phormium tenax* (from the Family Agavaceae) has been widely adopted for landscaping purposes, because it forms handsome architectural clumps of long, straplike leaves that have been used in traditional basketry. As a Maori herb, known as harakeke, it is used similarly to aloe vera, being applied topically to wounds and sores, burns and abscesses, ringworm, varicose ulcers, chilblains and rheumatic joints. It has also been used to normalize digestive disorders.

Galangal

Latin Name *Alpinia galanga* Zingiberaceae
Other common names **Blue ginger, Siamese ginger, Thai ginger**
Part used **Rhizomes**

Galangal (*Alpinia galanga*)

There are two types of galangal —
greater galangal, which is native to
Java, and lesser galangal, which can
be found in the coastal regions of
southern China. They are both grown
throughout Southeast Asia, Indonesia
and India.

Gardening

Greater galangal (*Alpinia galanga*) is
a rhizomatous perennial producing
several 6.5-ft. (2-m) stalks with
alternate sheathing leaves. The
flowers are followed by red three-
valved fruits. The white-fleshed
rhizomes have a characteristic spice
and pine fragrance, and are widely
used in Asian cooking. The flowers,
flower buds and cardamom-scented
red fruits are all edible. Lesser
galangal (*A. officinarum*), native to
Vietnam and China, is a smaller
plant with aromatic reddish brown
rhizomes that are used medicinally.

The related low-growing
Kaempferia galanga is also known
as lesser galangal and resurrection
lily, and it flowers at ground level. It
is used as a spice and medicinally.

Fingerroot (*Kaempferia
pandurata*), also called Chinese
keys, grows to 1.5 ft. (50 cm) and
has long, slender fingerlike storage
roots attached to the rhizome, which
is crisp, with a fresh lemony taste.
The Australian *Alpinia caerulea* has
ginger-scented rhizomes. The red
fruits of *A. oxyphylla* from southern
China, known as black cardamom
or sharp-leaf galangal or yi zhi, are
used in Chinese medicine.

Position ▶ Galangal requires
warm-temperate to subtropical
conditions, and grows best in rich,
moist, well-drained soils.

Propagation ▶ Galangal is an
annual crop, grown by seed or from
rhizome segments; cut them so
that each segment contains one or
two buds.

Maintenance ▶ Keep the soil moist.

Pests and diseases ▶ Rhizome
rot is the principal problem.

Harvesting and storing ▶
For fresh culinary use, dig up the
rhizomes in late summer or early
autumn. Store fresh galangal in a
cool, dark place for up to 2 weeks.
Dry the root about 10 months after
planting. Store dried slices in an
airtight container in a dry, dark place
for 2 to 3 years.

Herbal medicine

Alpinia officinarum. Part used:
rhizomes. In the past, galangal's
calming effects on the gut were
often used to relieve symptoms of
indigestion, including flatulence
and nausea. Like ginger, it was
reputed to be helpful in alleviating
seasickness.

For the safe and appropriate
medicinal use of galangal, consult
your healthcare professional. Do not
use galangal in greater than culinary
quantities if you are pregnant or
breastfeeding.

Cooking

Galangal's flavor is similar to
ginger's but is not as strong. Greater
galangal (*Alpinia galanga*) is the
type more often used in cooking,
especially in Thailand, but also in
Malaysia, Singapore, India and China.

Use the rhizome fresh, or in dried
slices (Before using dried slices, soak
them in hot water for 30 minutes.),
with fish and in soups (especially
the hot-and-sour ones of Southeast
Asia). It features in spicy condiments
such as sambals and in the Moroccan
spice blend ras el hanout. If galangal
is not available, substitute half the
quantity of grated fresh ginger.

Chewing John

Chewing John is the root of the
galangal plant. Chewed like
tobacco, it calms the stomach and
sweetens the breath, but it is also
associated with good luck: It is
said that if you spit the juice onto
the floor of a courtroom before
the judge enters, you'll win your
case. Other names for this root
are Little John or Low John in the
Deep South.

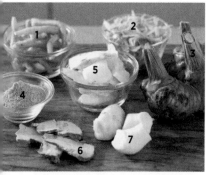

1. Fingerroot 2. Grated fresh root 3. Whole
root 4. Dried ground root 5. Sliced fresh root
6. Sliced dried root 7. Peeled fresh root

Garlic & onions

Latin Name *Allium* sp. Liliaceae
Parts used **Leaves, bulbs, bulbils, seed, flowers**

The Sumerians planted onions more than 5,000 years ago, while the ancient Egyptians had about 8,000 medicinal uses for them, and often placed them in their tombs. In culinary terms, however, onions are said to be the poor man's truffle.

Gardening

The alliums — approximately 700 species of them — include not only globe onions, eschallots, leeks, garlic, wild garlic and chives of various kinds, but also exotic forms, such as walking onions and potato onions. Many are so attractive they long ago made their way into the ornamental garden. Alliums are all either bulbous or rhizomatous in habit, characteristically with straplike or hollow leaves and simple umbels of star-shaped flowers emerging from a papery sheathing bract.

Garlic

Garlic (*A. sativum*) is divided into two groups: 'softnecks' (*A. sativum* var. *sativum*), which contain all the common garlic varieties, and 'hardnecks' (*A. sativum* var. *ophioscorodon*), which contain the remarkable rocambole (serpent garlic or Spanish garlic). It produces tall, sinuously looping stems with a head of bulbils (secondary bulbs that can grow into new plants) mixed with miniature plants. Belowground it forms a bulb of 4 to 14 cloves.
Ramsons or bear's garlic (*A. ursinum*) is an intensely garlic-scented species, and both the leaves and bulbils are used.
Russian garlic or giant garlic or sand leek (*A. scorodoprasum*) develops

a large basal bulb comprising several huge cloves.
Wild garlic or three-cornered leek (*A. triquetrum*) has garlic-flavored foliage, small garlic-flavored bulbs and nodding umbels of attractive starry white flowers.

Chives

Four culinary species of chives are widely grown for their foliage: fragrant garlic chives (*A. odorum*) from central Asia, with red-striped white petals; onion chives (*A. schoenoprasum*), with umbels of pink flowers; garlic or Chinese chives (*A. tuberosum*), with white flowers and deliciously garlic-scented, straplike foliage; and mauve-flowered, garlic-flavored society garlic (*Tulbaghia violacea*) in both a green and variegated leaf form.

Onions

Common globe onion (*Allium cepa*) is the best known of this aromatic tribe. Spring onions are any variety of onion that is pulled when just beginning to bulb.
Tree onion or Egyptian onion or walking onion (*A. cepa*, Proliferum Group) forms a basal bulb, while the flowers are replaced by a cluster of small bulbils that weigh the stalk to the ground, allowing the bulbils to take root.
Potato onion (*A. cepa*, Aggregatum Group) forms a large cluster of plump smallish onions at the base.
Shallots — or eschallots or scallions (*A. cepa*, Aggregatum Group) — form

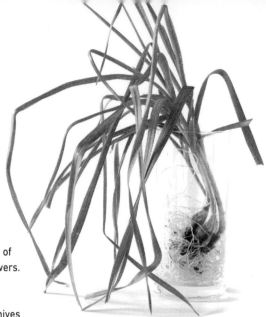

Garlic (*Allium sativum*)

an aboveground bulb that splits to form a cluster of bulbs with a delicate flavor.
Chinese onion or rakkyo (*A. chinensis*) is an Asian species cultivated for its crisp textured bulbs, which are popularly used raw, pickled or cooked.
Nodding onion or lady's leek (*A. cernuum*), a North American perennial, has an intense onion flavor in all parts.
Canada onion (*A. canadense*) forms crisp white bulbs and has deliciously onion-scented foliage.
Milder-flavored leeks (*A. porrum*) originate from the Mediterranean. Some excellent varieties include 'Musselburgh,' 'Giant Carentan' and 'Bleu Solaise.'
Garlic leek, sweet leek or Levant garlic (*A. ampeloprasum*) is perennial and develops a large basal bulb, which splits into several cloves.

Opposite page: 1. Green onions
2. Yellow (brown) onions
3. Green onions with their tops
4. Red onion 5. Spring onions

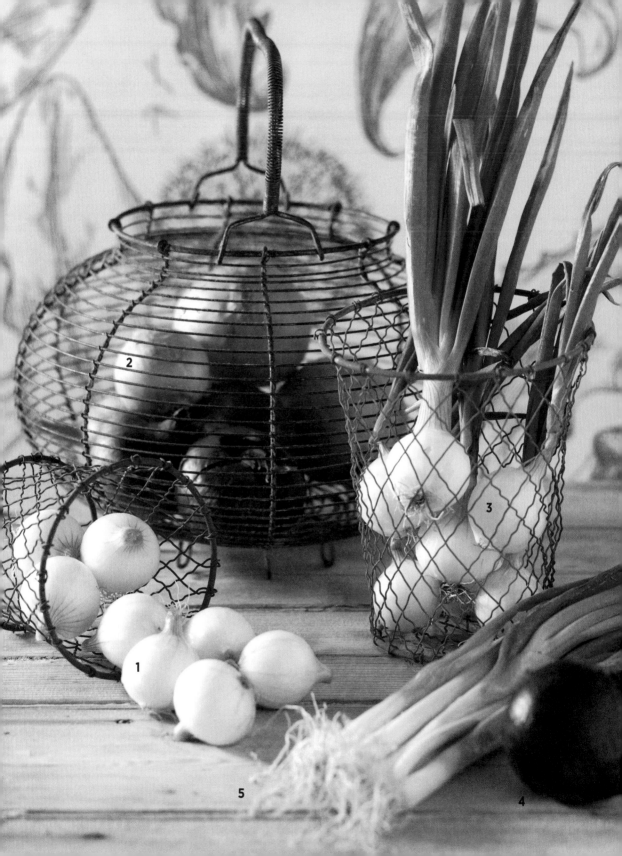

Garlic & onions *Continued*

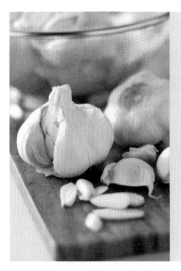

How to peel garlic

Peeling large quantities of garlic is rather tedious. If you're peeling garlic that is to be sliced or chopped, first thump the clove with the flat blade of a large knife. This will distort and crack the skin, making it easier to remove. If you want to use the cloves whole, use a commercially available gadget consisting of a small flexible rubber tube; place the unpeeled cloves in this and roll the tube on a work surface for a few seconds. When you tip out the contents, the cloves should be neatly separated from their husks.

Poor man's leek or Welsh onion (*A. fistulosum*) grows in the same manner as leeks but has hollow leaves. The plant divides at the base, forming a perennial clump.

Ramps or wood leeks (*A. tricoccum*) form scallionlike, onion and garlic-tasting bulbs.

Position ▶ All the principal *Allium* species require a well-tilled and weed-free soil, good drainage and a sunny position.

Propagation ▶ Plant onions by seed. In areas with a short growing season, grow them to the size of bulbils, or sets, in their first season, then plant them out to mature in the second season. Raise chives, cold-tolerant leeks and their relatives by seed. Propagate garlic by planting cloves vertically, with the pointed tip covered by about 1 in. (2.5 cm) of soil.

Maintenance ▶ Regular weeding is essential, particularly in the earlier stages of growth. Do not overwater.

Pests and diseases ▶ The main problems are downy mildew and black aphid. Garlic is susceptible to nematode (eelworm) attack.

As it is an accumulator, do not use chemicals. To clear the soil of nematodes, plant a prior crop of dwarf orange marigolds (*Tagetes patula*).

Harvesting and storing ▶ If growing species for their aromatic foliage, use them fresh. Harvest globe onions at any stage. When they've stopped growing, the tops of both onions and garlic fall over and wither. Choose a sunny day to pull the bulbs of both types, then leave them for a few days to dry out. Store in a dry, well-ventilated area to prevent fungal rots.

Herbal medicine

Allium sativum. Part used: bulbs. Regular consumption of garlic, a potent natural antibiotic, can help to prevent and treat infections of the lungs and is a traditional cure for coughs and colds. Garlic's antimicrobial effects also extend to the gut, and it can be helpful in the treatment of gastrointestinal infections. Furthermore, inclusion of garlic in the diet has also been shown to have a preventative effect against stomach and colorectal cancers.

Garlic produces a number of beneficial effects on the cardiovascular system, many of which have been confirmed by clinical trials. Garlic supplementation has been shown to lower cholesterol levels, prevent the hardening of arteries and lessen the risk of blood-clot formation. It can also help to reduce blood pressure as well as improve general circulation.

For the safe and effective medicinal use of garlic, see Sore throats, colds & flu, *page 174,* and High blood pressure & cholesterol, *page 202.* Do not use garlic in greater than culinary quantities if you are pregnant or breastfeeding.

Cooking

Garlic complements almost any savory dish, and goes well with most culinary herbs and spices. It is an essential ingredient in many cuisines, especially Asian, Mexican, Mediterranean, Middle Eastern and

---

Elephant garlic

Native to the Mediterranean and the Middle East, the giant cloves of elephant garlic (*A. ampeloprasum* 'Elephant') have a sweet flavor that is much less pungent than the garlic commonly used in cooking. The plant is actually a member of the leek family (one of its common names is perennial sweet leek). Eat the cloves raw or cook them like onions.

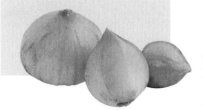

Remove any small green shoots from the center of a cut garlic clove, because these tend to make food taste bitter.

Caribbean. Even if you don't like the taste of garlic itself, a small amount will enhance the flavor of many dishes.

Garlic comes in white-, pink- and purple-skinned varieties, and in a range of sizes. Choose firm bulbs that are not sprouting, and that are tightly encased in their husks. Peeled cloves should be creamy white, not gray or yellow. Remove any areas of discoloration before using, as these will impart a rank taste to the dish.

When peeled, then sliced or chopped, the enzymes within a clove of garlic react on exposure to air to produce a strong, lingering, sulphurous aroma. The flavor of garlic is similarly strong and sharp, and gives the impression of heat on the palate. The more finely it is crushed or chopped, the stronger its aroma becomes. When cooked properly, the flavor is mellow and sweet. Try baking a whole head in foil, then squeeze out the contents of the cloves. This mellow, creamy paste is delicious spread on bread or cooked meats or stirred through mashed vegetables such as potato. Take care when cooking garlic; if it is cooked over too high a heat, it will burn, become bitter and taste unpleasant. Even a tiny amount of burned garlic will permeate and spoil a whole dish.

Garlic is used raw in aïoli (a French garlic mayonnaise) and tapenade

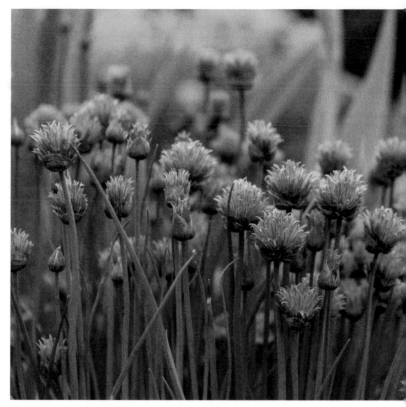

Chives bear pale purple to pale pink bell-shaped umbels of flowers in summer.

(olive paste). Crushed garlic mashed into butter is a delicious and simple sauce for cooked meats, or it can be spread on a sliced loaf or baguette, wrapped in foil and baked in a medium-hot oven for 10 minutes or so. Push slivers of garlic into slits in a joint of lamb or pork, or put a few cloves inside the cavity of a chicken before roasting.

Various processed forms of garlic are commercially available, including crushed pastes and dehydrated flakes, powders and granules. If you are using commercial garlic pastes in a recipe, you may need to make adjustments for the flavor of the salt and vinegar that are often added as preservatives. Garlic is also used in many commercial spice blends, including herb salt, garlic salt and pizza seasoning.

Chives

Depending on the variety, chives (*A. schoenoprasum*) have a mild onion or garlic flavor that goes well with sauces, stews, mashed vegetables such as potatoes, fish, poultry and egg dishes (especially scrambled eggs), and cream cheeses and salad dressings. The delicate flavor is easily destroyed by heat, so add chives during the last few minutes of cooking time, or scatter them on a finished dish to garnish.

Snip chives with scissors, rather than chop them with a knife. They are essential (along with chervil, parsley and tarragon) in the French herb blend called *fines herbes*. Snip chives finely and freeze them in ice-cube trays to preserve. The flowers make a pretty garnish.

Ginger

Latin Name *Zingiber officinale* Zingiberaceae

Part used **Rhizomes**

Ginger was highly recommended by none other than Confucius, who is reputed to have flavored all his food with it. It has many medicinal uses, including treating motion sickness and nausea.

Gardening

Native to tropical Asia, ginger is a rhizomatous perennial to about 35 in. (90 cm) high, producing many fibrous leaf stalks sheathed in alternating lanceolate leaves. The plump rhizomes, known as 'hands,' are pale yellow when freshly dug. The yellow flowers, with purple lips and green bracts, are arranged in dense, club-like spikes. They are followed by fleshy, three-valved capsules.

The spring shoots and flower buds of Japanese or myoga ginger (*Z. mioga*) are popular in Japanese cuisine, and cassumar ginger (*Z. cassumar*) is used in Southeast Asia.

Position ▶ It grows best in rich, moist, well-drained soil and requires warm temperate to subtropical conditions.

Propagation ▶ Grow ginger by seed or from rhizome segments, cut so that each segment contains one or two buds.

Maintenance ▶ Keep the soil moist.

Pests and diseases ▶ Rhizome rot is the principal problem.

Harvesting and storing ▶ For fresh culinary use, dig up the rhizomes in late summer or early autumn. If drying, do so about 10 months after planting.

Ginger root
(*Zingiber officinale*)

Herbal medicine

Zingiber officinale. Part used: rhizomes. Ginger has been clinically proven as a safe, effective remedy for the prevention and treatment of nausea. It can also benefit other digestive symptoms such as indigestion, colic and flatulence.

It is traditionally used to relieve various conditions associated with 'cold' symptoms as well as period pain, cold hands and feet, arthritis and rheumatism. It may also help protect the heart and blood vessels by preventing the formation of blood clots and lowering cholesterol levels.

Cooking

Young ginger is tender and sweet, with a spicy, tangy, warm to hot flavor. Older ginger is stronger, hotter and more fibrous. Japanese ginger (*Z. mioga*), known as gari, is widely used as a sushi condiment.

In Asian, Caribbean and African cuisine, ginger is an essential ingredient in curries, stews, soups,

Storing and preserving ginger

Select clean, plump, firm rhizomes, then wrap them tightly in foil and store in the vegetable crisper of the refrigerator for several weeks. For long-term storage, ginger may be pickled, preserved in sherry or other strong spirit, or crystallized. Store crystallized ginger or ginger in syrup in an airtight container in a cool, dry place. They will keep for up to 1 year.

salads, pickles, chutneys, marinades, stir-fries and meat, fish and vegetable dishes. Fresh ginger's uses are mostly savory; crystallized ginger is used in baked goods, or eaten on its own as confectionery, often sugar-coated.

Dried ginger is hotter than fresh ginger. Ground dried ginger is used in baking and in commercial spice mixtures. Both ground dried ginger and ginger essential oil are used in commercial food flavoring, while ginger extracts are used in cordials, ginger beer and ginger ale.

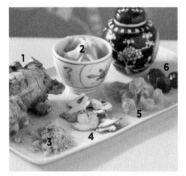

1. Whole ginger root 2. Pickled ginger
3. Ground dried ginger 4. Sliced dried ginger 5. Crystallized ginger 6. Glacé ginger

Ginkgo

Latin Name *Ginkgo biloba* Ginkgoaceae
Other common name **Maidenhair tree**
Parts used **Fruits, leaves**

The ginkgo dates back to the time of the dinosaurs, before the evolution of flowering plants. It may now be extinct in the wild, but is one of the most frequently prescribed herbs in Western herbal medicine.

Gardening

The sole remaining species of the once abundant and widely distributed plant order Ginkgoales, which dates back to the Jurassic and Triassic periods, ginkgo has long been cultivated in Japan and China as a sacred tree. The plant has fan-shaped notched leaves resembling those of the maidenhair fern, and makes an attractive ornamental tree. The species is dioecious, so the

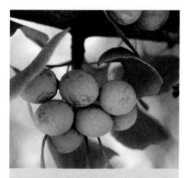

A seed of promise

Ginkgo has a longstanding association with improvement in brain function and mood, especially in older people. Human trials have shown positive effects on memory impairment and poor concentration as well as the treatment and prevention of symptoms of some types of dementia, including Alzheimer's disease.

unpleasant smelling plumlike fruit are formed only where male and female trees are grown together.

The 'fruits' are naked seeds, as true fruits only developed with the rise of the flowering plants. Within is a seed resembling an almond, prized in both China and Japan, which is boiled, roasted or baked before being cracked open. The tree is deciduous, coloring a clear gold in autumn.

Varieties ▶ Most varieties of ginkgo were selected for ornamental purposes. These include the fastigiate 'Princeton Sentry,' the dwarf 'Chi Chi' and 'Jade Butterfly,' and the excellent male clone, 'Autumn Gold.'

Position ▶ Ginkgo is fully hardy, suited to a cool climate, and prefers a sunny position and well-drained, fertile soil. It is very slow-growing.

Propagation ▶ You can propagate ginkgo by seed, and if you require fruit, plant a male with a female. Grow named varieties by grafting or by cuttings of semi-ripe wood in summer.

Maintenance ▶ These trees require little pruning.

Pests and diseases ▶ Ginkgo is virtually pest-free.

Harvesting and storing ▶ Harvest ripe fruits when they fall from the tree and extract the almond-like seed. Harvest the leaves and dry them as they begin to change color in autumn.

Herbal medicine

Ginkgo biloba. Part used: leaves. Extensive laboratory research has identified many pharmacological

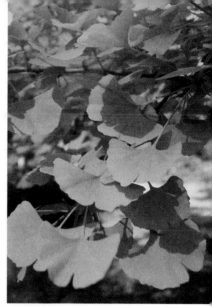

Ginkgo (*Ginkgo biloba*)

actions associated with ginkgo leaf, including potent antioxidant and anti-inflammatory effects, an ability to enhance blood flow through arteries, veins and capillaries, as well as a protective effect on many cells of the body against toxin damage. These properties explain the therapeutic application of ginkgo to a range of health conditions, many of them verified by human trials. (See box, left.)

Clinical studies in patients have shown ginkgo to be beneficial for the treatment of some circulatory disorders, including intermittent claudication, where poor blood flow to the legs results in symptoms of numbness, pain and cramping, and Raynaud's syndrome, where there is poor circulation to the hands and feet. Further clinical trials also indicate its use in the treatment of vertigo, tinnitus, asthma and premenstrual syndrome.

For the safe and appropriate use of ginkgo, see Memory & concentration, *page 187*, and Circulation problems, *page 200*. Do not use ginkgo if you are pregnant or breastfeeding.

Ginseng

Latin Name *Panax* **sp.** and *Eleutherococcus senticosus* **Araliaceae**
Part used **Roots**

Ginseng has been used in Chinese medicine for at least 5,000 years. Today it is widely recognized in Western medicine as an adaptogen, reducing the body's reaction to trauma and stress. The closely related Siberian ginseng and American ginseng have similar uses.

Gardening

Chinese (Asian or Korean) ginseng (*Panax ginseng*) is a long-lived deciduous perennial with branched taproots, from which spring long-stalked, divided leaves. Siberian ginseng (*Eleutherococcus senticosus*), which is part of the same plant family, is a deciduous shrub with thick roots, divided leaves and umbels of black berries.

Varieties ▶ American ginseng (*Panax quinquefolius*) is close in appearance and activity to Chinese ginseng, while Japanese ginseng (*P. japonicus*) is widely used in tonic drinks in Japan. Notoginseng (*P. pseudoginseng*) is a hemostatic herb.

Ginseng root
(*Panax ginseng*)

Position ▶ Plants grow in full sun to light shade, and need a moist, rich, well-drained soil. *Panax* species require mild summers and cold winters, deep shade and a slightly acidic soil.

Propagation ▶ Plants are seed grown, germinating rather erratically, so that seed is often stratified (see box, *page 40*). Propagate *Eleutherococcus* by seed, by softwood or hardwood cuttings, and by root cuttings.

Maintenance ▶ With forest-floor crops, little is required other than patience.

Pests and diseases ▶ Field-grown crops can attract a range of pests and diseases.

Harvesting and storing ▶ Harvest ginseng roots in autumn from plants that are usually 6 years or older. Use them fresh or peeled and dried.

Herbal medicine

Korean ginseng (*Panax ginseng*), American ginseng (*P. quinquefolius*), Siberian ginseng (*Eleutherococcus senticosus*). Part used: roots. Modern research has shown that these herbs improve the body's capacity to cope with stress, so they have become popular remedies for enhancing mental function and physical performance during times of overwork, fatigue, exhaustion or convalescence.

American ginseng has recently been successfully trialled as a treatment for reducing the incidence of upper respiratory infections. All three ginsengs have also been shown to lower blood sugar, and may be of

Withania

Although not related to the ginsengs, withania (*Withania somnifera*) is sometimes called Indian ginseng as a result of its ability to improve mood, mental capacity and physical strength during recovery from illness and times of stress. Withania also appears to have an adaptogenic-type effect on the body, as well as positive effects on immune function. However, in contrast to the ginsengs, withania has a mild sedative action and has traditionally been prescribed for some cases of insomnia. It is also high in iron, and can be a valuable remedy for treating anemia.

benefit in the treatment of diabetes. Although the ginsengs appear to be of benefit in a wide range of chronic illnesses, many clinical trials investigating these herbs have produced mixed results, perhaps due to the large variations in the quality, dose, preparation and duration of the different ginsengs used.

For the safe and appropriate use of Korean ginseng, see Tension & stress, *page 184*. For the safe and appropriate use of Siberian ginseng and withania, see Tiredness & fatigue, *page 186*. Do not use these herbs if you are pregnant or breastfeeding.

Gotu kola

Latin Name *Centella asiatica* syn. *Hydrocotyle asiatica* Apiaceae
Other common names **Arthritis herb, Asiatic pennywort**
Parts used **Whole plant, leaves**

The reputed extraordinary longevity of Professor Li Chung Yon, who is said to have died at the age of 256, outliving 24 successive wives, is attributed to drinking tea made with this Chinese "long-life herb," which is also an important Ayurvedic plant.

Gardening

Gotu kola is closely related to the pennywort (*Hydrocotyle* sp.) and more remotely to celery and parsley. The plant is a small, creeping, subtropical to tropical groundcover that spreads by stolons, in a similar manner to strawberries and violets, forming plantlets that root into the ground and eventually form a dense mat. Individual plants have basal rosettes of shiny, kidney-shaped, slightly fleshy, serrated, long-stalked leaves. The modest flowers are borne in umbels below the leaves. Its natural habitat is in damp places and along stream and pond margins.

Position ▶ Gotu kola is easily grown in a large pot or a dedicated garden bed filled with free-draining, sandy soil enriched with compost and kept moist. It can be grown in full sun or light shade. In cool-climate areas it should be grown under cover in winter. It tends to die back, but will reshoot in spring.

Propagation ▶ It can be propagated by seed, but is most easily grown from rooted sections of stolon with at least one plantlet attached.

Maintenance ▶ Regularly water and weed gotu kola as necessary.

Pests and diseases ▶ There are no significant problems.

Used in various skin rejuvenation products, gotu kola stimulates collagen production.

Harvesting and storing ▶
Harvest the leaves and use them fresh as required. Dry the leaves out of direct sunlight: Spread them out in a single layer or dry them under warm fan-forced air, then store them in an airtight container for medicinal use and for tea. You can also juice the leaves and add them sparingly to tonics.

The elixir of youth

According to official records of the Chinese government, Professor Li Chung Yon, a renowned scholar and herbalist, was born in 1677. The story goes that he was a vegetarian who used gotu kola and ginseng and took brisk daily walks while cultivating a calm and serene attitude to life (walking like a pigeon, sitting like a tortoise and sleeping like a dog). When he died in 1933, as reported by *The New York Times*, he apparently looked like a man in his prime, with his hair and teeth intact. He spent the first 100 years of his life studying and gathering wild herbs, and the latter part lecturing and educating people about herbs and longevity.

Gotu kola (*Centella asiatica*)

Herbal medicine

Centella asiatica. Parts used: whole plant, leaves. Gotu kola has been used therapeutically for centuries. Ayurvedic herbalists regard gotu kola as an effective nerve tonic that exerts a calming and strengthening effect on nerve and brain cells, helping to improve memory and reduce anxiety.

According to traditional Chinese medicine, gotu kola is believed to slow senility, act as a promoter of longevity and improve rheumatic problems.

Studies investigating the topical and internal use of gotu kola have confirmed an impressive burn- and wound-healing capacity, and a strengthening effect on veins, with notable improvement in varicose veins and other vein disorders.

For the safe and appropriate use of gotu kola, consult your healthcare professional. Do not use gotu kola if you are pregnant or breastfeeding.

Heartsease

Latin Name *Viola tricolor* Violaceae
Other common names **Johnny-jump-up, love-lies-bleeding, wild pansy**
Parts used **Flowers (culinary), aerial parts (medicinally)**

This pretty European wildflower, which has acquired an extraordinary number of names, is associated with thought in the language of flowers. Although it may not heal broken hearts, as once reputed, it does have a wide variety of herbal uses.

Gardening

Heartsease is an annual or short-lived perennial forming a spreading, low-growing herb, which flowers profusely in spring and summer with tiny pansylike flowers. It was one of the progenitors of the modern pansy, and the flowers vary considerably in their color patterns. They usually have a purple spur and upper petals, while the remaining three petals are variously colored purple, white and yellow with characteristic "pussy whisker" markings created by fine purple veins.The leaves are oval and coarsely toothed. The flowers are followed by three-valved capsules, which burst open to reveal densely packed, round brown seeds.

Varieties ▶ The variety 'Helen Mount' is a short-lived perennial with richly colored flowers of purple, lavender and yellow.

Position ▶ Heartsease prefers a moist, cool location in light dappled shade and slightly acidic soil. In the right position, it will reseed generously.

Propagation ▶ Raise plants from seed, then plant the seedlings in autumn and lightly cover with soil. They can also be successfully sown directly into the garden.

Maintenance ▶ A gentle clipping over the whole plant in summer will encourage it to bloom through autumn. The plants are fully cold-hardy.

Pests and diseases ▶ Heartsease encounters few problems.

Harvesting and storing ▶ For culinary purposes, harvest the fresh flowers at any time. The aerial parts of the plant are harvested for medicinal use, usually when in full flower. To dry the plants, hang them upside down in a well-ventilated place away from direct sunshine.

Herbal medicine

Viola tricolor. Parts used: aerial parts. Heartsease may have acquired its name from its traditional reputation as a beneficial remedy for heart conditions or a belief that it acted as a love potion.

However, these days heartsease is regarded as a remedy for the skin and is used to treat eczema and other skin conditions. It is commonly prescribed for such conditions in both infants and adults, and is administered either as an infusion or topically to the area in the form of a compress on the affected area.

When taken internally, the soothing and anti-inflammatory properties of heartsease are also useful for conditions of the lungs and urinary system, helping to alleviate the symptoms of bronchitis and cystitis.

For the safe and appropriate use of heartsease, consult your healthcare professional. Do not use heartsease if you are pregnant or breastfeeding.

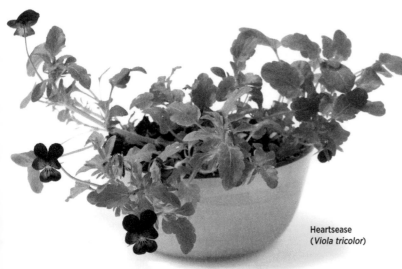

Heartsease
(*Viola tricolor*)

Salad in bloom

Many herbs, including heartsease, have edible flowers, which look very pretty in a salad. (Some flowers are poisonous, so be sure to check before use.) Mix a variety of salad greens with heartsease flowers (the green parts removed) and the flowers of nasturtium, borage, bergamot, fennel, rocket or calendula. Add a light dressing that won't overwhelm the delicate flavor of the flowers.

Hops

Latin Name *Humulus lupulus* Moraceae
Parts used **Strobiles (cones), shoots, flowers, leaves, vines**

Malted grains used for brewing beer are very sweet and do not keep well, so many bitter herbs, like hops, have been used to improve its flavor and help preserve it. Hops also has sedative properties, and can be used to make a relaxing decoction for the bath.

Gardening

Hops forms a perennial vine that reaches 33 ft. (10 m) each season. Only female plants produce the required small, conelike inflorescences called strobiles. The leaves resemble those of a grape vine and are used as a brown dye, while the vines are used for papermaking and basketry.

Varieties ▶ 'Aureus' is a popular ornamental variety, with light golden leaves that can be used for similar purposes. Early maturing 'Fuggle' is popular with home brewers in England.

Position ▶ Hops is very adaptable but prefers an open, sunny position and a moist, humus-rich soil.

Propagation ▶ Hops can be raised from seed. Only the female plants are required, so propagate either by root division in spring or from cuttings taken in summer.

Maintenance ▶ For the home garden, train hops on a tall tripod or pyramid support. In hop fields, vines traditionally are trained on tall poles. Clean away all dead material in winter.

Pests and diseases ▶ The major problems are downy mildew on leaves, and *Verticillium* wilt.

Harvesting and storing ▶ Young shoots are harvested in spring for culinary use. Strobiles are harvested in autumn and dried. Both the pollen and leaves can cause allergic responses.

Herbal medicine

Humulus lupulus. Part used: female flowers (strobiles). Hops is well known for its mild sedative properties and is commonly prescribed with other relaxing herbs for insomnia, particularly when there is difficulty falling asleep.

The heavily scented essential oil is believed to be responsible for the plant's relaxing effects on the nervous system; the flowers can be used in pillows placed by the bed to induce sleep. Hops' calming effects can also help in reducing anxiety.

Hops has a gently stimulating effect on sluggish digestion due to the presence of bitter compounds, and it is a useful remedy for gastrointestinal complaints, particularly when they are exacerbated by tension and stress. Hops also

Hops
(*Humulus lupulus*)

contains estrogen-like substances and is being investigated for its use in menstrual and menopausal problems.

For the safe and appropriate use of hops, see Insomnia, *page 188*. Do not use hops if you are pregnant or breastfeeding.

It is said George III cured his insomnia by sleeping on a pillow of dried hops.

Horseradish & wasabi

Latin Name *Armoracia rusticana* and *Wasabia japonica* syn.
Cochlearia wasabi Brassicaceae

Parts used **Root and leaves (horseradish); rhizomes (wasabi)**

The grated root of horseradish, cultivated in the eastern Mediterranean region for more than 3,500 years, is used as a pungent condiment and in medicinal preparations. Wasabi, native to Japan, has been cultivated since the 10th century and possesses a similar, very hot taste.

Gardening

Horseradish and wasabi both belong to the same botanical family, Brassicaceae.

Horseradish *Horseradish (Armoracia rusticana)* is a hardy perennial that forms a rosette of long leaves. The 30 or more strains in cultivation include 'Bohemian,' 'Swiss' and 'Sass,' and almost all of them are sterile. There are two ornamental forms — one is variegated with white, the other has purple-suffused leaves. Belowground, horseradish forms a taproot that expands in diameter in the second and third year.

Wasabi Native to Japan, wasabi or Japanese horseradish (*Wasabia japonica*) is a semi-aquatic perennial with long-stemmed, heart-shaped leaves. Its inflorescences of white cruciform flowers reach 16 in. (40 cm).

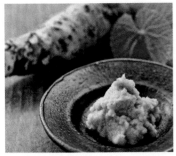

Peel and finely grate fresh wasabi root for use as a condiment.

There are a number of varieties, including 'Tainon No. 1' and 'Daruma,' but all form thick, knobbly rhizomes.

Position ▶ Horseradish requires a sunny position and a well-dug soil enriched with rotted compost. Grow wasabi in very clean, cool, slightly alkaline running water, with plenty of shade. The temperature should be between 50°F and 55°F (10°C and 13°C).

Propagation ▶ In spring, plant pencil-thin sections of lateral horseradish roots horizontally, or up to an angle of 30° from the horizontal. Cover with soil, and firm down. Propagate wasabi from offsets of the rhizome.

Maintenance ▶ Don't let horseradish dry out, or the roots will become bitter. Keep wasabi well-shaded, cool and watered.

Pests and diseases ▶ A number of leaf-eating insects can be a problem for horseradish. White rust, *Alternaria* and bacterial leaf spot may occur.

Harvesting and storing ▶ Dig up horseradish roots and use them fresh at any time in the second and third year; they are at their peak in flavor after the first frost. Store clean roots in sealed plastic bags in the refrigerator for up to 2 months.

Herbal medicine

Armoracia rusticana, Wasabia japonica. Part used: roots or rhizomes. The hot and pungent nature of these roots is due to the presence of compounds responsible for many of their medicinal properties.

Horseradish is antimicrobial and acts as a nasal, sinus and bronchial decongestant, making it a popular remedy for colds and respiratory tract infections. Its antiseptic properties and a diuretic effect have also been used to treat urinary tract infections. Wasabi is believed to have therapeutic effects similar to those of horseradish.

For the safe and appropriate medicinal use of horseradish, see Hay fever & sinusitis, *page 177.* Do not use these herbs in greater than culinary quantities if you are pregnant or breastfeeding.

Cooking

Young horseradish leaves can be eaten as a vegetable, but the root is the part most often used. Peel and grate it as needed, as it loses its pungency soon after grating, or when heated. Alternatively, grate the root (in a well-aired place to avoid the fumes), adding ½ cup (125 ml) white wine vinegar and ¼ teaspoon salt to each cup (250 ml) of pulp. Store, covered, in the refrigerator. Use as a condiment for beef or fresh or smoked fish. Wasabi, often in paste form, is served with sushi, sashimi, soba noodles and other Japanese dishes.

Horseradish (left) and wasabi

Horsetail

Latin Name **Equisetum arvense, E. hyemale** Equisetaceae
Other common names **Pewterwort, scouring rush**
Part used **Sterile stems**

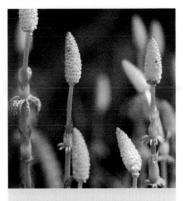

The forests where dinosaurs once roamed were full of giant horsetails, some the height of large trees, but the few that remain 350 million years later are small by comparison. An excellent source of silica, they were once used to scrub pots.

Gardening

Horsetails have slender, hollow, jointed stems with leaves that are reduced to scales. The plants have a deep root system and can spread by rhizomes. Horsetail produces spores in clublike terminal structures, reproducing by cell division of the fallen spores. Occasionally, livestock are poisoned after long-term grazing on horsetail, a condition known as equisetosis.

Horsetails are divided botanically into two major groups: the horsetails, which have whorled branches, and the scouring rushes, which are unbranched.

Varieties ▶ The field horsetail, bottle-brush or shave grass (*E. arvense*) grows to about 2.5 ft. (80 cm) and the sterile stems have whorled branches. The rough horsetail or Dutch rush (*E. hyemale*) produces upright unbranched stems to waist height.

Position ▶ Horsetails are primarily located around water sources, but the rhizomes allow them to move into drier areas. They prefer full sun to part shade and are fully cold-hardy.

Propagation ▶ You can grow horsetails in moist soil from small pieces of rhizome or divisions in spring; however, it can be a very invasive weed that is both difficult to

control and resistant to herbicides. It is a prohibited weed in Australia where it is under statutory control.

Maintenance ▶ None required.

Pests and diseases ▶ None of note.

Harvesting and storing ▶ Harvest the sterile stems in mid- to late summer and dry them.

Herbal medicine

Equisetum arvense. Part used: stems. Horsetail has notable astringent and tissue-healing properties due to its exceptionally high silica content. This herb has a particular affinity for the urinary tract and male reproductive system. Combined with its gentle diuretic action, horsetail is a favored remedy for treating mild inflammatory and infectious conditions of the urinary tract, bladder and prostate gland. Perhaps surprisingly considering its diuretic effects, it is also used in the management of incontinence and bedwetting in children.

Horsetail has long been regarded as an excellent herb for removing waste material from the body, and was used for arthritic and skin disorders where the presence of toxins was believed to exacerbate these conditions. Externally, a poultice of horsetail was used to staunch bleeding and promote the repair of slow-healing wounds.

For the safe and appropriate use of horsetail, consult your healthcare professional. Do not use horsetail if you are pregnant or breastfeeding.

Scouring rush

Rich in silica, horsetails were once every cook's blessing. The hardened longitudinal siliceous ridges on the stems were utilised in ancient Roman times through to the 18th century for scrubbing pots and pans. Horsetail stems were found to be particularly effective for cleaning and polishing pewterware, hence one of the plant's common names—pewterwort. The silica also provided a natural type of nonstick coating for cookware.

Horsetail (*Equisetum hyemale*)

Hyssop

Latin Name *Hyssopus officinalis Lamiaceae*
Other common name **Gratiola**
Parts used **Flowering spikes, leaves**

Grown as much for its beauty and ability to attract bees and butterflies as for its culinary and medicinal uses, hyssop is an ancient herb that was attributed with cleansing properties in biblical times, and for this reason was even used against leprosy.

Gardening

A semi-evergreen perennial subshrub to 2 ft. (60 cm), hyssop is multistemmed from the base, and has small linear leaves borne in whorls up the stems. In summer, the plant bears long slender spikes of lipped, rich blue, nectar-filled flowers borne to one side of the stem only.

Varieties ▶ A white-flowered variety called 'Alba' and a pink-flowered variety called 'Rosea' are also available. The dried flowers and leaves are used to make a tea for sore throats and bronchitis. Rock hyssop (*H. officinalis* 'Aristatus') is a dwarf compact form with purple-blue flowers.

Position ▶ Hyssop requires a sunny, well-drained position, and is not fussy about the soil.

Propagation ▶ You can easily propagate hyssop by seed sown in spring, or you can grow it from cuttings taken either in spring

or autumn. The plants require a minimum spacing of 2 ft. (60 cm), although the distance can be halved if you are using hyssop for hedging.

Maintenance ▶ To prevent plants from becoming "leggy," lightly prune after flowering and again in spring. Hyssop makes an excellent hedge that is comparable to that of lavender.

Pests and diseases ▶ Hyssop has few problems. It is used as a trap plant for cabbage white butterfly around brassicas and as a companion plant for grapes.

Harvesting and storing ▶ Harvest the leaves at any time and use them fresh, or dry them out of sunlight before storing them in airtight containers. When flowering starts, pick the inflorescences to use fresh, or dry them.

Herbal medicine

Hyssopus officinalis. Parts used: aerial parts. Hyssop possesses a remarkable range of medicinal properties. It is particularly suited to alleviating conditions of the respiratory tract and is associated

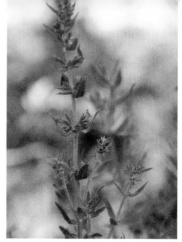

Hyssop (*Hyssopus officinalis*)

with antibacterial and antiviral activity, assisting the removal of catarrh and alleviating fevers. Hyssop is therefore often prescribed for colds, flu, feverish conditions, bronchitis and coughs.

Hyssop is also reputed to have a calming effect on the nerves and can assist with reducing anxiety. It has been used to help bring on delayed periods, particularly when the cause is due to tension and stress.

Modern research indicates that as a topical agent, hyssop may help combat herpes infections such as cold sores.

For the safe and appropriate use of hyssop, consult your healthcare professional. Do not use hyssop if you are pregnant or breastfeeding.

The bitter mint–tasting leaves are used to flavor rich foods such as wild game and pâté.

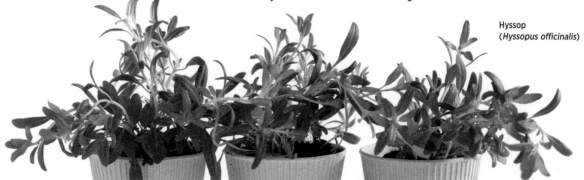

Hyssop
(*Hyssopus officinalis*)

Iris

Latin Name *Iris* sp. Iridaceae
Part used **Rhizomes**

The beautiful irises include several herbal species with rhizomes, known as orris root, which are used for a multitude of purposes, from perfumery (as a fixative) and herbal medicine to flavoring gin and chewing gum.

Gardening

Iris x *germanica* 'Florentina' and the Dalmatian iris (*I. pallida* 'Dalmatica') are used for commercial orris production. The early flowering 'Florentina' is a tall bearded iris with white, sweetly scented flowers. The species form of *I.* x *germanica*, which has also been used for orris, is known by names such as 'Old Purple Flag,' 'Germanica Ancien' and 'Florentina Blue.' The beautiful ceremonial white-flowered *I.* x *germanica* 'Albicans' is still planted on Muslim graves in the eastern Mediterranean.

Varieties ▶ *Iris pallida* has grape-scented flowers, but its variety, 'Dalmatica,' has tall-stemmed, pale lilac flowers. The blue flag (*I. versicolor*) has purple to violet flowers and tall, swordlike deciduous leaves; the plant can cause allergic responses. The yellow flag

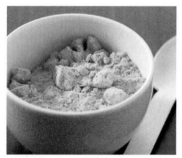

Dried orris root is used in homemade toothpastes and in potpourri.

(*I. pseudacorus*) has tall, swordlike deciduous foliage and tall, stemmed yellow flowers.

Position ▶ *Iris pallida* 'Dalmatica' and *I.* x *germanica* 'Florentina' are hardy, easily grown plants if provided with a well-drained soil and full sun. Grow both *I. versicolor* and *I. pseudacorus* in moist soil.

Propagation ▶ Grow *I. pallida* 'Dalmatica' and *I.* x *germanica* 'Florentina' from divisions of rhizomes that have at least one leaf fan attached. Cut back the fans to about 6 in. (15 cm), and plant the rhizomes horizontally so that only the lower half is buried in the soil.

Maintenance ▶ Control weeds.

Pests and diseases ▶ Rhizome rots occur in poorly drained or shaded plants.

Harvesting and storing ▶ In late summer, dig rhizomes, clean and dry them, and cure for 2 years to intensify the violet fragrance.

Herbal medicine

Iris versicolor. Part used: rhizomes. A close relative of the popular garden irises, blue flag has a long history of medicinal use in the treatment of skin problems such as acne and eczema. Traditionally these conditions are believed to be the result of an accumulation of toxins in the body, and blue flag appears to work by encouraging the liver, bowel and lymphatic system to remove waste material from the body more effectively.

Blue flag is often used in combination with other cleansing herbs, such as yellow dock and burdock, for these purposes.

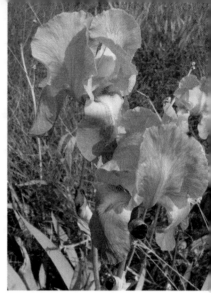

Iris (*Iris* sp.)

For the safe and appropriate use of blue flag, consult your healthcare professional. Do not use blue flag if you are pregnant or breastfeeding.

Around the home

Orris root, a grayish powder with the aroma of violets, is derived from the root of the Florentine iris. It is used less for its scent than for its fixative ability — that is, it slows the evaporation of essential oils and prolongs the life of potpourris. Orris root can be sprinkled around the edges of areas of carpet or under rugs to deter, although not kill, moths and destructive carpet beetles.

Heraldic emblem

The yellow flag (*I. pseudacorus*) is the *fleur de lis* of heraldry. In the 12th century, the French kings were the first to use an image of the flower on their shields, and later English kings used it to emphasize their claims to the French throne. Its resemblance to a spearhead is seen as an appropriate symbol of martial power and strength.

Jasmine

Latin Name *Jasminum* sp. Oleaceae
Other common name Jessamine
Parts used Flowers, roots

Many species of jasmine — the delicate floral emblem of Indonesia, Pakistan and the Philippines — are renowned for their superb sensuous scent, and the very valuable essential oil is produced in several countries for perfumery and aromatherapy.

Gardening

Common jasmine (*J. officinale*) is a frost-hardy, tall twining climber with compound leaves and five-petaled, intensely fragrant flowers fused into a tube at the base. Brought to Europe in the 16th century, it is now extensively cultivated commercially for its flowers in southern France, Spain, India, Egypt, China, Algeria and Morocco.

Varieties ▶ Fancy leaf forms include 'Argenteovariegatum,' 'Aureum' and 'Frojas.' Fragrant *J. x stepanense* is a pink-flowered hybrid. The large-flowered Catalonian jasmine, also known as royal jasmine, poet's jasmine or Spanish jasmine, is variously regarded as a variety of *J. officinale* 'Grandiflora,' or as the separate species, *J. grandiflora*.

Arabian jasmine (*J. sambac*) is used to make a fragrant tisane in China, the blossoms being hand-picked early in the morning and mixed with dried green or Oolong tea. Native to India, it forms an arching bush.

Double-flowered forms of *J. sambac*, favored for garlands and religious ceremonies, include the very double, miniature roselike 'Duke of Tuscany' (syn. *kudda-mulla*), the semi-double 'Maid of Orléans' and the smaller-flowered double 'Belle of India.'

Other common fragrant, white-flowered species include angel wing jasmine (*J. nitidum*), the pink-budded *J. polyanthemum*, Azores jasmine (*J. azoricum*), Canary Island jasmine (*J. odoratissimum*), *J. multiflorum* and *J. floribundum*. There are a number of yellow-flowered species, some fragrant, but they are not used herbally.

Position ▶ Plants prefer a well-drained soil enriched with rotted compost. Most species require warm to tropical climates but in colder areas can make excellent glasshouse plants.

Propagation ▶ Propagate jasmine from semi-ripened wood cuttings.

Maintenance ▶ In cold areas *J. sambac* and its varieties should be overwintered under protection, because they are unlikely to survive frost exposure. Trim *J. officinale* immediately after flowering.

Pests and diseases ▶ Jasmine plants grown in the open have few problems; however, those grown under glass can be attacked by whitefly, mealy bugs and spider mites.

Harvesting and storing ▶ Gather fully developed buds in the early morning and add the opening flowers to tea. You can dry them for herbal use. Lift the roots of *J. sambac* in autumn and dry them for medicinal use.

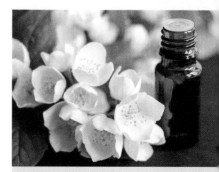

Jasmine essential oil

The delicate, star-shaped flowers of this evergreen vine are distilled to form an essential oil with a rich, warm floral scent that is important in perfumery. It blends well with other "floral-style" oils, such as rose, and is particularly helpful in preparations for dry, irritated or sensitive skin. The oil is also used in aromatherapy as an antidepressant and relaxant.

The name "jasmine" comes from the Persian "yasmin," which means "gift from God."

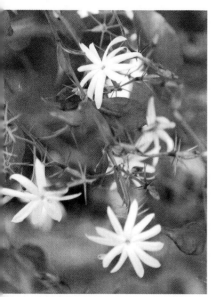

Angel wing jasmine (*Jasminum nitidum*)

Opposite page: Common jasmine (*Jasminum officinale*)

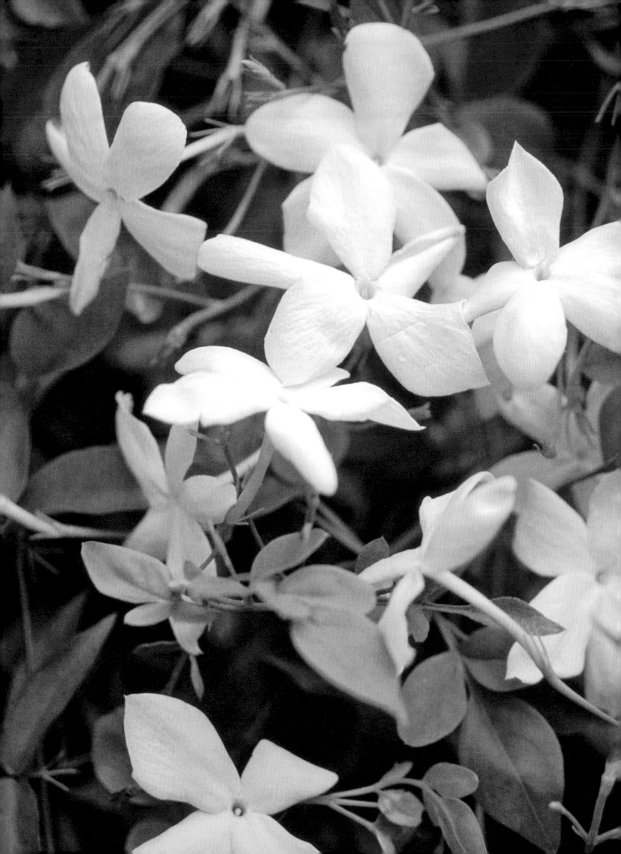

Lavender

Latin name *Lavandula* sp. Lamiaceae
Part used **Flowers**

Popular around the world, fragrant lavender is becoming one of the most important botanicals with a wide range of medicinal uses, earning it the title of the Swiss Army knife of herbal medicine." Fresh or dried, lavender also has many applications around the home, and the essential oil is used in homemade air fresheners and cleaning products.

Gardening

There are about 30 species of lavender, which can be found from the Canary Islands eastward into western India, and they are divided into six sections, of which four are significant as herbs: Lavandula, containing true lavender (*L. angustifolia*) and its subspecies — woolly lavender (*L. lanata*), spike lavender (*L. latifolia*) and hybrid lavender (*L. x intermedia*); Stoechas, containing *L. stoechas* together with its various subspecies and green lavender (*L. viridis*);

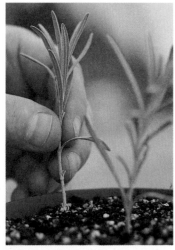

Propagate varieties of lavender by cuttings taken in summer.

Dentata, containing French or fringed lavender (*L. dentata*) and its varieties and hybrids; and *Pterostachys* species, characterized by branched inflorescences and pinnate or bipinnate leaves. All have fragrant foliage.

True lavender *L. angustifolia* syn. *L. vera*, *L. officinalis*, or 'English' lavender, occurs in the wild on dolamitic soils at altitudes of 1,500 ft. to 5,000 ft. (500 m to 1,500 m). Like all lavenders, it is a woody-based subshrub and will rarely exceed 2.5 ft. (74 cm cm) in height. It has unbranched flowering stems.

Excellent dwarf varieties include 'Rosea,' 'Compacta' syn. 'Nana Compacta,' 'Folgate' and 'Munstead.' Medium-height varieties include 'Hidcote,' 'Miss Katherine,' 'Pacific Blue,' 'Sarah,' 'Summerland Supreme,' 'Melissa,' 'Twickel Purple,' 'Tucker's Early Purple' and 'Ashdown Forest.' The taller varieties include 'Alba' and the twice-flowering 'Irene Doyle.'

Essential oil gathered from wild harvested lavender in France is greatly prized, particularly therapeutically. The very fragrant camphor-free essential oil from high-altitude grown seedling or clonal (single variety) lavender is highly valued in the perfumery industry, herbal medicine and aromatherapy. Lavender has been grown in France on a large scale for the perfume trade since the 17th century.

The varieties grown for essential oil production include the great 'Maillette,' 'Matheronne,' 'Fring,' 'Heacham Blue,' 'No. 9' and 'Norfolk J2.'

Both fresh and dried flowers are used in cooking (including

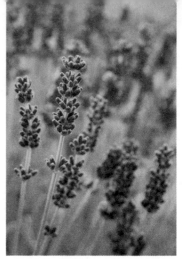

Lavender (*Lavandula angustifolia*)

herb mixtures such as *herbes de Provence*) and craftwork, for which the finest variety is 'Super-Blue.' Make sure that any flowers you use for culinary purposes have not been sprayed with garden chemicals.

Spike lavender Sometimes called *Nardus italica*, spike lavender (*L. latifolia* syn. *L. spica*) is endemic to Spain, France, Italy and the Balkans, and grows in the wild at much lower altitudes than *L. angustifolia*.The plant has a lavender and camphor scent, and the flowering stems have paired lateral branches. It is the source of oil of aspic (*oleum spicae*).

Intermedia lavenders In the overlap zone on mountainsides where both *L. angustifolia* and *L. latifolia* grow, natural hybridization occurs, resulting in plants with intermediate characteristics. They are larger and stronger-growing than true lavender, more tolerant of humidity and yield twice the volume of essential oil compared with true lavender.

Selected hybrids of *L. x intermedia* are the major producers of lavender essential oil worldwide. The oil contains perceptible camphor and is valued at approximately half that of true lavender. It is widely used for personal and household toiletries.

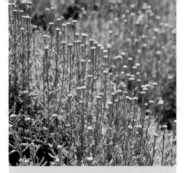

Intermedia lavenders may be identified by their paired flowering side branches.

The most popular variety for essential oil production is 'Grosso,' although 'Abrialii,' 'Super,' 'Sumian' and 'Provence' are used, too. The flowers are also dried. Many fine landscape varieties found among the Intermedias include 'Alba,' 'Dutch White,' 'Grappenhall,' 'Hidcote Giant,' 'Impress Purple,' 'Seal,' 'Silver Edge' and the double-duty 'Provence.'

Woolly lavender L. *lanata* has leaves that are heavily felted with hairs, and long spikes of scented flowers. It is very resentful of rain and will not tolerate wet feet. It is best grown in large pots in full sun.

Several hybrids are popular for gardens, including 'Richard Gray,' 'Silver Frost' and 'Sawyers,' which is stronger than the species, with long spikes of bright violet flowers and silver foliage.

Stoechas lavenders These lavenders have compressed flower spikes shaped rather like a pineapple surmounted by flaglike sterile bracts. All of them are suited to low-altitude warm-climate gardens, including those near the sea. The Italian or Spanish lavender (L. *stoechas*) has short flowering stems (peduncles), while Portuguese lavender (L. *stoechas* subsp. *pedunculata*) is distinguished by long stems.

Excellent varieties include 'Major,' 'Kew Red,' 'Marshwood,' 'Somerset Mist,' 'Avonview' and 'Butterfly' syn. 'James Compton.' The 'Bee' and 'Bella' series developed by Bob Cherry in New South Wales in Australia and sold worldwide are remarkable breeding breakthroughs.

Green lavender (L. *viridis*) has green foliage, and green inflorescences with cream flowers and green sterile bracts. 'Beverley' differs in having white sterile bracts. Fringed lavender (L. *dentata*) has fragrant inflorescences similar to L. *stoechas*, but the narrow linear leaves are evenly rounded-dentate. Varieties include 'Ploughman's Blue,' the green and cream variegated 'Linda Ligon' and the hybrid 'Goodwin Creek Gray.'

Pterostachys lavenders These include a number of desirable landscape species, including L. *buchii*, Canary Islands lavender (L. *canariensis*), jagged lavender (L. *pinnata*), fernleaf lavender (L. *multifida*) and the electric blue-flowered L. *maroccana*.

Position ▶ All lavenders require excellent drainage and full sun. They are better grown fairly hard, and a slow-release fertilizer or a light application of organic compost is recommended. They are all suited to being grown in large pots.

Propagation ▶ Varieties are propagated by cuttings, but species are seed sown in spring.

Maintenance ▶ Prune lavenders annually, preferably in early spring.

Cotton lavender

Cotton lavender (*Santolina chamaecyparissus*), also known as santolina, has a compact habit that makes it ideal for a low hedge or edging a path. Its grey, toothed aromatic leaves have a similar scent to lavender and are very useful for repelling moths. Add the dried leaves to moth-repellent sachets and place dried bunches with stored blankets and other woollens. Silverfish also hate santolina.

True and Intermedia lavenders can be shaped during harvesting. Never cut back hard into old wood, or the plants may die.

Pests and diseases ▶ Lavenders are generally free of pests as well as diseases.

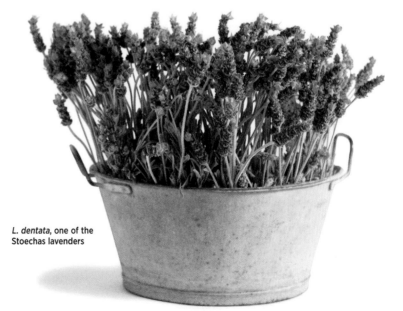

L. *dentata*, one of the Stoechas lavenders

Lavender Continued

Harvesting and storing ▶
Harvest True and Intermedia lavenders in midsummer when spikes are one- to two-thirds open. Tie lavender stems in bunches and hang them upside down to dry; strip them of their flowers. The oil is steam distilled.

Herbal medicine

Lavandula angustifolia. Part used: flowers. An age-old remedy for calming and soothing the nerves, improving moodand relaxing muscles, beautifully scented lavender and its essential oil are commonly used for inducing a restful sleep, relieving depression and anxiety and for other disorders relating to a nervous or tense state, including stomach upsets.

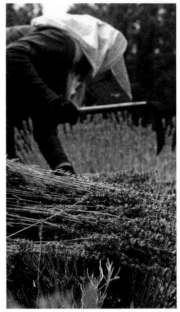

In Europe lavender is harvested from July to September, often by hand.

Lavender flowers can be taken as an infusion or added to a bath to soothe and aid in relaxation. Apply undiluted essential oil to relieve the sting of insect bites or to prevent cuts and grazes from becoming infected. You can add essential oil to massage oil to help relieve muscle tension and headaches.

For the safe and appropriate internal use of lavender, consult your healthcare professional. For its topical uses, see Depression & anxiety, *page 185,* and First aid, *page 194.* Do not use lavender if you are pregnant or breastfeeding, except under professional supervision.

Lavender essential oil is antiseptic and antibacterial, ideal for blemished skin.

Around the home

If you could choose only one herb for household use, lavender would have to be at the top of the list. Apart from its pretty flower and much loved scent, lavender is antibacterial, antibiotic, antiviral, antiseptic, deodorizing and insect repelling, which means that you can use it in the living room, kitchen, bathroom, laundry, nursery and patio, as well as in your wardrobes and drawers, on your pets and on your skin.
● Use both the dried flowers and leaves to make moth-repellent sachets and lavender bags — they both contain the aromatic oil that insects hate.
● Infuse distilled white vinegar with the flowers and leaves, fresh or dried, for an inexpensive and very effective spray for cleaning and disinfecting a variety of surfaces.
● Add drops of lavender essential oil to environmentally friendly unscented kitchen and laundry cleaning products for a fresh, natural scent.
● Dampen a wool ball and add a few drops of lavender essential oil. Drop it into your kitchen pantry or vacuum cleaner bag to eliminate stale odors.

Cooking

Lavender's culinary applications are limited, although the flowers are edible. They are used in the Moroccan spice blend ras el hanout and in the French herbes de Provence. Lavender goes well in sweet dishes containing cream, such as ice cream. It can be added to shortbread and icings and used in jams and jellies. Crystallize the flowers as edible cake decorations.

A history of epic proportions

Reputed to have been brought from the Garden of Eden by Adam and Eve, lavender has a history that is almost as old as humankind itself. The ancient Egyptians dipped shrouds in lavender water, while the Romans scented their public baths with it – hence its name, from the Latin word *lavare,* meaning 'to wash.' Under its biblical name 'spikenard,' it was popularly supposed to have been used by the Virgin Mary to perfume Jesus's swaddling clothes, by Mary Magdalene to anoint Jesus's feet, and was also favored in the Middle Ages by apothecary monks, who used it to treat everything from labor pains to demonic possession.

Lemon Balm

Latin Name *Melissa officinalis* Lamiaceae
Other common names **Bee balm, common balm, melissa, sweet balm**
Part used **Leaves**

Lemon balm smells like sweet lemon and is used in herbal teas, wines and liqueurs as well as in many eau-de-cologne formulations, including Carmelite water. Handfuls of the leaves, which contain a lemon-scented oil, were once used to polish wooden furniture.

Gardening

Lemon balm is a hardy perennial that bears some resemblance to its close relations, the mints. It is multi-stemmed, growing to about 2.5 ft. (74 cm), with ovate, regularly toothed green leaves. The insignificant lipped flowers are lemon yellow, and borne in clusters on the upper parts of the stems.

Varieties ▶ While the common form of balm has a fresh lemon fragrance, there are varieties with related but different scents,

From nymph to bee

Lemon balm's association with bees goes back to ancient times. According to Greek mythology, Melissa was one of the nymphs who hid Zeus from his father Cronus, feeding him milk and honey. Once Zeus ruled Olympus, he changed her into a queen bee.

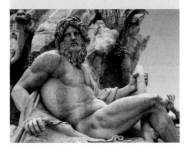

including 'Lime,' with a true lime fragrance; 'Liqueur'; and 'Citronella,' which mimics the scent of citronella oil and is said to act as an insect repellent. Two attractive color variations are available: 'Variegata' is a gold-splashed form, and 'All Gold' has pure golden foliage in spring.

Position ▶ Lemon balm is an unfussy plant, but prefers full sun to partial shade and a well-drained but moist soil. It also grows well in pots.

Propagation ▶ Lemon balm is a perennial usually grown from seed, although it is easy to raise from cuttings taken in spring and autumn, or from rooted divisions. Grow named varieties from tip cuttings, which will root easily, or by layering.

Maintenance ▶ If you do not want seedlings, or you desire a new flush of foliage, cut back the whole plant, including the flowering heads. Cut back 'All Gold' regularly to maintain its color. Remove any plain green shoots from both 'All Gold' and 'Variegata.'

Pests and diseases ▶ Lemon balm is prone to powdery mildew, particularly in areas with little air circulation.

Harvesting and storing ▶ Harvest the fresh foliage as required. To dry, cut the plant down to about 3 in. (7.5 cm) in mid- to late afternoon, secure the stems in small bunches with rubber bands, and hang upside down in a well-ventilated area out of direct sunlight. Strip off the dried leaves and store them in airtight containers in a cool place.

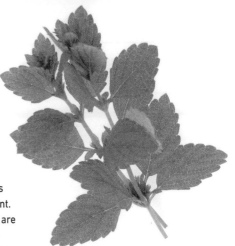

Lemon balm (*Melissa officinalis*)

Herbal medicine

Melissa officinalis. Part used: leaves. Lemon balm's mild sedative and mood-enhancing effects are commonly used to treat sleep disorders, restlessness, anxiety and depression.

It is also suited to afflictions of the gastrointestinal tract and can help with flatulence, spasm and nausea, particularly when these are aggravated by periods of stress and tension.

Scientific studies have shown that lemon balm has antiviral effects, and topical preparations of the herb have been used to relieve the symptoms of cold sores, which are caused by the herpes virus.

For the safe and appropriate use of lemon balm, see Tension & stress, *page 184*. Don't use lemon balm if you're pregnant or breastfeeding, except under professional supervision.

Cooking

Lemon balm's lemon scent and lemon-and-mint flavor go with most foods complemented by either of those flavors. Use the leaves in tea, salads, cordials, fruit dishes, wine and chilled summer drinks or in stuffings for poultry or fish.

Lemon grass

Latin Name *Cymbopogon citratus* Poaceae
Part used **Stems**

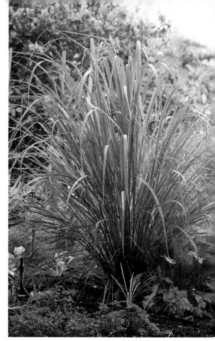

Lemon grass (*Cymbopogon citratus*)

Lemon grass, a tall tropical grass with a powerful lemon fragrance, is widely used for cooking in Thailand, Vietnam and other Southeast Asian countries. It makes a vitamin A–rich tea, and the essential oil is used in many commercial toiletries.

Gardening

A number of the 56 *Cymbopogon* species are fragrant, but the herb most commonly called lemon grass is West Indian lemon grass (*C. citratus*), one of several species that share this scent. Its narrow, leafy stalks grow in large clumps that reach 3.5 ft. (1 m) or more.

East Indian lemon grass or Cochin lemon grass (*C. flexuosus*) is also widely grown for its essential oil. Ceylon citronella (*C. nardus*) and Java citronella (*C. winterianus*) share the lemon-related scent of citronella.

Palmarosa, geranium grass or rosha grass (*C. martinii*) smells delightfully of rose geranium when crushed. The closely related ginger grass (*C. martinii* var. *sofia*) has a harsher scent.

Position ▶ This herb is best suited in a sunny position, well-drained soil, warm growing conditions — ideally between 69°F and 100°F (18°C and 38°C) — and high humidity. In cooler areas it is best grown in a large pot and overwintered indoors.

Propagation ▶ To propagate, carefully divide the clump. Raise other species, mentioned above, by seed. Feed with seaweed fertilizer.

Maintenance ▶ Water plants regularly.

Pests and diseases ▶ Crown rot can occur in plants grown in poorly drained or flooded soils.

Harvesting and storing ▶ Harvest stems as required. Cut the upper green part into segments and dry it out of direct sunlight, then store it in airtight containers and use it for tea. For cooking, wrap the white bulbous lower portion in plastic wrap and store in the refrigerator for several weeks.

Herbal medicine

Cymbopogon citratus. Part used: stems. Lemon-grass tea was traditionally used to treat digestive upsets and to alleviate stomachache, cramping and vomiting. It was also used for a number of other disorders, including cough, fevers, high blood pressure and exhaustion.

Lemon grass has also traditionally been regarded as having pain-relieving effects and has been used internally as an infusion for nerve and rheumatic pain. Applied as a topical remedy, lemon grass and its essential oil can ease the pain and discomfort of headaches, abdominal pain, aching joints and muscles and neuralgia.

For the safe and appropriate medicinal use of this herb, consult your healthcare professional. Do not use lemon grass in greater than culinary quantities if you are pregnant or breastfeeding.

Cooking

The strong citrus flavor of lemon grass goes well in Southeast Asian cooking and is often teamed with chillies and coconut milk. Lemon grass is also an excellent addition to Western cooking, particularly in fish and seafood dishes. Use the lower white part of the fresh stems and slice finely crosswise to avoid a fibrous texture in the finished dish. If using a whole stem or large pieces, bruise first to release the flavor and remove before serving.

Natural protection

A natural insect repellent, lemon grass offers some protection from fleas, ticks, lice and mosquitoes. The essential oil can be used in an oil burner. Alternatively, combine a few drops with equal amounts of eucalyptus oil in a water spray and lightly spritz over outdoor furniture on summer evenings. Or, light a candle made with citronella, a close relative of lemon grass.

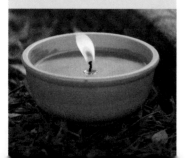

Lemon verbena

Latin Name *Aloysia citriodora* syn. *Lippia citriodora*, syn. *A. triphylla* Verbenaceae
Other common names **Herb Louisa, lemon beebrush**
Parts used **Leaves, flowers**

The deliciously fresh, refined and intense lemon fragrance of this herb, which is native to Peru and Argentina, has long been prized for use in tisanes, liqueurs, cooking, potpourri and perfumery.

Gardening

Lemon verbena is a shrub with arching branches and pointed leaves arranged in whorls of three around the stems. In summer the bush produces large terminal panicles of tiny, four-petaled, white or pale lavender flowers.

Position ▶ It requires full sun, and a free-draining loam with nearly neutral pH.

Propagation ▶ Propagate by semi-ripe tip cuttings.

Maintenance ▶ Lemon verbena is cut back by frost, so it should be winter mulched in cool climates. In heavy frost areas grow it in a pot and bring it under protection during winter dormancy. Trim to shape. Bushes often leaf out very late in spring; don't discard them prematurely.

Pests and diseases ▶ Under greenhouse conditions, lemon verbena is prone to whitefly and spider mites.

Harvesting and storing ▶ Leaves can be harvested at any time to use fresh or for air-drying.

Herbal medicine

Aloysia citriodora syn. *Lippia citriodora* syn. *A. triphylla*. Parts used: aerial parts. Lemon verbena is used as a digestive aid for symptoms of flatulence and colic. It is thought to help with insomnia and nervous agitation. Lemon verbena is also prescribed for feverish conditions.

For the safe and appropriate use of these herbs, consult your healthcare professional. Do not use these herbs if you are pregnant or breastfeeding.

Around the home

Lemon verbena makes an ideal filling for a herbal sleep pillow. Or you can use it with other lemony leaves, such as lemon-scented geranium, lemon thyme, and lemon balm to make a room-freshening, citrus-scented pot-pourri. Place the mixture in a bowl or push it into sachets to slide down the sides and backs of lounge cushions or inside cushion covers.

Cooking

The leaves are best used fresh and young. Use sparingly; otherwise the flavor can overwhelm the food and be reminiscent of lemon-scented soap. Lemon verbena is a common ingredient in many herbal teas, imparting a wonderfully fragrant flavor, and can be substituted for lemon grass in Asian recipes.

The leaves are used to give a lemon flavor to fruit salads and other fruit dishes, desserts and drinks. Infuse them in custard-based sauces for desserts, or finely chop and add to Asian dishes, poultry and stuffings.

Add whole leaves to apple jelly, and chopped young leaves to fruit salads. With its digestive and relaxant properties, the tea is ideal for drinking after dinner.

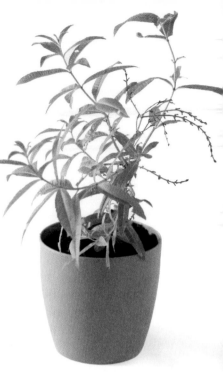

Lemon verbena (*Aloysia citriodora*)

Licorice

Latin Name *Glycyrrhiza glabra* Papilionaceae
Parts used **Taproot, rhizomes**

In 1305, Edward I of England taxed imports of continental licorice to pay for repairs to London Bridge. Domestic crops became concentrated around Pontefract, where Dominican monks planted licorice in the 14th century.

Gardening

Licorice is a graceful, arching, deciduous perennial to about 5 ft. (1.5 m). It has a thick, deep taproot and spreads underground via extensive stolons. Aboveground it has pinnately compound leaves and loose spikes of purple flowers. Licorice grows particularly well on the rich alluvial plains of Turkey which together with Spain and Greece, is still a leading world supplier.

Varieties ▶ There are three recognized botanical varieties:

Fit for an emperor

Pontefract, or pomfret, cakes became a popular sweet in England in the 16th century. These soft, flat discs made with licorice, gum arabic and sugar were stamped with a stylized image of Pontefract Castle. They are still made and loved, along with another English favorite, the distinctive multicolored licorice allsorts. It is said that Napoléon Bonaparte always carried licorice lozenges, which were based on pontefract cakes.

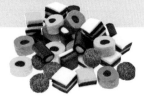

Spanish or Italian licorice (*G. glabra* var. *glabra*), Russian licorice (*G. glabra* var. *glandulifera*) and *G. glabra* var. *violacea*. Other species used in a similar way are Chinese or Mongolian licorice (*G. uralensis*) and Manchurian licorice (*G. pallidiflora*).

Position ▶ Licorice prefers a rich, deep, sandy loam and a sunny position.

Propagation ▶ New crops are propagated by rhizome segments planted in spring, but can also be propagated by seed. Portions of rhizome left in the soil at harvest time will generate new plants.

Maintenance ▶ Keep weeds at bay.

Pests and diseases ▶ There are no significant problems.

Harvesting and storing ▶ Both the taproot and the rhizomes can be used. They are usually dug when 3 years old and air-dried before being ground and then processed.

Herbal medicine

Glycyrrhiza glabra. Part used: roots. Licorice root is one of the most scientifically researched herbal medicines of our time and investigations are confirming many of its traditional uses, which date back to ancient times. A common ingredient in many respiratory remedies for its soothing effects and ability to expel mucus, licorice is used to treat coughs, bronchitis and catarrhal lung conditions.

A compound called glycyrrhizin, which is responsible for the herb's licorice taste, is known to be responsible for the healing effects of licorice on gastrointestinal ulcers and inflammatory conditions of

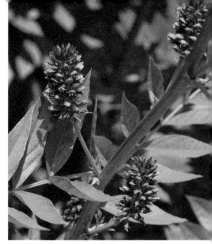

Licorice (*Glycyrrhiza glabra*)

the digestive system. It also acts as a tonic for the adrenal glands, so licorice is often prescribed as a supportive remedy in times of stress and exhaustion.

For the safe and appropriate use of licorice, consult a healthcare professional. Do not use licorice if you are pregnant or breastfeeding.

Natural beauty

This herb is considered an effective natural lightener for brown age spots. For the best result, use it for mild discoloration and pair it with a natural fruit peel containing vitamin C and alpha hydroxy acids to slough off dead skin.

Cooking

Licorice root is one of many spices and herbs used in Chinese master stocks, adding to their intensity and depth of flavor. Add the chopped root sparingly (it can be bitter) when stewing fruit.

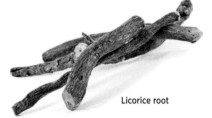

Licorice root

Lime

Latin Name *Tilia cordata* syn. *T. parvifolia, T. x europaea* Tiliaceae
Other common names **Linden, tilia**
Part used **Flowers**

Called the "tree of life" due to its many medicinal uses, in the Medieval Period lime was associated with the Virgin Mary and was planted for its fragrant healing flowers and to provide shade in monastery gardens.

Gardening

Small-leafed lime (*T. cordata*) is a small-to-medium deciduous tree to 33 ft. (10 m) with glossy, dark green, heart-shaped leaves. In midsummer, it bears clusters of pale yellow flowers, heavy with fragrance, which attract bees to their copious nectar. Hives placed around flowering trees yield a prized fragrant honey. While *T. cordata* is the principal species harvested, other species used herbally include *T. x europaea* and *T. platyphyllos*. *Tilia* is occasionally confused with the citrus fruit species known as lime (*Citrus aurantiifolia*).

Lime is also known as the linden tree in Germany and *tilleul* in France.

Position ▶ *Tilia* prefers a moist neutral to alkaline soil and a sunny open position.

Propagation ▶ It can be propagated by fresh ripe seed or by stratification of stored seed planted in spring (see box *page 40*) and also by suckers.

Maintenance ▶ *Tilia* species tend to sucker. Either remove these, or pot them and, when established, plant elsewhere.

Pests and diseases ▶ Aphids and caterpillars on leaves can be a problem, although rarely so in Mediterranean areas. Look out for gall mite, too.

Lime (*Tilia cordata*)

Harvesting and storing ▶ The petals drop rapidly to allow the fruits to swell so, over a short time interval, harvest flower clusters together with a few attendant young leaves at the peak of flowering. Spread out the flowers and thoroughly air-dry them before storing.

Herbal medicine

Tilia cordata, T. platyphyllos. Parts used: flowers, bracts. Lime flowers are a common ingredient of many herbal teas that are prescribed to help induce a restful sleep, especially in children. The plant has a sedative and calming effect on the nerves and muscles, and can help to reduce restlessness, tension and anxiety.

Lime flowers are a specific remedy for certain circulatory disorders. They have both relaxing and restorative effects on the blood vessel walls, and have been used to counteract high blood pressure, especially when it is associated with nervous tension. The flowers can also be helpful in the treatment and prevention of atherosclerosis (hardening of the arteries).

Regarded as one of the most important diaphoretic herbs in European medicine, lime flowers are beneficial in feverish conditions such as colds, influenza and other respiratory infections.

For the safe and appropriate use of lime flowers, see High blood pressure & cholesterol, page 202. Do not use lime flowers if you are pregnant or breastfeeding.

Celebrating lime blossom

Linden trees are popular ornamentals in Europe, where the flowering tips are harvested at their peak and air-dried for use in lime blossom tea, a particularly popular tisane in France. The center of production is Buis les Baronnies, a medieval town that each July celebrates an annual lime blossom festival, together with their annual harvest sales.

Lovage

Latin Name *Levisticum officinale* Apiaceae
Other common names **Bladder seed, Cornish lovage, garden lovage, Italian lovage, love parsley**
Parts used **Leaves, seeds, roots**

Lovage has an intense celery flavor that's perfect for winter dishes, but it is far easier to grow than celery. Traditionally used in aphrodisiacs and love potions, these tall plants provide generous harvests and have a wide range of medicinal uses.

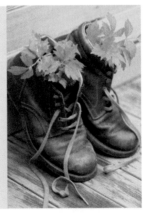

Lovage (*Levisticum officinale*)

Gardening

Lovage is native to the eastern Mediterranean and is the only species in its genus, although it is closely related to both angelica and celery. This hardy perennial plant, with large, frondlike, glossy compound leaves divided into diamond-shaped leaflets, can grow to 6 ft. (1.8 m). The tiny yellow flowers, borne in umbels, are followed by oval seeds (fruits), that can be used like celery seeds in cooking. The plant dies down completely in winter, emerging early in spring.

Position ▶ Lovage requires a rich, moist but well-drained soil, and light shade where summers are hot.

Propagation ▶ It is propagated by seed, which remains viable for 3 years, or by division in spring. The plants benefit from generous quantities of compost.

Maintenance ▶ Remove older, yellowing leaves, and consider cutting back older plants to about 1 ft. (30 cm) high to encourage fresh foliage growth in midsummer. In a mixed herb garden, mark the position of lovage, because it is fully deciduous.

Pests and diseases ▶ Lovage is rarely affected, but young leaves may be damaged by leaf miner or slugs.

Harvesting and storing ▶ For cooking, pick the leaves as required, but if you intend to use them for

Lovage is sometimes called 'Maggi plant' because its flavor is reminiscent of Maggi bouillon cubes.

essential oil extraction or medicinal preparations, pick them before flowering. Harvest when ripe. Dig the roots after the plant dies down, usually in the third year. You can dry all parts of the plant and also freeze the leaves in sealed plastic bags.

Cooking

Called *céleri bâtard*, or false celery, by the French, lovage is used as an ingredient in many commercial bouillons, sauces, stocks and condiments; its seeds are added to liqueurs and cordials as well as to breads and sweet pastries. Blanch the stems in the same manner as rhubarb, or eat them raw in salads. You can also candy the stems and eat them as confectionery, or use the leaves in cooking to provide an intense, celery-like flavoring.

Love ache

As its common name indicates, lovage, or love ache as it was once called, was traditionally used as an aphrodisiac and an ingredient in love potions and charms. On a more practical note, however, medieval travelers once lined their boots with lovage leaves to absorb foot odors, while a decoction of lovage root and foliage makes an effective body deodorant. Perhaps lovage was less a love potion than a deodorant, making close physical contact more appealing in a period when people rarely washed.

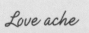

Mallow & hollyhock

Latin Name **Althaea officinalis, Malva sp. and Alcea sp. Malvaceae**
Other common name **Hollyhock (cheeses)**
Parts used **Roots, leaves, flowers, seeds**

Hollyhock reportedly reached Europe from China via the Holy Land, hence its original name of holy mallow or holyoke. The mucilaginous marsh mallow is widely used medicinally, while the ornamental musk mallow was once used for magical protection.

Gardening

Mallow and hollyhock contain similar mucilaginous compounds.

Mallow A perennial with finely hairy, gray-green, coarsely toothed leaves, marsh mallow (*Althaea officinalis*) has small, five-petaled pink flowers on stems to 4 ft. (1.2 m).

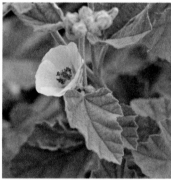

Marsh mallow (*Althaea officinalis*)

Musk mallow (*Malva moschata*) is a European perennial with kidney-shaped basal leaves and contrasting, much-divided leaves on the upper stems. The leaves and profuse pink (pure white in the variety 'Alba') flowers are musk-scented.

Hollyhock Hollyhock (*Alcea rosea*) forms a large basal rosette of large, long-stalked, rough-textured leaves, which may be broad and palmately lobed or, in the ancient yellow-flowered Antwerp hollyhock

(*A. ficifolia*), fig leaf–shaped. The tall flowering stems can reach 3 m, and the single or double flowers — in shades of lemon, apricot, white, pink, red or purple — are borne in racemes.

Varieties ▶ The black hollyhock 'Nigra' is the darkest maroon single. All mallows have disk-shaped, nutty-flavored seeds.

Position ▶ All species prefer a well-drained, moist soil and a sunny position; hollyhocks will thrive in an alkaline soil.

Propagation ▶ All species are propagated by seed sown in spring.

Maintenance ▶ Stake both hollyhocks and musk mallow in summer. Cut plants down in late autumn.

Pests and diseases ▶ All members of the Malvaceae family are prone to rust (*Puccinia malvacearum*) and are also a food source for some butterfly larvae.

Harvesting and storing ▶ Gather flowers and leaves to use fresh or dried. Dig up and dry marsh mallow roots when they are 2 years old.

Herbal medicine

Althaea officinalis. Parts used: leaves, roots. Rich in mucilaginous compounds, the leaves and roots of the marsh mallow have a soothing effect and are both used to treat irritated and inflamed conditions of the respiratory tract, including irritable cough, bronchitis and sore throat.

With a higher amount of mucilage, the root is regarded as the more effective remedy for inflammatory conditions of the gut, such as

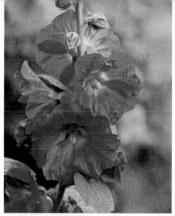

Hollyhock (*Alcea rosea*)

stomach and intestinal ulcers, gastroenteritis and ulcerative colitis. The root is also used as a topical agent in mouthwashes for inflammation of the mouth and throat and as an ointment to soothe eczematous skin conditions.

Malva sylvestris. Parts used: leaf, flower. Due to similar mucilaginous compounds, mallow has been used for similar purposes to marsh mallow, although it is considered less potent. Like marsh mallow, it is used for respiratory and gastrointestinal conditions, characterized by inflammation and irritation, that benefit from the plant's soothing properties.

For the safe and appropriate use of marsh mallow, see Sore throats, colds & flu, *page 174.* Don't use these herbs if you are pregnant or breastfeeding.

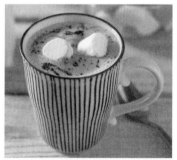

Confectionery marshmallow was once made from the mucilage in the roots of marsh mallow.

Marjoram & oregano

Latin Name *Origanum* sp. Lamiaceae
Parts used **Leaves, flowers**

The Greeks called these fragrant-leafed herbs "Brightness of the Mountain," and it is impossible to imagine the cuisines of the Mediterranean and Aegean without their strong, warm aromatic taste.

Gardening

Origanum is a genus that is fraught with taxonomic difficulties, and there are more than 30 species from the Mediterranean and the Middle East. Confusingly, marjoram and oregano are common names that are often used interchangeably.

Sweet or knot marjoram (*O. marjorana* syn. *Marjorana hortensis*) has gray-green leaves with a mouthwatering fragrance. Although usually treated as an annual, it is a short-lived perennial in mild climates. A hardier hybrid, *O. x marjoricum*, may be sold incorrectly as 'Italian Oregano.'

Spartan oregano (*O. minutiflorum*) is frequently included in dried oregano mixes from Turkey. It resembles a diminutive gray-leafed sweet marjoram that has undergone relaxation therapy.

Pot marjoram or Turkish oregano (*O. onites*) is a cold-tender, strongly aromatic species from Greece. Selections of *O. vulgare* are often incorrectly sold under this name.

Common oregano (*O. vulgare*) contains six subspecies. *O. vulgare* subsp. vulgareis the mild-flavored wild marjoram with clustered heads of pink flowers and deep burgundy bracts that attract bees, but lacks any appreciable flavor. It is often sold as oregano. Cultivars of *O. vulgare* subsp. *vulgare* include the very attractive golden oregano,

Sweet marjoram (*Origanum marjorana*, left) and common oregano (*Origanum vulgare*)

'Aureum,' sometimes sold as 'golden marjoram,' which makes a superb aromatic groundcover for full sun, and 'Jim Best,' which is a vigorous gold and green variegated variety. *O. pulchellum* is a name attached to forms of *O. vulgare* with purple bracts.

Greek oregano (*O. vulgare* subsp. *hirtum*) has a deliciously strong fragrance. The very mildly aromatic *O. vulgare* subsp. *virens* and *O. vulgare* subsp. viridulum are both called wild marjoram.

Lebanese oregano, Syrian hyssop or white oregano (*O. syriacum*) forms a tender perennial subshrub with gray-green foliage. Ezov, the biblical hyssop, was almost certainly *O. syriacum*. A hybrid with *O. vulgare*, sold as *O. maru*, has greater cold resistance.

Russian oregano (*O. vulgare* subsp. *gracile*) has an aroma that is similar to Greek oregano.

Algerian oregano (*O. vulgare* subsp. *glandulosum*) is rarely seen outside its native land but is a good culinary herb.

Za'atar

Za'atar is an Arabic term for a number of aromatic herbs, often varying according to the region and also the local flora. While the term most often refers to origanums, za'atar species also include conehead thyme (*Thymbra capitata*), za'atar hommar (*T. spicata*), true thyme (*Thymus* sp.) and Satureja species such as *S. cuneifolia* and *S. thymbra*. The seasoning mixture called 'za'atar' usually includes toasted sesame seeds and coarse salt, and is used on vegetable and meat dishes and also sprinkled on bread before baking.

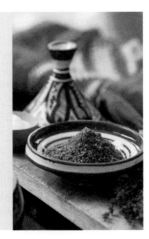

Ornamental origanums Many species and hybrids of *Origanum* are grown simply for their beauty and fragrance. They include 'Herrenhausen,' 'Country Cream,' the aromatic and strangely beautiful Dittany of Crete (*O. dictamnus*) and *O. creticum*, a very aromatic species, the source of the essential oil *oleum origani*.

Position ▶ *Origanum* species are found in the wild in sunny, well-drained and often stony places. They thrive in full sun and are stronger flavored if grown with tough love.

Propagation ▶ Raise the species from seed in spring, and ornamental varieties by cuttings.

Maintenance ▶ Once the plants are established, do not overwater them. Cut back old growth in spring.

Pests and diseases ▶ Origanums are very resistant to both.

Harvesting and storing ▶ You can harvest the foliage fresh but the flavor is enhanced if you dry it in bunches in a dark, dry, warm, well-ventilated place for several days. When dry and crisp, rub the leaves off the stems and store in an airtight container.

Herbal medicine

Origanum vulgare. Parts used: leaves, flowers. An infusion of the herb is a useful remedy for feverish conditions and also for treating coughs, colds and influenza due to its ability to improve the removal of phlegm from the lungs and relax the bronchial muscles. Traditionally, oregano is also regarded as an herb for the gut; it relieves flatulence and improves digestion as well as treats intestinal infections due to a strong antiseptic effect.

The essential oil of oregano has been shown to possess potent antimicrobial and antioxidant properties, primarily due to the presence of the constituents thymol and carvacrol. Some commercial oregano oil products have been used to treat a range of conditions, including respiratory and gastrointestinal infections, although substantial clinical evidence proving its efficacy is lacking.

Origanum marjorana syn. *Marjorana hortensis*. Parts used: leaves and flowers. Medicinally, sweet marjoram is used predominantly in the form of its essential oil, which is applied topically to ease headaches, sore muscles and rheumatic pain. As an external remedy it can also relieve catarrhal conditions of the lung, digestive colic, flatulence and period pain.

For the safe and appropriate medicinal use of these two herbs, consult a healthcare professional. Do not use these herbs in greater than culinary quantities or the essential oils of these herbs internally or externally if you are pregnant or breastfeeding.

Cooking

Oregano has a more pungent scent than marjoram, with a stronger flavor. The hotter and drier the climate, the more aroma and flavor avariety will have.

Sweet marjoram is the type used in cooking. Its aroma is damaged by heat, so use it in uncooked or lightly cooked dishes, or add it at the end. Oregano is a more robust herb and can withstand longer cooking.

Both herbs go well with lemon, garlic, wine, meats, fish, salads, Greek and Italian dishes, beans, eggplant, capsicum and tomato-based dishes and sauces. They are also used in commercial mixed herbs.

Marjoram and sausage pasta

10.5 oz. (300 g) rigatoni
9 oz. (250 g) sausages
2 tablespoons olive oil
1 large red onion, roughly chopped
3 cloves garlic, finely chopped
1 small eggplant, diced
3 small zucchini, diced
2 cups (500 g) tomato pasta sauce
1 tablespoon chopped fresh marjoram or oregano
1.5 oz. (40 g) black olives
9 oz. (250 g) cherry tomatoes
2 tablespoons chopped fresh parsley
fresh marjoram leaves, for garnish
grated parmesan, to serve

Cook pasta in boiling water until al dente, about 10 minutes. Drain. Grill sausages until brown. Cool slightly; cut into thick slices. Heat oil in saucepan over moderate heat. Fry onion until starting to color, about 3 minutes, Add garlic and sausages; cook a few minutes. Increase heat; add eggplant and zucchini; cook, stirring, 5 minutes, until eggplant begins to soften. Add tomato pasta sauce, stir in marjoram and season to taste. Cover and simmer, stirring occasionally, 15 minutes, or until eggplant is tender. Stir in olives and tomatoes. Cover and cook a further 5 minutes. Combine pasta and sauce in a large bowl. Stir in parsley. Sprinkle with marjoram leaves and parmesan. Serves 4.

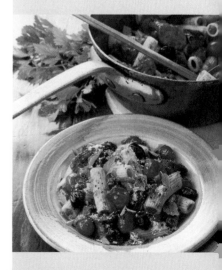

Meadowsweet

Latin Name *Filipendula ulmaria* syn. *Spiraea ulmaria* Rosaceae
Other common names **Bridewort, lady of the meadow,**
     meadow queen, queen of the meadow
Parts used **Flowers, leaves**

With its fragrant and beautiful flowers, meadowsweet was considered one of the most powerful and sacred herbs of the Druids. In medieval times, it was a very popular strewing herb, a favorite of Elizabeth I, who ordered it used in her bedchamber.

Gardening

Meadowsweet forms a basal clump of pinnate leaves, and bears dense, frothy, tall corymbs of almond-scented, creamy white flowers to 4 ft. (1.2 m) in summer. (Corymbs are flower clusters with the appearance of a flat or rounded top.) The leaves smell like wintergreen when crushed. The plant occurs in moist meadows and around fresh water, and is widely distributed across Asia and Europe.

Varieties ▶ Ornamental but herbally active varieties include the particularly desirable double-flowered 'Flore Pleno'; 'Grandiflora,' with large flowers; 'Aurea,' with golden foliage; and 'Variegata,' with cream-variegated leaves. Dropwort (*F. vulgaris*) is a closely related plant, once employed as a diuretic. It has similar flowers, although the individual leaflets are re-pinnately divided. The beautiful North American species *F. rubra* is larger, with pink- to rose-colored flowers.

Position ▶ Hardy meadowsweet will grow in full sun, provided the soil is very moist. It prefers a well-enriched, alkaline soil.

Propagation ▶ Propagate the species by seed in autumn, or by stratified seed (see box *page 40*) and plant in spring. Both the species and named varieties can be propagated by division in spring.

Maintenance ▶ Every 3 or 4 years, lift and divide meadowsweet in autumn.

Pests and diseases ▶ Check for mildew toward the end of the growing season.

Harvesting and storing ▶ Cut and dry flowers when in full bloom and use fresh for culinary use, or dried for herbal use. Harvest and dry leaves at the same time.

Herbal medicine

Filipendula ulmaria syn. *Spiraea ulmaria*. Parts used: flowers, leaves. Meadowsweet is considered one of the most important digestive remedies, indicated for many conditions of the gut, particularly those associated with inflammation and excess acidity. Meadowsweet has a balancing effect on acid production in the stomach as well as a soothing and healing effect on the upper digestive tract. It is prescribed commonly for acid reflux, indigestion, gastritis and stomach ulcers.

Meadowsweet contains aspirin-like compounds that are responsible for its pain-relieving and anti-inflammatory properties. These compounds can also help to bring down fevers, so this herb is often recommended for the treatment of colds and flu. The plant's medicinal effects make it an effective remedy for helping to alleviate joint and muscle pain.

For the safe and appropriate medicinal use of meadowsweet, see Indigestion, *page 178*. Do not use meadowsweet if you are pregnant or breastfeeding.

Cooking

The flowers are used to flavor jams, stewed fruits and wine as well as mead and the non-alcoholic Norfolk Punch.

Meadowsweet was once used in garlands for brides and as a strewing herb at weddings.

The source of aspirin

In 1827, salicin was isolated from meadowsweet's salicylates-containing leaves, then synthesized to acetyl salicylic acid (aspirin) by Felix Hoffman in Germany in 1899. His employer, Bayer AG, named the drug aspirin after an old botanical name for meadowsweet, *Spirea ulmaria*. The herb is considered less irritating to the stomach than the purified drug.

Meadowsweet
(*Filipendula ulmaria*)

Mint

Latin Name *Mentha sp.* Lamiaceae
Part used **Leaves**

True mints come in an amazing range of flavors and fragrances. While everyone is familiar with spearmint and common mint, there are many more mouthwatering varieties, including apple, chocolate, lime, grapefruit, lemon and ginger.

Gardening

Spearmint (*Mentha spicata*) has terminal spikes of lavender-colored flowers. There are many named clones, some with typical spearmint fragrance, such as the very sweet 'Provence Spearmint.' Others have a peppermint, fruit-and-mint or even lavender fragrance.

Curly spearmint (*M. spicata* var. *crispa*) has ornamental fluted and curled foliage with a true spearmint scent. The large and slightly crinkly leafed variety, 'Kentucky Colonel,' is very close to the common garden mint of Australia and England. 'Moroccan' mint is a neat form with a very sweet flavor.

Peppermint (*M. x piperita*) is a virtually sterile natural hybrid of water mint (*M. aquatica*) and spearmint (*M. spicata*). The most commonly cultivated clones are 'Black' (var. *piperita*), with an inflorescence resembling water mint; 'Mitcham,' the best selection of black peppermint; and white peppermint (var. *officinalis*), with a spearmintlike inflorescence. Other varieties include the quite delicious 'Chocolate' mint and 'Grapefruit.'

Water mint (*M. aquatica*) has a strong peppermint-like scent. The best-known variety is 'Eau de Cologne' or 'Bergamot,' with a strong and delightful true scent of eau-de-cologne. The whole plant is deep green suffused with purple.

A natural hybrid between corn mint (*M. arvensis*) and spearmint (*M. spicata*), *Mentha x gentilis* has a long inflorescence with clusters of lavender-colored flowers in the axils of the lanceolate leaves. Two varieties are 'Red-stemmed Applemint' ('Madalene Hill') and 'Ginger.'

Apple or pineapple mint (*M. suaveolens*) is a sweetly fruit-scented species with finely hairy leaves. Commercially they are sold as 'Apple' mint or 'Pineapple' mint (the variegated form).

Woolly or Bowle's mint (*M. x villosa* var. *alopecuroides*) is a vigorous, tall-growing species with broadly oval furred leaves, often sold as 'Apple' mint, but it is distinguished by the dense, pointed terminal clusters of lavender flowers.

Japanese peppermint or North American cornmint (*M. canadensis*) is piercingly peppermint-scented.

Pennyroyal (*M. pulegium*) is a creeping mint that forms dense mats. Its small smooth leaves are powerfully hot mint-scented and the inflorescences have clusters of lavender flowers. The American pennyroyal is Hedeoma pulegioides.

Corsican mint (*M. requinii*) is a strongly mint-scented ornamental that forms a very dense groundcover of tiny emerald green leaves, well suited to moist areas or cultivation in large pots.

Rau ram (*Persicaria odorata* syn. *Polygonum odoratum*) is an easily grown perennial, ideal for pot culture in a lightly shaded position. Although not of the mint family, it is also called Vietnamese mint and is used in Asian cooking. Its pointed, lance-shaped opposing leaves are green marked with deep brown and burgundy.

Position ▶ The ideal conditions are moist, rich soil and half to full sun.

Propagation ▶ You can easily propagate mints from cuttings or by dividing clumps.

Spearmint (*Mentha spicata*)

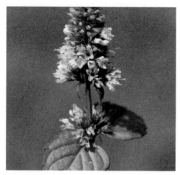
Peppermint (*Mentha x piperita*)

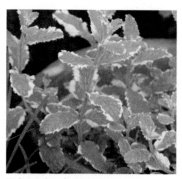
Variegated apple mint (*M. suaveolens* 'Variegata')

Mint *Continued*

Maintenance ▶ If your mint is proving invasive, grow it in large pots.

Pests and diseases ▶ Some mints, mainly varieties of *M. spicata*, are prone to a rust disease, Puccinea menthae. The mint flea beetle can cause leaf fall and browning; caterpillars are also a problem.

Harvesting and storing ▶ Mints dry well in a warm, airy place away from direct sunlight. Store crumbled leaves in an airtight container. Harvest foliage to use fresh as required.

Herbal medicine

Mentha x *piperita*. Part used: leaves. Peppermint produces notable relaxing effects on the gut and can help to relieve indigestion, nausea, gas and cramping. Clinical trials have verified a therapeutic effect of the herb on many of the symptoms of irritable bowel syndrome, including diarrhea, constipation, bloating and abdominal pain, especially when taken in the form of enteric-coated peppermint oil capsules.

Topically, peppermint essential oil has a pain-relieving effect, which can be valuable in alleviating the discomfort of joint and muscle pain and headaches. When it is inhaled, it can also help to reduce feelings of nausea and act as a nasal decongestant.

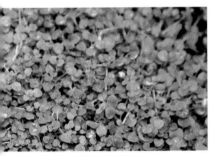

Pennyroyal (*M. pulegium*)

For the safe and appropriate medicinal use of peppermint, see Wind, bloating & flatulence, *page 180*; Nausea, *page 179*. Do not use peppermint in greater than culinary quantities, and do not use the essential oil if you are pregnant or breastfeeding.

Around the home

Peppermint and pennyroyal (*M. pulegium*) are both natural insect repellents that are easy to grow.

● Sprinkle cotton balls with peppermint essential oil and leave them where rodents enter.

● Add a few drops of peppermint essential oil to a damp rag and wipe on cabinet interiors to deter ants and cockroaches.

● To make a personal insect repellent, mix 1 part lavender, 1 part eucalyptus, 1 part peppermint essential oils with 3 parts unscented moisturizer or sweet almond oil, and rub into the skin.

● To deter fleas, sprinkle dried pennyroyal under your dog's bedding or put a spot of oil on its collar. Don't use pennyroyal on cats or pregnant dogs, because it is toxic.

Cooking

Lovely though its flavor is, fresh mint can overwhelm milder flavors and is best used with a light hand. Dried mint is less assertive and is favored in eastern Mediterranean and Arab countries.

In general, mint does not complement other herbs well, except parsley, thyme, marjoram, sage, oregano and coriander. It goes well with yogurt, and is used in Vietnamese food and in some Indian dishes. The coriander and

Rau ram
or Vietnamese mint
(*Persicaria odorata*)

lemon taste of Vietnamese mint is refreshing in salads.

Spearmint is the ordinary garden mint, and the most common culinary type. It is a classic flavoring for roast lamb and its accompaniments, and also goes well with potatoes, peas and salads.

Peppermint has a particularly strong flavor and aroma. It makes a pleasant digestive tea. The oil is used in ice cream, confectionery and liqueurs.

Mint jelly

1 lb. (500 g) green apples, cored and roughly chopped
½ oz. (15 g) roughly chopped fresh mint leaves
1½ cups (375 ml) white wine vinegar
1 lb. (500 g) jam-setting sugar
½ oz. (15 g) finely chopped fresh mint leaves, extra

Place apples, mint and vinegar in medium saucepan; cook, uncovered, until apples are very tender. Purée apples; drain through a sieve (don't push them through, but allow the liquid to run through so jelly doesn't become cloudy). Return liquid to saucepan; add sugar. Return to boil, boiling for 10 minutes. Remove from heat, stir through extra mint. Pour into clean container; refrigerate 6 hours, or until set. Makes about 2 cups (600 g).

Nettle

Latin Name **Urtica dioica** Lamiaceae
Parts used **Leaves, roots**

While the famous 17th-century herbalist Culpeper noted with unusual levity that nettles "may be found by feeling, in the darkest night," arthritis sufferers once whipped themselves with stinging nettles to relieve their pain — not a treatment for the faint-hearted.

Gardening

The stinging nettle (*Urtica dioica*) is a cold-tolerant herbaceous perennial growing to 4 ft. (1.2 m), with coarsely toothed, oval leaves armed with stinging hairs. Tiny green male and female flowers are borne on separate plants, the pendulous branched inflorescences emerging directly from the upper nodes of the square stems. The spreading roots are yellow. The young leaves are rich in minerals (particularly potassium, calcium, silicon and iron) and also contain vitamin C. Roman nettle (*U. pilulifera*) finds similar uses.

Classified into five subspecies, all of which have similar uses, *U. dioica* is indigenous to much of the temperate Northern Hemisphere. As an introduced plant, it is widespread in the temperate Southern Hemisphere.

Position ▶ Nettles prefer full sun to light shade and thrive in a rich, moist soil that is high in nitrogen.

Propagation ▶ Plant seed in spring or, if you are brave, by division of plants in spring.

Maintenance ▶ Nettles can become invasive plants.

Pests and diseases ▶ While nettles are quite disease-free, they are a valuable food supply for the caterpillar stage of a number of butterfly species.

Harvesting and storing ▶ In addition to spring picking, harvest in midsummer and again in autumn, and always wear gloves to protect your hands. Dig up the roots in autumn and air-dry them with the tops out of direct sunlight.

Herbal medicine

Urtica dioica. Parts used: Leaves, roots. Nettle leaf is a traditional blood-purifying remedy. It has a gentle diuretic effect and encourages the removal of toxins from the body. It is used medicinally to treat arthritic conditions and certain skin disorders such as eczema, which some herbalists believe can benefit from a detoxifying action.

The leaf is also associated with anti-allergic properties, and herbalists often prescribe it for symptoms of hay fever and skin rashes.

Modern research has shown that nettle root may inhibit overgrowth of prostate tissue, and clinical trials have provided some compelling evidence that therapeutic use of the root may improve the urinary symptoms associated with disorders of the prostate gland, such as frequent urination and weak flow.

For the safe and appropriate use of nettle, consult a healthcare professional. Do not use nettle in greater than culinary doses if you are pregnant or breastfeeding.

Cooking

The young leaves were once widely used in the spring diet to revitalize the body after winter. For culinary purposes, use leaf tips from plants less than 4 in. (10 cm) high, since these have yet to develop the stinging compounds. Nettle leaves may be cooked as a vegetable, in similar ways to spinach, or added to soups or to vegetable, egg or meat dishes. A tisane can be made from the leaves. Do not eat nettles raw. Also note that older leaves are high in calcium oxalate and should not be eaten at all.

Nettle (*Urtica dioica*)

Cornish yarg

A handmade semihard cheese with a creamy taste, Cornish yarg is wrapped in nettle leaves after pressing and brining. The leaves are carefully arranged by hand to form a pleasing pattern and also to attract natural molds in various colors that aid in the ripening process, adding a subtle mushroom taste. Remove yarg from the refrigerator about an hour before serving.

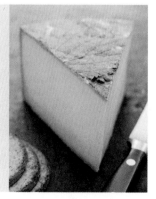

Parsley

Lain Name *Petroselinum* sp. Apiaceae/Umbelliferae
Parts used Leaves, stalks, roots, seeds; root of Hamburg parsley

Parsley has widespread culinary, medicinal and cosmetic uses, and is also used as a dye plant. It was once used as fodder for the chariot horses of the Ancient Greeks. Native to the southeastern Mediterranean, parsley is now cultivated in temperate climates throughout the world and is one of the most popular herbs for growing at home, both in gardens and containers.

Curly parsley (*Petroselinum crispum* var. *crispum*, pot) and flat-leaf parsleya (*Petroselinum crispum* var. *neapolitanum*)

Gardening

Parsley is a biennial crop, forming a dense rosette of leaves in the first year and flowering in its second summer, when the foliage becomes bitter.

There are three distinct types of parsley. Probably the most familiar is curly parsley (*P. crispum* var. *crispum*). The many excellent varieties include 'Triple Curl' and 'Green River.' The plain-leaf types, known as Italian or French or flat-leaf parsley (*P. crispum* var. *neapolitanum*), have flat leaf segments. In Italy, the true Italian parsley is considered to be 'Catalagno,' which is usually listed elsewhere as 'Giant Italian.' Hamburg or turnip-rooted parsley (*P. crispum* var. *tuberosum*) is grown more for its delicately flavored tap root than its leaves, although they can also be used. Japanese parsley or mitsuba (*Cryptotaenia japonica*) is in the same family. Its flavor is a mixture of celery, angelica and parsley.

Position ▶ Parsley prefers full morning sun to partial shade, and well-composted, well-drained but moist soil. It tolerates fairly acidic to alkaline soil, but if the soil is very acidic, incorporate lime before planting.

Propagation ▶ This herb is grown only from seed and takes 3 to 8 weeks to germinate. You can speed up this process by soaking the seed in warm water overnight before planting into trays or pots. Alternatively, pour freshly boiled water along seed drills just before planting. Cover seed very lightly with soil. Transplant seedlings into the garden (or thin seedlings sown directly into the garden) to around 10 in. (25 cm) apart. Parsley self-seeds under suitable conditions. In cold climates, a cloche will warm the soil and allow for earlier planting of seedlings, or even protect a winter crop.

Maintenance ▶ Water regularly or parsley will flower ('bolt') in its first season. Cutting out the emerging flowering stalks will frustrate this process to some extent.

Pests and diseases ▶ Generally easy to grow, parsley can be attacked by pests of closely related members of the same family — for instance, celery fly and carrot weevil. Septoria leaf spot can also be a problem. In Hamburg parsley, crown rot can occur after prolonged rain.

Harvesting and storing ▶ New growth comes from the center of the stem, so harvest leaves from around the outside of plants. Wrap in a plastic bag and store in the freezer. Parsley is not a good herb for drying, as it loses much of its flavor. Collect seeds when pale brown. They ripen progressively from the outside of the inflorescence inward. Hang bunches of ripening seed heads upside down inside paper bags. Harvest the roots at the end of the second season and air-dry them.

Herbal medicine

Petroselinum crispum var. *crispum*. Parts used: leaves, roots, seeds. The leaves are a good source of vitamin C, and both the leaf and root are well known for eliciting considerable diuretic effects in the body. Parsley has been used to treat fluid retention, urinary tract disorders and arthritic conditions of the joints, including gout, an inflammatory condition usually affecting a single joint, such as a big toe.

Parsley has a calming effect on the gut, alleviating flatulence and colic, and also a gentle stimulatory action, encouraging appetite and improving digestion. It can also have a notable stimulating effect on the uterus and has been used to encourage menstruation — but should not be used for this purpose if pregnancy is a possibility.

For the safe and appropriate medicinal use of parsley, consult your healthcare professional. Do not use parsley in greater than culinary quantities if you're pregnant or breastfeeding.

Cooking

Flat-leaf parsley is generally considered to have the best flavor, while curly parsley has a pleasing crunchy texture. Use either one as a garnish or in salads, vegetable and egg dishes and sauces

Parsley is essential to many traditional flavoring mixtures, particularly in French cooking. Bouquet garni, a small bunch of pungent fresh herbs for slow cooking, is most often comprised of a bay leaf, sprigs of parsley and sprigs of thyme. Other mixes include persillade (finely chopped parsley and garlic). Sprinkle them on a dish near the end of its preparation to retain its flavor.

The edible root of Hamburg parsley is used in soups and stews and can be roasted or boiled in the same way as other root vegetables.

Mitsuba is used in Japanese cooking, in soups, salads, slow-cooked dishes and fried foods. Blanch the leaves briefly to tenderize them or add to food at the last moment to preserve the delicate flavor.

Emerald risotto

For a delicious-tasting and attractive emerald-green herb risotto, cook a classic risotto recipe using arborio rice, chicken or vegetable stock and white wine, but add a handful of chopped baby spinach leaves when the rice is almost cooked. Once the rice is fully cooked (it should be a creamy, dropping consistency), stir in a generous amount of finely chopped fresh parsley and coriander. Season to taste.

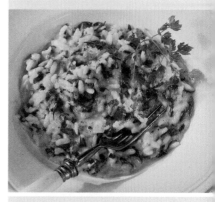

Chimichurri sauce

Parsley is used in many herb and spice mixes around the world. Try this Argentinian sauce with meat hot off the barbecue.

In a jar, combine 6 cloves garlic, 2 tablespoons fresh oregano leaves and a handful of parsley leaves, all finely chopped. Add 1 tablespoon red onion, chopped, a pinch of dried chilli flakes, 1 teaspoon ground black pepper, 5 fl. oz. (150 ml) olive oil, 6 tablespoons red wine and salt, to taste. Seal jar, shake well. Leave 4 hours for flavors to develop.

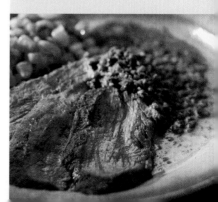

The source of Peter Rabbit's remedy

According to Greek myth, parsley sprang from the blood of a Greek hero, Archemorus, the forerunner of death, while English folklore has it that parsley seeds go to the Devil and back seven times before they germinate, referring to the fact that they can be slow to sprout. It is also claimed that only witches can grow it. On a more lighthearted note, however, parsley is traditionally a curative, a fact that Beatrix Potter weaves into *The Tale of Peter Rabbit* when Peter eats too much in Farmer McGregor's vegetable patch: "First he ate some lettuce and some broad beans, then some radishes, and then, feeling rather sick, he went to look for some parsley."

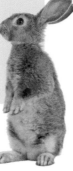

Passionflower

Latin Name *Passiflora incarnata* Passifloraceae
Other common names **Maypops, purple passionflower,
  wild apricot, wild passionflower**
Parts used **Dried aerial parts (especially leaves), ripe fruits, flowers**

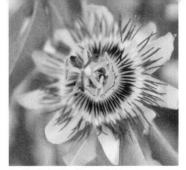

Passionfruit (*Passiflora edulis*)

To Spanish missionaries in South America, the passionflower represented the Passion of Christ: the three stigmas symbolized the nails, the corona the crown of thorns, the five stamens the wounds, and the 10 petals the Apostles (except Judas Iscariot and Peter).

Gardening

There are about 400 species of passionflowers. Many are ornamental, tendrilled climbers; some produce delicious fruit. Most require warm-temperate to tropical conditions, although *P. incarnata* is one of the most tolerant of cooler conditions. Deciduous in colder areas, it can survive occasional winter freezes.

A common wildflower in the southern United States, it was used as a tonic by Native Americans, and was first noted by a Western doctor in 1783. The leaves are palmately divided with 3 to 5 smooth, textured, pointed lobes with serrated margins. The fragrant large flowers are lavender-colored, with a white center and a deeper purple, threadlike corona. The fruits, ovoid yellow berries when ripe, are about 2 in. (5 cm) long.

Position ▶ It prefers a light, acidic soil and a warm, sunny position. In cooler areas, it is an excellent greenhouse plant.

Propagation ▶ Sow passionflower seed in spring when the soil has warmed. Or propagate by semi-ripe stem cuttings in summer, or by layering.

Maintenance ▶ Provide a trellis or other support, and mulch plants well. Shape and prune the vine as necessary in spring.

Pests and diseases ▶ Passionflower vines are mainly pest-free and, although *Passiflora* is an important food source for the caterpillar stage of some butterflies, they cause no permanent damage.

Harvesting and storing ▶ Harvest the aerial parts in mid- to late summer and air-dry for medicinal preparations. For culinary use, pick the fruits at the "dropping" stage.

Herbal medicine

Passiflora incarnata. Part used: leaves. Medicinally, passionflower can be of immense benefit in conditions in which nervous tension and stress are prominent factors. This herb has a calming effect on the mind and body, and is commonly prescribed for insomnia in adults and children, especially when there is difficulty falling asleep.

Results of preliminary human trials have provided supportive evidence for the traditional use of passionflower for treating anxiety disorders. It's also interesting to note that further research has elucidated a potential role as a supportive remedy during withdrawal from addiction to narcotic drugs.

The relaxing and antispasmodic effects of passionflower can also be applied in the treatment of digestive symptoms, nervous headaches and neuralgic pain that are exacerbated by stress and tension.

For the safe and appropriate medicinal use of passionflower, refer to Insomnia, *page 188*. Do not use passionflower if you are pregnant or breastfeeding.

Cooking

The seeds and pulp of ripe fruits have a tangy flavor, and are eaten raw or used in fruit salads and other desserts, curds, jams, jellies and fruit drinks. The popular cocktail Hurricane is made with passionfruit syrup, rum and lime juice.

*Opposite page: Passionflower
(Passiflora incarnata)*

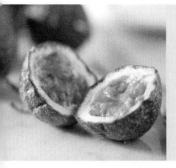

Passionfruit cordial

Spoon the pulp of 8 passionfruit into a mixing bowl. You need about ¾ cup (180 ml) pulp. Add 1 teaspoon vanilla extract, 1 cup (230 g) sugar and ¼ cup (60 ml) freshly squeezed lemon juice. Stir well. Pour into a clip-lock bottle and refrigerate. Keeps for 1 week. Pour into a jug. Add 4 cups (1 l) chilled club soda. Serves 8.

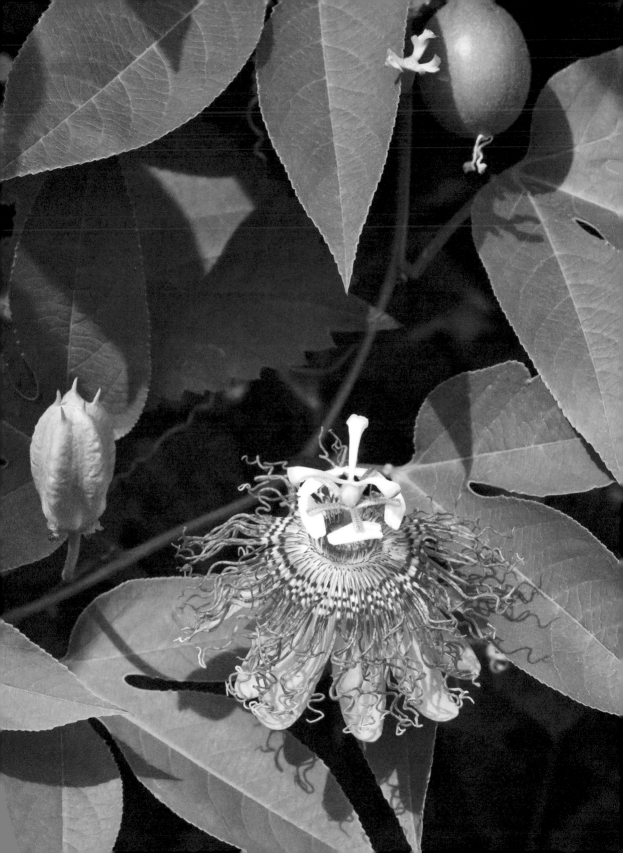

Peony

Latin Name *Paeonia lactiflora* syn. *P. albiflora, P. officinalis,*
P. suffruticosa syn. *P. moutan* Paeoniaceae
Other common names **Bai shao, Chinese peony, white peony** (*P. lactiflora*)
Parts used **Roots, flowers**

Once the favored flower of Chinese emperors, peonies were first mentioned as a medicinal herb in about 500 ce. However, the medicinal use of the three peonies mentioned here are restricted to qualified practitioners.

Gardening

The Chinese peony (*P. lactiflora*) is a herbaceous perennial. It has erect stems with lobed leaves and very large, scented flowers, which in the wild are white and single. Cultivated plants grow to 3.5 ft. (1 m), are fully hardy, can be red, pink or purple and are usually double.

The tree peony (*P. suffruticosa*), found from Western China to Bhutan, forms a branched upright shrub to 6.5 ft. (2 m) with slash-cut and lobed leaves. The terminal flowers are very large and slightly fragrant.

Common peony (*P. officinalis*) is a herbaceous perennial with many erect stems to 2.5 ft. (74 cm), bipinnate leaves composed of ovate-lanceolate segments, and large terminal flowers that are single, fragrant, usually purple-crimson and hermaphroditic.

Varieties ▶ Common peony varieties include 'Alba Plena' and 'Rosea Plena.'

Position ▶ Peonies prefer cold winters and a deep, rich, moist (and in the case of *P. officinalis*, slightly alkaline) soil.

Propagation ▶ Plant fresh seed in autumn, or stratify older seed (see box *page 40*), then plant it in spring. You can also divide plants in late autumn or spring, take root cuttings in winter or semi-ripe stem cuttings.

Maintenance ▶ Peonies require heavy feeding, and their roots resent disturbance. Remove dead wood in spring.

Pests and diseases ▶ These plants are susceptible to Botrytis, peony wilt (caused by a blight fungus), leaf spot, nematodes (eel worm) and honey fungus.

Herbal medicine

Paeonia lactiflora. Part used: roots. In traditional Chinese medicine, white peony root nourishes the blood and is a key remedy for the treatment of conditions of the female reproductive system.

Laboratory studies have shown white peony possesses moderate hormonal activity. Herbalists prescribe this herb, often with licorice, to regulate the menstrual cycle and relieve pain. This combination is used to treat irregular, heavy, delayed or absent bleeding, period pain, premenstrual syndrome, fibroids and polycystic ovarian syndrome.

White peony can also have a relaxing effect on muscles, and it may lower blood pressure due to its ability to dilate blood vessels and improve circulation. Traditionally and in combination with other herbs, white peony has also been used to ease muscle cramps and reduce intestinal griping, enhance memory and concentration, relieve night sweats and treat angina.

For the safe and appropriate use of white peony, consult your healthcare professional. Do not take white peony if you are pregnant or breastfeeding.

Cooking

The flowers of *P. officinalis* are used to scent tea, and the seeds were once used as a spice.

The peony is named after Paeon, physician to the Greek gods.

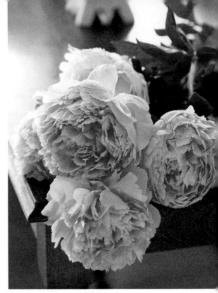
Peony (*Paeonia lactiflora*)

Gender bias

The old herbalists recognized two different leaf forms of *P. officinalis* as "male" and "female" peonies, which were used for male and female complaints, respectively. The "female" peony had leafier foliage, scented dark purple flowers and black seeds, while the "male" peony had purple-red flowers and black and crimson seeds.

Perilla

Latin Name **Perilla frutescens** syn. *P. ocimoides* Lamiaceae
Other common names **Beefsteak plant, Chinese basil, shiso**
Parts used **Leaves, flower spikes, seed**

Perilla is a popular, spicily aromatic culinary herb that is used fresh in salads and for pickling and flavoring. The colorful and curly leafed forms are increasingly popular as an ornamental bedding annual.

Gardening

Perilla is a hardy, branched annual to 4 ft. (1.2 m) with broadly ovate, serrated leaves, which vary in color from green to red and purple. The leaf edges may be curled (a form previously called *P. crispum*), while the tiny white to purple flowers are borne in dense spikes about 4 in. (10 cm) long.

Varieties ▶ 'Green Cumin' and 'Purple Cumin,' both readily available, have cumin- and cinnamon-scented leaves. 'Aojiso' has green ginger-scented leaves, often used with sashimi. 'Red' or 'Akajiso' has rich, deep red to purple leaves. The large-leafed 'Kkaennip' or Korean perilla is used in salads, as a food wrap and preserve, and the seeds for culinary flavoring. 'Thai' perilla has a strong, delicious flavor.

Position ▶ Perilla flourishes in moist, well-drained soils enriched with compost.

Propagation ▶ Plant seed in spring when the soil has warmed.

Maintenance ▶ Pinch out the initial flower spikes to encourage bushy growth.

Pests and diseases ▶ This herb has few problems.

Harvesting and storing ▶ Harvest the leaves in summer and use them fresh or dried. Harvest flower spikes when they are fully developed, and the seed in autumn.

Herbal medicine

Perilla frutescens. Parts used: leaves, seeds. Both the leaves and seeds of perilla have been used for centuries in traditional Japanese medicine (a system known as Kampo), and also by Chinese herbalists for similar therapeutic purposes. Perilla is commonly prescribed with other herbs for the treatment of respiratory conditions, including colds, flu and coughs, and to ease symptoms caused by poor digestive function, such as lack of appetite, nausea and bloating. Perilla is also used successfully for the management of hay fever and dermatitis. It is a key ingredient in the Kampo herbal formula known as Saibokuto, a popular remedy that is used for a number of allergic conditions.

Laboratory research has confirmed substantial anti-allergic as well as anti-inflammatory effects of perilla extracts. Clinical trials have produced promising results for the use of oral preparations of perilla for the relief of hay fever symptoms, including watery, itching eyes. Additional studies have also recorded improvements in the symptoms of allergic dermatitis with the use of a topical perilla cream.

For the safe and appropriate medicinal use of perilla, see Hay fever & sinusitis, *page 177*. Don't use perilla in greater than culinary quantities if you are pregnant or breastfeeding.

see Hay fever & sinusitis, *page 177*.

Japanese cuisine

In Japan the fresh red leaves of perilla are used in salads or as a garnish or wrapping for dishes such as sushi. The leaves are also used to color and flavor pickled plums and ginger, while the seeds are sprouted for use in salads, or pickled as a condiment for Japanese dishes. Different varieties of perilla are also used in Indonesian, Vietnamese and Korean cuisine.

Cooking

The red variety of perilla is more often used for culinary purposes than the green. (Be aware that excessive handling of the leaves can cause dermatitis.) A volatile oil in the leaves of *P. frutescens* contains a compound that is 2,000 times sweeter than sugar and is used as an artificial sweetener in Japan.

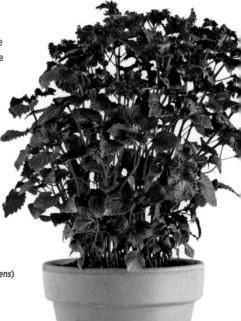

Perilla (*Perilla frutescens*)

Plantain

Latin Name *Plantago major, P. lanceolata, P. asiatica*
 syn. *P. major* var. *asiatica, P. psyllium* Plantaginaceae
Other common names **Greater plantain, rat-tail plantain** (*P. major*)
Parts used **Leaves** (*P. major, P. lanceolata*); **seeds, seed husks**
 (*P. psyllium, P. ovata*)

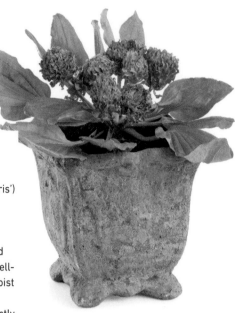

Rose plantain (*Plantago major 'Rosularis'*)

Common plantain is considered a weed by many gardeners, but it has long been valued in folk medicine, and continues to find herbal uses. There are also some equally useful and very ornamental varieties for the garden.

Gardening

Common plantain (*P. major*) is an evergreen perennial that forms a basal rosette of stalked, broadly ovate leaves to 6 in. (15 cm), from which emerge cylindrical spikes of tiny green flowers to 8 in. (20 cm). Ribwort plantain (*P. lanceolata*), with ribbed lanceolate leaves, is used interchangeably with *P. major* in herbal medicine. Asian plantain (*P. asiatica* syn. *P. major* var. *asiatica*) bears flower spikes to 20 in. (50 cm).

Psyllium (*P. psyllium*) is an annual with inflorescences that release tiny seeds. Blond psyllium (*P. ovata*) is also widely used; black psyllium (*P. indica*) and golden psyllium (*P. arenaria*) to a lesser degree.

Varieties ▶ The inflorescences of rose plantain (*P. major* 'Rosularis') resemble double green roses. 'Rubrifolia' has purple leaves, and 'Variegata' is marbled white.

Position *P. psyllium, P. ovata* and *P. asiatica* prefer full sun and a well-drained soil. *P. major* prefers a moist situation with light shade.

Propagation ▶ Plant seed directly in spring after the soil has warmed.

Maintenance Weed regularly.

Pests and diseases ▶ In dry weather, powdery mildew is a problem for *P. major*.

Harvesting and storing ▶ Cut the leaves and dry them for herbal use, as required. Collect seed when ripe, as soon as the dew has dried, and dry them also.

Herbal medicine

Plantago lanceolata, P. major. Part used: leaves. Due to plantain's mucilaginous compounds, it has a soothing effect on the lungs, reducing inflammation and irritation, and helping to remove catarrh. Plantain is also used for its healing effect on peptic and intestinal ulcers, gastritis and colitis.

Plantain can be used as a mouth-wash or gargle for inflammatory conditions of the mouth and throat, and as an ointment it can be applied to hemorrhoids, cuts and bruises to aid healing.

Plantago psyllium, P. ovata. Parts used: seeds, husks. Psyllium is an excellent bulk laxative. The soluble fiber contained in the seeds absorbs water, making bowel movements easier and more regular.

Clinical trials have confirmed its benefit in the treatment of chronic constipation and irritable bowel syndrome. Psyllium can also be used in cases of anal fissures, recovery from anal/rectal surgery and haemorrhoids where a softer stool is needed to ease the passing of stools.

Its content of soluble fiber also makes psyllium a valuable part of any cholesterol-lowering program. The fiber binds to cholesterol in the gut, enabling it to be excreted from the body.

For the safe and appropriate use of plantain, consult a healthcare professional. For the use of psyllium, see Constipation & hemorrhoids, *page 181, and Detox, page 183.* Do not use these herbs if you are pregnant or breastfeeding, except under medical supervision.

A sacred herb

One of the Nine Sacred Herbs of the Anglo-Saxons, plantain was believed to cure headaches. The *Lacnunga*, a collection of medical texts written in the 11th or 12th century, relates this story of the god Woden: '...out of the worm sprang nine poisons. So Woden took his sword and changed it into nine herbs. These herbs did the wise lord create and sent them into the world for rich and poor, a remedy for all...'

Poppy

Latin Name *Papaver rhoeas, P. somniferum; Eschscholzia californica* Papaveraceae
Parts used **Aerial parts (Californian poppy only); latex (opium poppy only)**

Cultivated for 5,000 years, poppies were once symbolic both of the earth goddess and of Ceres, the goddess of cereals. Opium poppy is the source of some of our most important painkillers, morphine and codeine, but also of dangerously addictive heroin.

Gardening

The opium poppy (*P. somniferum*) is a hardy annual that grows to about 4 ft. (1.2 m) with large, coarse, toothed, silvery green foliage and tall flowering stems bearing four-petaled flowers that may be white, pink, lavender or red, followed by a globose capsule with an operculum that opens to scatter the ripe seed. The wall of the green capsule oozes bitter white latex when wounded.

Opium poppy cultivation is strictly controlled in many countries; however, a number of ornamental forms are widely grown, including the 19th-century red and white 'Danish Flag,' double 'peony' forms and the very old 'Hen and Chickens,' which has a ring of tiny flowers encircling each large flower.

The European annual red or field poppy (*P. rhoeas*) has four silken, bright red petals, sometimes with a black blotch in the center. It was used to breed ornamental Shirley poppies.

Californian poppy (*Eschscholzia californica*), which is related to true poppies, is a heat- and drought-resistant annual, native to the western United States, with the subspecies *mexicana* extending south into the Sonoran Desert. The blue-green, finely divided leaves form a basal rosette and the many flower stalks bear single silken, four-petaled flowers in lemon to orange.

Position ▶ All poppies, including Californian poppy, require a well-drained soil and sunny position.

Propagation ▶ To sow poppy seeds evenly during spring, mix them with dry sand.

Maintenance ▶ Weed regularly.

Pests and diseases ▶ Powdery mildew can be a problem.

Harvesting and storing ▶ Harvest and dry the petals immediately after the flowers fully open. Collect seed from ripe capsules and dry them.

Remembrance Day

In the World War I battlefields around Flanders in Northern Europe, red or field poppies bloomed everywhere in the ravaged earth. Since then, they have become a symbol of Armistice or Remembrance Day on November 11th of each year.

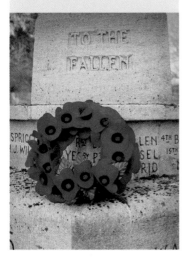

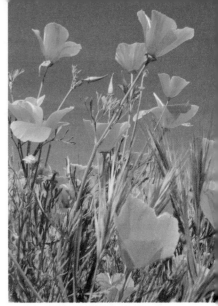

Californian poppy (*Eschscholzia californica*)

Herbal medicine

Eschscholzia californica. Parts used: aerial parts. The aerial parts of Californian poppy were used by Native Americans as a painkiller, and have been incorporated into Western herbal medicine as a valuable pain-relieving and relaxing herb. It is used for treating insomnia, anxiety and over-excitability, and may be a useful remedy for aiding relaxation during times of tension and stress.

Californian poppy alleviates many types of pain, including headaches, nervous cramping of the bowel, and rheumatic and nerve pain.

Substances known as alkaloids are responsible for the plant's sedating and painkilling properties, and are similar to those found in opium poppy, from which morphine and codeine are derived. However, the alkaloids that are found in Californian poppy have a far gentler therapeutic effect and are also regarded as non-habit forming.

Papaver rhoeas. Part used: petals. Despite being closely related to the opium poppy, the red or field poppy possesses none of its counterpart's

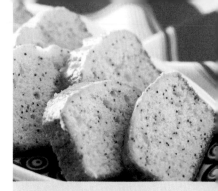

Opium poppy

Opium derived from the latex of the unripe seed capsules of the opium poppy (*P. somniferum*) was once a traditional herbal medicine as well as a legal recreational drug, but we now know that opiates are addictive and associated with serious adverse effects. In the Western world, opium is a heavily regulated and licensed product used to produce morphine and codeine. Morphine and codeine provide exceptional pain relief as pharmaceutical drugs, but still carry a risk of dependency with overuse.

Poppy seeds, the source of poppy oil, are harmless flavorings for baked goods.

potent narcotic effects. Instead, it is used as a reliable traditional remedy for soothing respiratory conditions that are associated with irritable coughing and the presence of catarrh. Red poppy is regarded as mildly sedating and can be useful for alleviating poor or disturbed sleep.

For the safe and appropriate use of Californian and red poppy, consult your healthcare professional. Do not use these herbs if you are pregnant or breastfeeding.

Cooking

Poppy seeds are not narcotic and are widely liked for their flavor and crunchy texture. They are popular in baked goods, such as breads, cakes, pastries, muffins and bagels. In India, the seeds are ground and used to thicken sauces. The seeds also feature in Jewish and German cooking.

Lemon poppy-seed cake

⅓ (43 g) cup sugar
1 egg
3 tablespoons canola oil
3 tablespoons orange juice
½ teaspoon lemon essence
⅔ cup (85 g) plain flour
¾ teaspoon baking powder
1/8 teaspoon salt
1 teaspoon poppy seeds
⅓ cup (43 g) confectioner's sugar
2 tablespoons lemon juice

1. Preheat oven to 180°C. Grease and flour a 9 x 5 x 3 in. loaf tin.
2. In a small bowl, combine sugar, egg, oil, orange juice and lemon essence. Combine flour, baking powder and salt; add to egg mixture and mix well. Stir in poppy seeds.
3. Bake 30–35 minutes or until a skewer inserted into the centre comes out clean. Cool for 10 minutes before removing from pan to a wire rack to cool completely.
4. For a glaze, whisk confectioner's sugar and lemon juice in a small bowl until smooth; drizzle over cake.

Serves 6

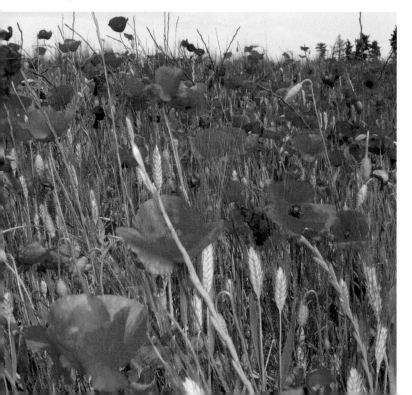

Red poppies, also known as field poppies (*Papaver rhoeas*).

Primrose and cowslip

Latin Name *Primula vulgaris, P. veris* Primulaceae
Another common name **Paigle (cowslip)**
Parts used **Leaves, flowers, roots**

Cowslips were once known as cowsloppes, in the belief that they grew in cow droppings, or as the "keys of St Peter," who supposedly dropped the keys from heaven, causing cowslips to spring up where they fell. Traditionally, it was believed that if you nibbled on cowslips, you would see fairies.

Gardening

Primrose (*P. vulgaris*) is a perennial forming a basal rosette of oblong, rugose leaves, from which spring a number of stalked, solitary flowers with a sweet, fresh fragrance. The flowers are five-petaled and pale golden yellow (rarely white), with a central cleft in each petal. The foliage

Strewing herbs

In the Middle Ages, strewing herbs were used instead of, or mixed with, rushes or straw as a floor covering. They helped to mask unpleasant odors, deter household pests and, it was believed, protect against disease.
   According to Thomas Tusser's *Five Hundred Good Points of Husbandry* (1573), the 21 strewing herbs comprised 'Bassell [basil], Bawlme [lemon balm], Camamel [chamomile], Costemary [costmary], Cowsleps and paggles [cowslips], Daisies of all sorts, Sweet fennel, Germander, Hysop [hyssop], Lavender, Lavender spike, Lavender cotten [santolina], Marjorom, Mawdelin, Peny ryall [pennyroyal], Roses of all sorts, Red myntes, Sage, Tansey, Violets, Winter savery.'

of cowslips closely resembles that of primroses, but the smaller, golden yellow, sweetly scented flowers are borne in clusters at the top of each flowering stem, well above the leaves. According to the English herbalist John Gerard, writing in the 16th century, a tisane made from the flowers was drunk in the month of May to cure the "frenzie."

Varieties ▶ Primrose varieties that are mentioned in Tudor and Elizabethan herbals, and are still available, include 'Jack in the Green,' with a much enlarged persistent rufflike calyx; 'Hose in Hose,' with a second flower emerging from the first; and the very attractive fully double varieties such as 'Alba Plena,' 'Double Sulphur' and 'Miss Indigo.'

Position ▶ Primroses require a moist, rich soil and light shade, while cowslips prefer a well-drained drier site in full sun or light shade.

Propagation ▶ Propagate cowslips and primroses by seed or by division. Stratify the seed for 10 weeks to break dormancy (see box, *page 40*). Because of habitat loss and over-harvesting of these plants, do not gather them in the wild.

Maintenance ▶ Mulch the plants. Break up any clumps and replant well-rooted divisions every 2 years.

Pests and diseases ▶ Leaf-eating insects can damage plants. Rust may infect leaves, and *Botrytis* can kill plants.

Harvesting and storing ▶ Gather leaves and flowers in spring to use fresh, and for use in preserves and wine. Before storing, air-dry flowers, leaves and roots (lifted in autumn).

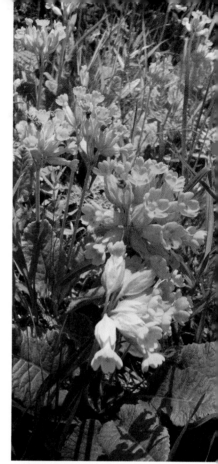

Cowslip (*P. veris*)

Herbal medicine

Primula veris, P. officinalis. Parts used: flowers, roots. Both the flowers and roots of cowslip have been used medicinally over time. The flowers are more commonly associated with relaxing and sedative properties and are used to treat insomnia and restlessness. They can also act as a valuable supportive remedy in times of stress and tension.

Cowslip is also traditionally used to alleviate catarrhal congestion and irritable coughs associated with some respiratory disorders, such as bronchitis.

For the safe and appropriate use of cowslip, consult a healthcare professional. Do not use cowslip if you are pregnant or breastfeeding.

Purslane

Latin Name *Portulaca oleracea* Portulacaceae
Parts used **Leaves, stems**

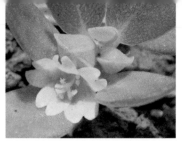

Rich in vitamins A, C and E, purslane is considered one of the future 'power foods.'

In centuries past, purslane was held up as a cure for "blastings by lightning or planets." Like a number of "weeds" condemned in modern gardens, this succulent herb was once appreciated as a salad, pickle and sautéed vegetable. It is now coming back into culinary fashion.

Gardening

Purslane is an annual that grows to about 3 in. (7 cm) high and up to 1.5 ft. (45 cm) wide, with soft trailing branches and wedge- to spoon-shaped, succulent green leaves. The ephemeral flowers are inconspicuous, five-petaled and yellow, while the seeds are tiny, spherical and black. Cultivated purslane is sometimes sold as var. *sativa*. The leaves are tender and fleshy, with a slight crunchy texture. Purslane has been used both as a food and a medicine in the Mediterranean basin, India and China for thousands of years.

Varieties ▶ There is a golden-leafed variety (var. *aurea*) with reddish stems.

Purslane
(*Portulaca oleracea*)

Position ▶ Purslane is found very widely in well-drained soils, growing in full sun to light shade.

Propagation ▶ Plant the seeds after the soil warms in spring. Barely press them into the soil, which should be kept moist. Left uncovered, they will germinate rapidly. During the growing season, trailing branches will root where they touch the ground; detach the rooted tips and plant them out. In an area with a long growing season, you can sow monthly.

Maintenance ▶ For a tender, abundant crop, keep the soil moist at all times. An occasional light application of liquid seaweed fertilizer at the recommended rate is also helpful.

Pests and diseases ▶ Slugs may be a problem.

Harvesting and storing ▶ Harvest fresh plants before flowering, or the flavor will deteriorate. Dry them for decoctions.

Cooking

Purslane has a slightly sour, salty, lemony spinach flavor and has been eaten for thousands of years in India, where it grows wild. It is the leaves that are most commonly used, but the roots, flowers and seeds are also edible.

The plant contains mucilage, giving the palate a glutinous sensation and also serving to thicken such dishes as soups and sauces. Blanching reduces both the mucilage and the jellylike leaf texture.

Purslane was popular in England in the Elizabethan era and is once again finding favor as a culinary herb. You can cook it in a similar manner to spinach. In French cooking, the fleshy leaves are used raw in salads, or cooked in equal amounts with sorrel to make the classic soup *bonne femme*. They are sometimes included in fattoush, a Middle Eastern salad. In Asia, purslane is used in stir-fries. Aboriginal Australians used the seeds to make seed cakes.

Purslane makes an excellent pickle, using wine or apple cider vinegar spiced with garlic, chili and whole peppercorns.

Purslane soup

½ lb. (250 g) purslane, chopped
3.5 lb. (50 g) butter
4 cups (1 l) stock
½ lb. (250 g) potatoes, peeled and sliced
3 tablespoons cream
fresh purslane, to garnish

Cook purslane with butter in covered pan. Add stock, cook until potato is tender, then purée in a blender. Stir in cream, then garnish with fresh purslane.

Red clover

Latin Name *Trifolium pratense* Fabaceae
Other common names **Meadow honeysuckle, meadow trefoil, purple clover, wild clover**
Parts used **Flowers, young leaves**

Red clover has been an important agricultural forage and fertility-improving crop since the Middle Ages. The plant contains phytoestrogens and is increasingly important as a medicinal herb, particularly for menopausal symptoms.

Gardening

Red clover is a short-lived European perennial now widely grown as a valuable forage crop. In common with other clovers, nitrogen-fixing bacteria in its root nodules assimilate atmospheric nitrogen into the plant and significantly improve soil fertility. The plants form a creeping groundcover with stalked trifoliate leaves, each leaflet marked with a central pale arrowhead. The stalked inflorescences are dense and club-shaped, composed of many pink to purple pea flowers, which are rich in nectar.

Closely related species include lucerne or alfalfa (*Medicago sativa*), and fenugreek (*Trigonella foenum-graecum*). The latter is an important spice, particularly in Indian curry

powders. Medicinally, it is used under professional supervision to help manage blood sugar in patients with diabetes, and as a cholesterol-lowering agent. See Spices, *page 132*.

Varieties ▶ There are about 300 species of clover, including the beautiful crimson clover (*T. incarnatum*), an important forage crop that is also used in herbal crafts and planted for roadside erosion control, and white clover (*T. repens*), which is likewise an excellent fodder crop. It also has similar culinary uses to red clover, and is used as a tisane (flowers only).

Position ▶ Red clover prefers a light soil, good drainage, a cool to mild spring and full sunlight.

Propagation ▶ Sow seed in spring.

Maintenance ▶ Keep plants weed free.

Pests and diseases ▶ Powdery mildew can be a problem during dry weather.

Harvesting and storing ▶ Harvest red clover up to 3 times in a growing season. Harvest the leaves when young; use the flowers fresh or dried.

Herbal medicine

Trifolium pratense. Parts used: flowers, isolated isoflavone compounds. Red clover flowers have been used traditionally, both internally and externally, as a remedy for the treatment of chronic skin conditions such as eczema and psoriasis, particularly in children. Taken as an infusion or syrup of the flowers, red clover also alleviates

White clover
(*Trifolium repens*)

the coughing associated with some respiratory conditions, such as bronchitis.

These days, the most common medicinal application for red clover centers around the use of isolated compounds known as isoflavones that come from the leaves and flowers. These compounds have been shown to possess mild oestrogenic activity, and clinical studies suggest that they can alleviate many of the symptoms associated with menopause.

For the safe and appropriate use of red clover, consult a healthcare professional. Do not use red clover if you are pregnant or breastfeeding.

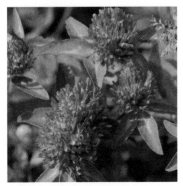

Red clover (*Trifolium pratense*)

The shamrock

In the teachings of St. Patrick, the clover's trifoliate leaves (from the Latin *tri*, meaning "three," and *folium*, "leaf") symbolized the Holy Trinity — the doctrine that God is the Father, Son and Holy Spirit — and became the shamrock of Ireland. Although the Celtic harp is the official symbol of Ireland, the shamrock is the popular symbol of St Patrick's Day.

Rocket or arugula

Latin Name *Eruca sativa* syn. *Eruca vesicaria* subsp. *sativa* Brassicaceae
Other common names **Italian cress, Roman rocket, rucola, rugula**
Parts used **Leaves, flowers, seeds**

Native to the Mediterranean Basin and eastward to Turkey and Jordan, rocket has been popular as a salad green since ancient Roman times for its peppery, smoky, meaty flavor. Even now, it is still sometimes known as Roman rocket.

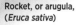

Rocket, or arugula,
(*Eruca sativa*)

Gardening

Rocket (*Eruca sativa*) is an annual plant resembling an open lettuce, with deeply pinnately lobed leaves that are aromatic and peppery, and contain similar isothiocyanate compounds to horseradish (*Armoracia rusticana*) and wasabi (*Wasabia japonica*); see Horseradish & Wasabi, *page 60*. The leaves add flavor to other salad greens, while the piquantly flavored, four-petaled white flowers can be added to salads. The small round seeds are borne in siliquas (which are seed capsules that separate when ripe).

Tall rocket or tumbling mustard (*Sisymbrium altissimum*), London rocket (*S. irio*) and Mediterranean rocket or smooth mustard (*S. erysimoides*) all have a peppery flavor. Sweet rocket or dame's violet (*Hesperis matronalis*), sometimes confused with rocket, is a popular old-fashioned garden flower that resembles a tall single stock with purple or white evening-scented flowers.

Plants that are sold as wild rocket or wild arugula or *Ruchetta selvatica* or roquette sauvage are usually *Diplotaxis tenuifolia* syn. *Brassica tenuifolia*, a species with yellow flowers and leaves that resemble a more slender version of rocket. The flavor is more intense.

Position ▶ Plant rocket in full sun in the cooler months, but in midsummer provide some light shade. Rocket is quite unfussy otherwise, thriving in average garden soil, while wild arugula requires similar conditions.

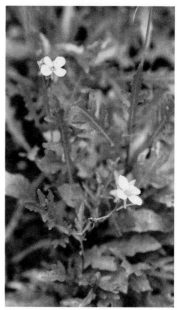

Wild rocket (*Diplotaxis tenuifolia*)

Grown in the Mediterranean area since Roman times, rocket has only been cultivated commercially since the 1990s.

Propagation ▶ Sow rocket in successive plantings each month, from spring to autumn, because it tends to run to flower fairly easily. If it doesn't self-seed in your garden, carry out monthly plantings to maintain your supplies.

Maintenance ▶ Weeding, providing shade protection in midsummer and regular watering are required.

Pests and diseases ▶ Flea beetles can be a problem, and some butterfly larvae may eat leaves.

Harvesting and storing ▶ Pick rocket leaves before flowering. Harvest the flowers as required for fresh use, and collect seeds when ripe.

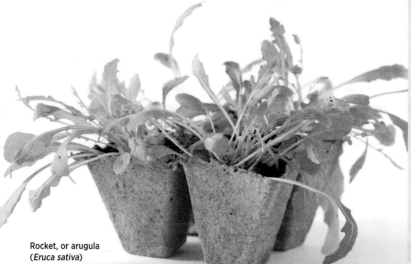

Rocket, or arugula
(*Eruca sativa*)

Cooking

A member of the same plant family as cabbage and broccoli, rocket has a tangy, peppery flavor when grown during the cool spring and autumn months, but a stronger, mustardlike taste if harvested during summer.

The leaves are best gathered before flowering, after which they become more bitter. Wash rocket well and store it in the refrigerator in the same way you would lettuce.

This salad herb goes well with other salad leaves to make a mixed salad or mesclun (see Salad greens in the box, right); the younger leaves tend to have a milder flavor, but old leaves can be bitter.

Rapidly sauté or steam rocket for use in pasta and risotto dishes, stir-fries, soups and sauces, or to replace basil in pesto. Rocket needs only the briefest cooking. Add a scattering of the fresh herb as a traditional topping for pizzas at the end of baking.

The Ancient Romans used rocket seeds to flavor oil and to concoct aphrodisiacs. The seeds make excellent sprouts and are also pressed for oil.

High in vitamin C and iron, rocket stimulates the appetite and assists digestion.

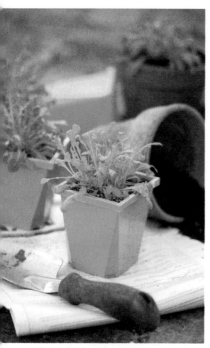

Plant rocket in spring and autumn. In summer, you'll need to provide some shade.

Roman salad

The Romans considered rocket an aphrodisiac but their recipe for a mixed salad of rocket, witlof, cos lettuce, lavender and tender mallow leaves with cheese and dressing is sufficiently seductive in its own right. A modern take on this salad is rocket simply dressed with good olive oil, balsamic vinegar and some shavings of Parmesan cheese.

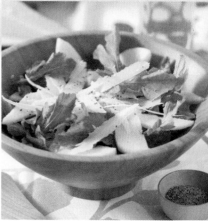

Salad greens

For a salad with more color, flavor and nutritional value, try combining a selection of salad greens. Rocket, mizuna, watercress and curly endive are all more nutritious than lettuce. In combination, they have a slightly bitter taste.

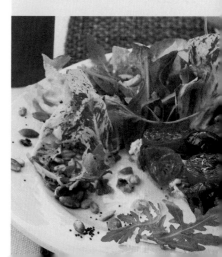

Rose

Latin Name ***Rosa*** **sp. Rosaceae**
Parts used **Petals, rosehips**

The edible petals of herbal roses make delicious conserves and are used in salads and desserts, while the petals of some varieties yield the fabulously expensive and richly fragrant attar of roses used in perfumery. Both the rosehips and petals find many uses in cosmetics.

Gardening

Herbal roses, not modern ones — fragrant and beautiful though they are — are the roses of choice for cooking, fragrance and herbal medicines.

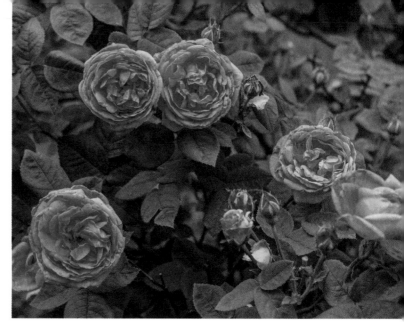

Centifolia roses

The Wars of the Roses

The 'Apothecary Rose,' Rosa gallica 'Officinalis,' may have been introduced from the Middle East into Western Europe by the Crusaders. In England it became the symbol of the House of Lancaster in the Wars of the Roses (1455–1487). The opposing House of York adopted the ancient semi-double Alba rose, 'The White Rose of York' (*R. alba* 'Semi-plena'), while the Jacobites chose the fully double form, which became known as the Jacobite Rose (*R. alba* 'Plena'). At the end of the wars, Henry VII, the father of Henry VIII, combined them into the Tudor Rose, usually depicted as a double rose with white on red, one of the symbols of the House of Tudor.

'Apothecary Rose' The most famous herbal rose is *R. gallica* 'Officinalis,' sometimes called the 'Rose of Miletus,' the 'Rose of Provins,' the 'Red Rose of Lancaster' and 'Champagne Rose'; (see also The Wars of the Roses and 'Rosa Mundi').

The 'Apothecary Rose' was cultivated in vast fields around the famous town of Provins, 30 mi. (50 m) southeast of Paris, from the 13th to the 19th century. Unlike other roses, the fragrance in the petals is strongly retained after drying. The petals are tonic and astringent, and were used by many physicians, including the great Arab doctor Avicenna.

In Provins, the petals of 'Officinalis' were manufactured into conserves, jellies, syrups, cordials, pastilles, fragrant perfumes, salves, creams and candles, all products still favored today.

'Officinalis' was grown in monastery gardens throughout Europe. The petals, either administered as a tea or a syrup, were used to treat the common cold, inflammation of the digestive tract and hysteria. A decoction was used to treat sprains, chapped lips and sore throats.

Other long-favored roses for the herb garden include the Gallica roses 'Tuscany' ('Old Velvet'), 'Belle Isis,' 'Duchesse de Montebello' and 'Belle de Crécy,' together with the Centifolia rose 'Reine des Centfeuilles.'

Attar of roses Today, the major producers of rose products and the extremely expensive perfume concentrate attar (otto) of roses are Iran and Bulgaria. Both regions grow the Damask rose (*R. x damascena*), 'Ispahan' and 'Gloire de Guilan' being favored in Iran and 'Kazanlik' syn. 'Trigintipetala' in Bulgaria. The area around Grasse in France still produces attar, which is derived mainly from the very fragrant 'Old Cabbage Rose' (R. centifolia). A small amount comes from the Alba rose and the Damask rose 'Quatre Saisons.'

Position ▶ The herbal roses prefer full sun, although the Alba roses are the most shade tolerant of all roses.

The charming Rosa gallica 'Versicolor' or 'Rosa mundi' ('rose of the world') is named for Rosamund Clifford, the reluctant mistress of Henry II, King of England in the 12th century. An ancient sport of 'Officinalis,' it bears semi-double deep pink blooms up to 3.5 in. (9 cm) across, with pale pink to white irregular stripes.

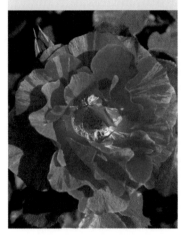

roses such as 'Frau Dagmar Hastrup' and 'Alba' are remarkably disease-resistant.

Harvesting and storing ▷

Harvest herbal roses when they have just opened, on sunny mornings as soon as the dew has dried. To dry, spread the flowers on screen-covered frames out of direct sunlight. Harvest the hips when fully colored and dry in the same way as the flowers.

Herbal medicine

Rosa canina. Part used: Rosehips. The hips of dog rose contain notable levels of vitamin C, and can be taken as a tea or syrup in winter to help fight off common colds and flus. Because of their slightly drying nature, rosehips have also been used to reduce symptoms of diarrhoea.

Medicinal preparations of rosehip, mainly in powdered form, have been the focus of recent scientific research for the treatment of osteoarthritic conditions. The results of clinical trials suggest that it may reduce symptoms of pain and stiffness.

For the safe and appropriate medicinal use of rosehips, consult your healthcare professional, and also see Pregnancy, *page 210*.

In Britain, during World War II, wild rosehips were harvested to make a vitamin C supplement for children.

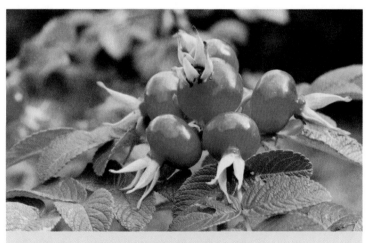

Rosehips

The single-flowered varieties of Rugosa rose (*R. rugosa*), with their abundant, repeat-flowering habit, and tolerance of cold and seaside locations, bear clusters of plum-size hips that are excellent for use in syrups and teas. Rosehip oil, also known as *rose mosqueta*, is very rich in essential fatty acids and has multiple benefits for the skin. This oil, an antioxidant and astringent that contains flavonoids and carotenoids, is prepared from the hips of both *R. canina* and *R. eglanteria*.

Propagation ▷ Most of the herbal roses flower only once a year but extremely abundantly over a month. 'Quatre Saisons' is repeat flowering. Rugosa roses are highly repeat flowering over a long season. All respond to the incorporation of well-rotted compost, but avoid using modern fast-release fertilizers.

Maintenance ▷ Old roses are very tough and need not be pruned or sprayed. If you wish to prune them for shaping, do so immediately after flowering ceases because they flower on ripe wood. Apply mulch in summer.

Pests and diseases ▷ The varieties mentioned above recover rapidly from any attack and can be grown without sprays, while rugosa

Rose *Continued*

Do not use rosehips in greater than culinary quantities if you're pregnant or breastfeeding, except under the supervision of a professional.

Rose oil was traditionally used to anoint British monarchs during the coronation ceremony.

Natural beauty

Rosewater distilled from the petals is a fragrant and mildly astringent tonic for the skin; it is especially useful for chapped skin and may also be used in soothing preparations for eye infections, such as conjunctivitis.

The essential oil has anti-aging effects and may be used in preparations for dry and sensitive skins as well as to reduce the appearance of fine wrinkles.

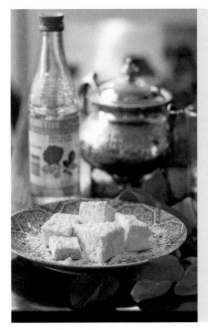

Around the home

The incredible fragrance of rose petals make for a great potpourri. Place potpourri sachets in a closet or drawer to freshen clothing, linens and towels or display petals with some essential rose oil in jars or vases.

Cooking

The hips (fruits) and petals of some varieties of roses — including *R. canina*, *R. x damascena* and *R. gallica* — are edible. Crystallized the petals and use for decoration to make rose petal jar or, (with the bitter "heel" at the base of the petals removed, add to salads.

Rosehips are high in vitamin C and can be made into jams, jellies or a syrup that serves as a dietary supplement for babies.

Ras el hanout, the Moroccan spice blend, has many variations, some of which contain dried rose petals and flower buds.

Turkish delight

Rosewater, a by-product of the distilling process that makes rose oil from rose petals, is an important flavoring in Middle Eastern cooking. It is used for some Asian and Middle Eastern sweets, including Turkish delight, and the rasgullas and gulab jamuns of Indian cooking. Turkish delight is a sticky, jellylike but firm sweet, made from starch and sugar. It is traditionally flavored with rosewater and generously dusted with icing sugar; other flavors include lemon and mint. The sweet was introduced to the West in the 19th century, when a British man, who was fond of it, shipped some home.

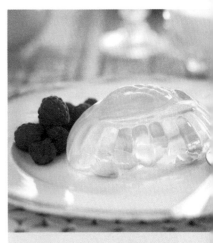

Rose petal jelly

4 gelatine sheets (or 2 heaped teaspoons powdered gelatine)
2 cups (500 ml) sparkling wine
⅔ cup (145 g) caster sugar
1 tablespoon rosewater
18 small rose petals, carefully washed
raspberries and cream, to serve

1. Soak gelatine leaves in cold water to soften (about 2–3 minutes).

2. Heat ½ cup (125 ml) sparkling wine and the sugar in large saucepan over medium heat, stirring until sugar dissolves.

3. Add gelatine leaves to sugar mixture, stirring to melt gelatine. Remove from heat to cool. Stir through remaining sparkling wine, rosewater and rose petals.

4. Pour mixture into individual glasses or a lightly oiled mould. Refrigerate at least 8 hours, or until set. Serve jelly with raspberries and cream.

Serves 2

Opposite page: The beautiful *Rosa canina* is a source of rosehip oil, which has benefits for the skin.

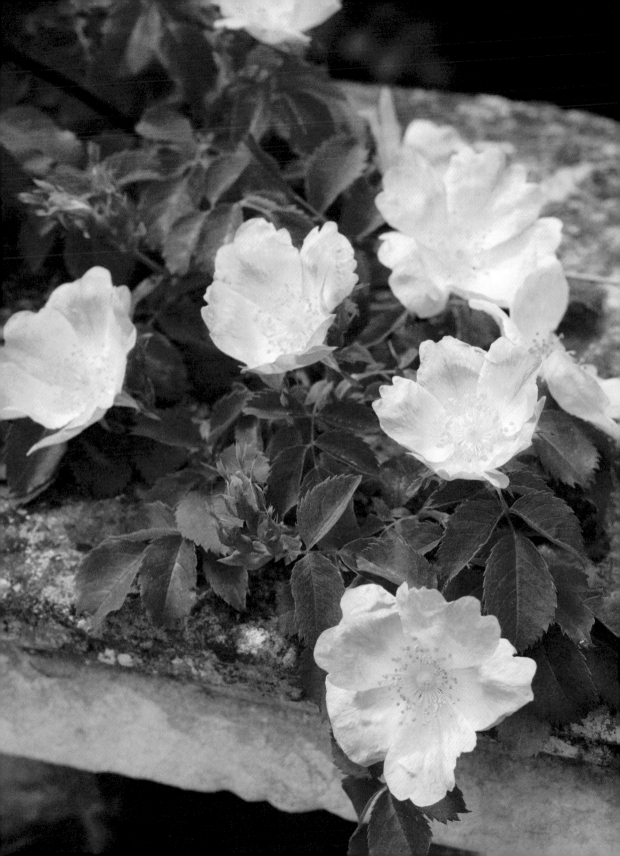

Rosemary

Latin Name *Rosmarinus officinalis* Lamiaceae
Other common names Compass plant, dew of the sea, incensier, Mary's mantle
Parts used **Leaves, flowering tops**

Few herbs are as universally grown and loved as rosemary. There are a number of varieties available and rosemary has many garden uses, from hedging, spillovers and pots to groundcovers and topiary. The refreshing resinous scent and flavor of its evergreen foliage is indispensable in cooking.

Gardening

Rosmarinus means "dew of the sea," and in the wild this herb is most commonly found growing on sea cliffs around the Mediterranean. Despite their different forms and colors, all the rosemary varieties offered in nurseries belong to one species, *R. officinalis*. There are two other species that are both rare — *R. eriocalyx* and

R. tomentosus, from southern Spain and northwestern Africa, which have not entered general cultivation. Rosemary flowers vary from pale to rich blue, violet, mauve, pink or white. The form varies, from rounded bushes and prostrate varieties to columnar varieties up to 10 ft. (3 m) tall. The majority are well suited to culinary uses. All are evergreen with small, dense, narrow, pointed leaves.

Varieties ▶ Recommended tall varieties include 'Tuscan Blue' syn. 'Erectus,' with large leaves; the delightfully scented 'Portuguese Pink,' with pink flowers; and 'Sawyer's Selection.'

Among the most intensely blue-flowered bush forms are 'Collingwood Ingram' syn. 'Majorca' and 'Benenden Blue,' 'Salem,' 'Blue Lagoon,' 'Severn Sea,' 'Corsican Blue,' the violet blue-flowered 'Miss Jessup's Upright,' 'Suffolk Blue,' the excellent 'Herb Cottage' and the strong-growing, superbly fragrant 'Gorizia,' introduced into general cultivation by Tom DeBaggio from the city of Gorizia in northern Italy.

Pink-flowered bush forms include 'Pink,' 'Majorca Pink' and 'Provence Pink,' while white-flowered forms include 'Wendy's White' syn. 'Upright

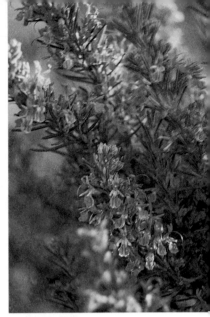

Scholars in ancient times wore rosemary garlands during exams to improve their concentration.

White,' 'Sissinghurst White' syn. 'Albus' and 'Nancy Howard.'

Semi-prostrate forms ideal for trailing over walls include the glossy-leafed, mid-blue 'Lockwood de Forest,' 'Fota Blue,' the very fine-leafed 'Mason's Finest,' sky-blue-flowered 'Prostratus,' 'Santa Barbara,' 'Huntington Carpet' and the beautiful 'Shimmering Stars,' with pink buds and blue flowers.

Variegated leaf forms currently available include 'Genges Gold,' 'Gilded' syn. 'Aureus' and the white-margined 'Silver Spires.' The varieties 'Arp,' 'Severn Sea' and 'Madeleine Hill' syn. 'Hill Hardy' are more cold-resistant than most.

Position ▶ This plant requires full sunshine and excellent drainage.

In World War II, rosemary leaves and juniper berries were burned in French hospitals to kill germs.

Rosemary (*Rosmarinus officinalis*)

Rosemary is tolerant of a range of pH, from moderately acid to moderately alkaline soil, although the latter results in more compact growth and intense fragrance. In colder areas, grow plants in pots outdoors, then take them into the greenhouse in winter. Rosemary is excellent for seaside plantings.

Propagation ▶ Propagate rosemary by tip cuttings taken in early autumn or spring. Rosemary seed germinates poorly, and plants do not come true to variety.

Maintenance ▶ Regular light pruning helps to shape plants. Bushes respond well to clipping and shaping, and make excellent topiaries. Correct mulching is essential, because organic mulches tend to hold moisture near the main stem as well as the lower foliage, encouraging a number of fungal rots. For this reason, gravel, coarse gritty sand or small pebbles are the most suitable mulch.

Pests and diseases ▶ Overwatered potted rosemary is very prone to root rot, often first seen as

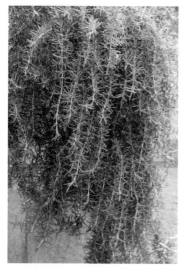

Prostrate rosemary is ideal for hanging baskets.

browning of the leaf tips. Porous clay pots are preferable to plastic because they allow the soil to drain properly. Regular light trimming allows good aeration of the foliage and inhibits fungal wilts. Other problems, largely associated with overwintering plants in greenhouses, include spider mites, white flies and mealybugs.

Harvesting and storing ▶ In milder climates, take clippings of rosemary any time of the year, then air-dry in a well-ventilated place. When completely dry, strip the whole leaves from the stems and store in airtight bottles. Major harvesting should be done before flowering. Gather fresh flowers to use as a garnish on salads and desserts.

Herbal medicine

Rosmarinus officinalis. Parts used: leaves, flowering tops. The medicinal properties of rosemary as a tonic and stimulant to the nerves and circulation make it a popular remedy for combating general fatigue and depression, and for improving poor circulation. Rosemary also enhances memory and concentration by increasing blood flow to the head.

While rosemary can be taken as an infusion, the essential oil is commonly used for these conditions. A few drops can be added to a vaporizer or diluted in a little vegetable oil and applied topically for its beneficial effects.

Used externally, rosemary essential oil can be applied in a diluted form to relieve muscle cramps and arthritic joint pain. It also has a reputation for preventing premature baldness and stimulating hair growth.

Rosemary is regarded as a traditional digestive remedy and, when taken as an infusion, it can help

to ease cramping, bloating and gas, and may ease "liverish" symptoms, such as headaches and poor digestion of fats.

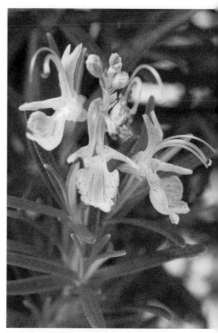

You can crystallize the flowers of rosemary with egg white and caster sugar.

An herb of goodness

Rosemary has a strong association with the Virgin Mary. It is said that, when the Holy family was fleeing from Herod's soldiers, Mary spread her blue cloak over a white-flowering rosemary bush to dry, but when she removed the cloak, the white flowers had turned blue in her honor. Also associated with ancient magical lore, rosemary was often called 'Elf Leaf,' and bunches of it were hung around houses to keep thieves and witches out and to prevent fairies from entering and stealing infants.

Rosemary *Continued*

For the safe and appropriate medicinal use of rosemary, consult your healthcare professional. Also, see Memory & concentration, *page 187,* for external use. Do not use rosemary in greater than culinary quantities if you are pregnant or breastfeeding.

Around the home

Rosemary is one of the main ingredients in the famous antiseptic Vinegar of the Four Thieves, *page 106,* and can be used in a number of ways around the home.

Hungary water

Until the invention of eau-de-cologne, this recipe was Europe's favorite fragrance, but it also became popular as a cure-all remedy for everything from dizziness, rheumatism, stomach cramps and headaches to indigestion and lack of appetite. The story of its invention is unclear, but it is thought that, in the 13th century, a hermit gave the recipe to Queen Isabella of Hungary, whose legs were crippled with rheumatism. Daily bathing in this water was said to have restored her legs and also her youthful beauty. Later additions to the formula included thyme, sage, mint and marjoram.

In this Hungary water recipe, a "handful" is the number of 1-ft. (30-cm) lengths of herb stems that can be encircled by the hand.

5 qt. (4.5 l) brandy or clear spirit
1 handful flowering rosemary tops
1 handful lavender
1 handful myrtle

Cut the herbs into 1-in. (2.5-cm) lengths and leave to macerate for a minimum of 2 weeks before filtering.

- Make a simple rosemary disinfectant by simmering a handful of leaves and small stems in water for 30 minutes. Strain and pour into a spray bottle.
- Disinfect and deodorize hairbrushes and combs by soaking them in a solution of 1 cup (250 ml) hot water, 1 tablespoon bicarbonate of soda and 5 drops rosemary essential oil.
- Use dried rosemary in moth-repellent sachets and in potpourri.
- Use a rosemary rinse on your dog to deter fleas after washing.
- Wash your pet's bedding, then add a few drops of rosemary essential oil to the final rinse. Or, spritz your pets with rosemary disinfectant as they dry themselves in the sun after a bath.

Rosemary tea makes a fragrant final rinse for darkening brunette hair.

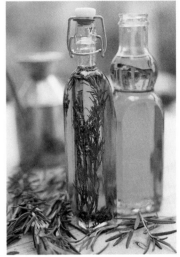

Infusion of rosemary with oil.

Cooking

The bruised leaves of rosemary have a cooling pinelike scent, with mint and eucalyptus overtones, and the strong taste can overwhelm other flavors if used too generously. It complements similarly strong flavors such as wine and garlic; starchy foods (bread, scones, potatoes); rich meats such as lamb, pork, duck and game; vegetables such as eggplants, zucchini and brassicas; and is also used in sausages, stuffings, soups and stews, or steeped in vinegar or olive oil to flavor them.

The leaves have a rather woody texture, so use them finely chopped. Alternatively, use whole sprigs, or tie leaves in a square of muslin, and remove just before serving. Dried rosemary has a flavor similar to that of fresh, but its very hard texture may not soften, even on long cooking.

Rosemary is popular in Italian cookery. Make a simple and delicious pizza topping with thinly sliced potatoes, crushed garlic and chopped fresh rosemary leaves.

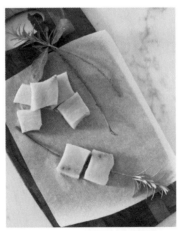

Rosemary stems, stripped of most of their leaves and used as skewers for fish, meat or vegetables cooked on the barbecue, will impart their flavor.

Opposite page: A basketful of fresh herbs, including thyme, oregano, sage, rosemary and lavender.

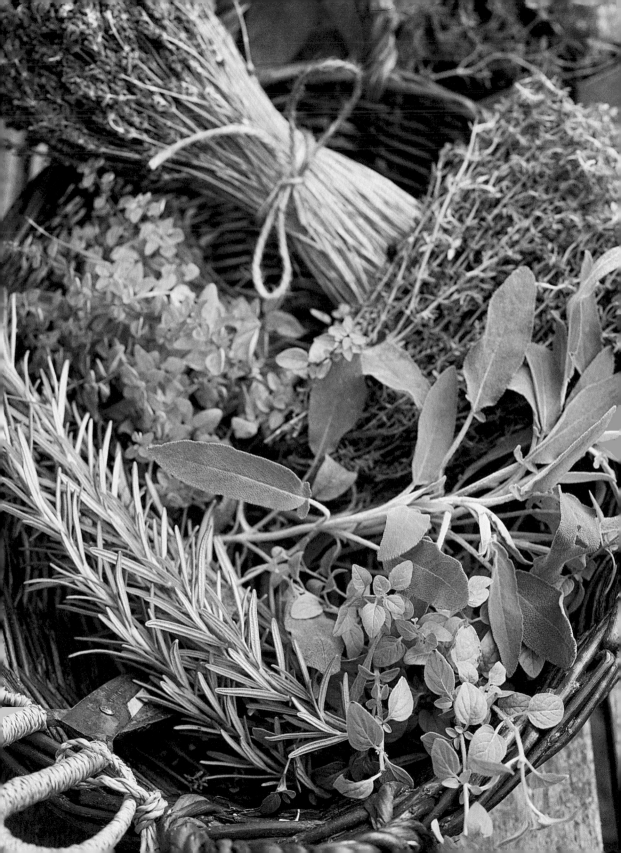

St. John's wort

Latin Name *Hypericum perforatum* Clusiaceae (Guttiferae)
Part used **Flowering tops**

Traditionally, golden-flowered St. John's wort was hung over entrances and cast on midsummer fires as an herb of great protection and purification. Today, it is still the symbol of midsummer solstice celebrations in Europe.

Gardening

Hypericum is a very large genus of about 400 species. *H. perforatum* is a hardy, partially woody perennial, an upright growing, unpleasant smelling, clumping plant that can reach 39 in. (1 m) high. Its small, smooth, oval leaves have numerous tiny oil glands, borne in opposite pairs along the stems. The small golden yellow flowers are borne in large dense cymes in midsummer. The small, ovoid seed capsule contains round black seed. The crushed flowers ooze a red, bloodlike pigment containing hypericin. Do not confuse St. John's wort with the many ornamental *Hypericum* varieties grown in gardens.

Position ▶ This plant is easy to grow in a well-drained, moist to fairly dry soil in full sun to light shade. It's recommended for ornamental meadows, but considered a weed toxic to livestock; it's under statutory control in Australia and New Zealand.

Propagation ▶ Sow seed as soon as it is ripe in autumn (under protection in colder areas), or in the following spring. Germination can take up to 3 months. You can also divide the runners either in autumn or spring.

Maintenance ▶ It is a strong grower requiring little tending.

Pests and diseases ▶ None worth noting.

Harvesting and storing ▶ Harvest the flowering heads in early summer, when buds commence opening, and dry them.

Herbal medicine

Hypericum perforatum. Part used: flowering tops. Traditionally used for treating nerve pain, including neuralgia and sciatica as well as psychological disorders such as anxiety and depression, St. John's wort continues to be used for these conditions but these days is best known for its antidepressant activity.

St. John's wort has been proven to be effective against mild to moderate depression in a large number of clinical trials. It was found to have similar effectiveness to other antidepressant medication but with fewer side effects. Two compounds, hypericin and hyperforin, are believed to work in a similar manner to pharmaceutical antidepressants, and many preparations using St. John's wort are produced to contain a fixed level of these constituents.

Clinical trials of St. John's wort also suggest a beneficial use for treating mood symptoms of menopause and premenstrual syndrome, for obsessive compulsive disorder and also for seasonal affective disorder.

Laboratory studies have shown that St. John's wort possesses anti-inflammatory, pain-relieving and antiviral activity. A tea or extract taken internally as well as the external use of the red oil prepared from the flowers can relieve sciatica, shingles, cold sores, genital herpes and rheumatic pain. Topically, the oil is also a valuable wound- and burn-healing remedy.

For the safe and appropriate use of St. John's wort, see Depression & anxiety, *page 185*. Do not use St. John's wort if you are pregnant or breastfeeding.

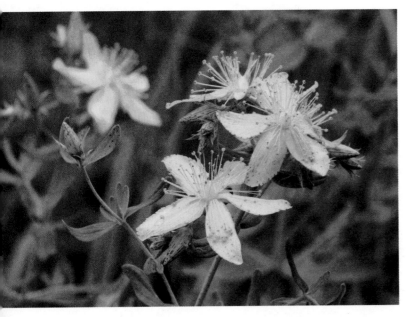

St. John's wort (*Hypericum perforatum*)

Sage

Latin Name **Salvia sp. Lamiaceae**
Parts used **Leaves, roots, seeds, flowers**

There are more than 700 species of salvias, many of them spectacular when in flower, and a number with leaves that are variously scented with pineapple, grapes, tangerine, grapefruit, anise, honey melon or fruit salad. Salvia flowers attract butterflies and nectar-sipping birds.

Gardening

Common or garden sage (*S. officinalis*) is one of the best-known culinary herbs, but there are also many ornamental species, all with small, lipped flowers in delightful shades, from white to dark purple.

A subshrub native to the Dalmatian Coast, common sage has silver-gray elliptical leaves and spikes of attractive lavender, pink or white flowers. It is a pleasantly pungent culinary herb, which also aids digestion.

In addition to the common form of garden sage, there are handsome broadleaf varieties, such as 'Berggarten,' and colored-leaf forms, such as the purple-leafed 'Purpurea'; the cream-, pink- and purple-variegated 'Tricolor'; and gold- and green-variegated 'Icterina.'

Three-leafed sage (*S. fruticosa*), native to Greece and Turkey, closely resembles garden sage except that most leaves are subtended by a basal pair of leaflets. The dried leaves are often sold as 'garden sage.' A hybrid between this species and garden sage, known as 'Newe Ya'ar,' is cultivated commercially in Israel.

Spanish sage (*S. lavandulifolia*), also known as lavender sage, resembles a narrow-leafed garden sage. It has a lavender-and-sage fragrance, and its oil is extracted for toiletries.

Clary sage or muscatel sage (*S. sclarea*), a biennial, is one of the most beautiful sages, forming a large rosette of broadly ovate, pebble-textured leaves and sending up tall dense spikes of large pink flowers. The leaves add a muscatel flavor to a diverse range of liqueurs, vermouths and wines, while the essential oil is used in perfumery. In water, the seeds become mucilaginous, and were once used to remove specks from the eyes.

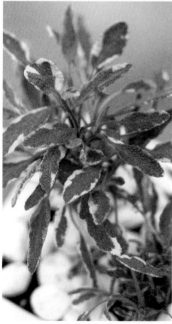

Variegated sage (*S. officinalis* 'Tricolor') makes a striking addition to the herb garden.

Common sage (*Salvia officinalis*)

White sage (*S. apiana*) is a silver-leafed, rosette-shaped subshrub native to southwestern North America. The leaves are used by Native Americans as a flavoring, medicinally to reduce mucous formation and salivation, and for smudge sticks in purification ceremonies.

The golden chia (*S. columbariae*), an annual, is native to the southwestern United States. Like chia (*S. hispanica*), which was cultivated as an important staple crop by the Aztecs until colonization by the Spanish, it produces tiny oily seeds that are gluten-free, very rich in omega-3 fatty acids (alpha-linolenic acid), and high in anti-oxidants, vitamins, minerals and fiber. A third chia, *S. polystachya*, is also nutritionally valuable.

Diviner's sage (*S. divinorum*) exists only in cultivation and has been

Sage *Continued*

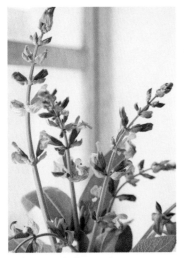

Potted salvias in flower make a pretty display, but are not suited to long-term indoor life.

Vinegar of the Four Thieves

This herbal vinegar is a strong insect repellent that can be used on your skin as well as on socks and shoes to discourage ticks and mites. Dilute it 50:50 with water if you are spraying it onto your skin and test it on a small patch of skin before using. In a glass jar, combine 8.5 cups (2 L) apple cider vinegar and 2 tablespoons chopped garlic with 2 tablespoons each of the following herbs: rosemary, rue, sage, lavender, wormwood and peppermint. Steep the mixture in a sunny spot for about 2 weeks, shaking the jar daily. Strain out the herbs, and retain the liquid. Add several cloves of crushed garlic, and seal again. Leave to soak for 3 days. Strain out the garlic fiber and discard. Label the jar and store it in a cool place. Do not use this vinegar if you are pregnant, and do not use it on small children.

used for many centuries by Mazatec shamans in Oaxaca, Mexico, to create visionary experiences and promote spiritual healing. Despite sensationalized media reports, it is neither LSD-like in action nor a "party drug."

It is generally understood to be non-addictive, and toxicological studies have shown it to be non-toxic. The plant is a prohibited substance in Australia, South Korea, Belgium, Italy and Denmark.

Fragrant-leafed species Some of these species find culinary uses. Pineapple sage (*S. elegans* syn. *S. rutilans*) has slender spikes of red flowers and pineapple-scented leaves used to flavor drinks and garnish desserts.

Others include its variety 'Honey Melon'; fruit salad or peach sage (*S. dorisiana*), with large, lush spikes of rose-pink flowers and broad fruit-scented leaves; and the very fragrant California species, Cleveland sage (*S. clevelandii*).

Found on several Greek islands, apple sage (*S. pomifera*) forms fruitlike semi-transparent galls that are candied and eaten as delicacies.

Position ▶ With few exceptions, the Salvia genus, particularly the gray-leafed species, requires a sunny, well-drained position. Salvias generally make poor indoor plants and become easily infested with white fly and scale. *S. officinalis* prefers alkaline conditions.

Propagation ▶ Sages are propagated from seed, or by tip cuttings or division for named varieties.

Maintenance ▶ Most shrubby salvias respond well to gentle pruning or pinching back, particularly

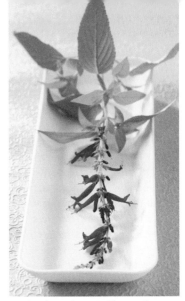

Use the pineapple-scented leaves of pineapple sage (*S. elegans* syn. *S. rutilans*) to flavor drinks.

> *"The desire of sage is to render man immortal."*
>
> From a medieval manuscript

after flowering. Do not heavily fertilize these plants.

Pests and diseases ▶ Pick caterpillars off by hand. Sudden wilting indicates poor drainage and root rot.

Harvesting and storing ▶ Harvest fresh leaves and flowers for culinary use at any time. Dry individual leaves and sprigs before flowering; spread them out in a well-aired place, then store in airtight containers.

Herbal medicine

Salvia officinalis. Part used: leaves. Sage is an anti-inflammatory and antimicrobial remedy, and is frequently used as a mouthwash and gargle for sore throats, gum infections, tonsillitis and mouth ulcers. It appears to have a drying effect on excessive sweating and is a popular herb for the treatment of night sweats associated with menopause. Sage also has a beneficial effect on the mind, improving memory, concentration and mood; results of a recent clinical trial suggest that it may have a positive effect on the symptoms of Alzheimer's disease.

Salvia miltiorrhiza. Part used: roots. In traditional Chinese medicine, dan shen is described as a remedy that "moves blood." Modern research has mostly focused on its beneficial effects on the circulatory system and the heart. The results of some clinical trials indicate potential use for the treatment of angina and high blood pressure. Laboratory studies have shown liver-protective effects and may explain dan shen's traditional

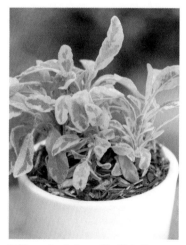

Golden variegated sage (*S. officinalis 'Icterina'*) can be used instead of common sage in cooking.

use in treating acute and chronic liver conditions.

For the safe and appropriate medicinal use of sage, see Menopause, *page 208*. For the safe and appropriate use of dan shen, consult your healthcare professional.

Do not use dan shen if you are pregnant or breastfeeding. Do not use sage in greater than culinary quantities if you're pregnant or breastfeeding.

Around the home

Sage, like so many herbs, is rich in essential oils, antiviral, anti-bacterial, deodorizing and antifungal, and this is reflected by its old French name, *toute bonne*, or "all is well." Use the leaves to make Herb vinegar spray and insect-repellent sprays. Alternatively, simply put a few drops of essential oil on a damp cloth when you're wiping down bathroom and kitchen surfaces.

Sage is also a moth-repellent — use it in dried herb or essential oil form to repel clothes moths and pantry moths. In the garden, plant sage to repel cabbage moth.

Cooking

Of the many types, which all differ widely in flavor, common sage (*S. officinalis*) is the one most often used for cooking. The aroma is highly pungent, while the flavor, which intensifies on drying, is savory, with camphorous overtones.

Sage goes with starchy, rich and fatty foods such as duck, with poultry and pork (and stuffings for them), red meats, beans, eggplant, tomato-based sauces, casseroles and soups, and also in commercially prepared stuffing mixes and Italian dried mixed herbs. You can also use deep-fried leaves as a garnish.

Best used with a light hand in long-cooked dishes, sage is popular in Italy, less so in France. In the Middle East, it is used in salads. Sage tea is popular in many European countries. In Dalmatia, where sage grows wild, the flowers are used to make honey.

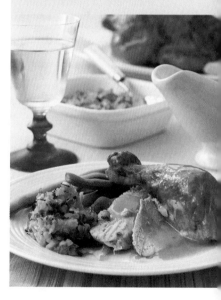

Salad burnet

Latin Name *Sanguisorba minor* syn. *Poterium sanguisorba,*
Pimpinella sanguisorba Rosaceae

Other common names **Burnet bloodwort, Di Yu, pimpernel (greater burnet)**

Parts used **Leaves, roots**

The ferny leaves of salad burnet have a scent reminiscent of fresh cucumber. The plant is sufficiently pretty to have been recommended by Sir Francis Bacon, the 16th-century English philosopher, for growing along alleys (paths) with thyme "to perfume the air most delightfully."

Gardening

Salad burnet (*S. minor*), a dainty, hardy, evergreen perennial to 1.5 ft. (45 cm), forms a low basal rosette of pinnate leaves with many paired, toothed, oval leaflets. Borne on tall, slender stalks, the tiny green, wind-pollinated flowers with deep red anthers are borne in dense globose heads.

Salad burnet's close relative, greater burnet (*S. officinalis* syn. *Poterium officinalis*), is similar to salad burnet in form but larger in all respects. The tiny, deep red flowers are borne in denseclub-shaped spikes to 3.5 ft. (1 m).

Position ▶ These plants prefer full sun to partial shade, and a well-drained, moist, slightly acid to alkaline soil that contains compost.

Propagation ▶ Propagate both species by sowing seed in either spring or autumn. Plants that are allowed to flower will self-seed, producing particularly healthy plants. Space seedlings about 1 ft. (30 cm) apart for salad burnet, and about 1.5 ft. (45 cm) apart for greater burnet.

Maintenance ▶ Cut emerging flower stems for increased leaf production.

Pests and diseases ▶ No pests or diseases worth noting.

Harvesting and storing ▶ Harvest leaves for medicinal use before flowering. For fresh use, harvest leaves as required. Lift roots in autumn for drying.

Herbal medicine

Sanguisorba officinalis syn. *Poterium officinalis*. Parts used: leaves, roots. Greater burnet has a very long tradition of use in Western and Chinese medicine. The plant is astringent due to the presence of some unusual tanins, together with gums and glycosides. It is used externally in treating minor burns and scalds, sores and skin infections, and to staunch bleeding.

In traditional Chinese medicine, the dried root is also sometimes applied internally for the treatment of bleeding hemorrhoids.

Cooking

Salad burnet is an ingredient in several sauces, including ravigote, which is used in French cooking and goes well with cold roast chicken or seafood. Add young leaves of salad burnet to salads, chilled summer soups and to soft cheeses. Also use as a garnish or infused in vinegar. This herb does not dry well, but the leaves can be frozen in ice-cube trays.

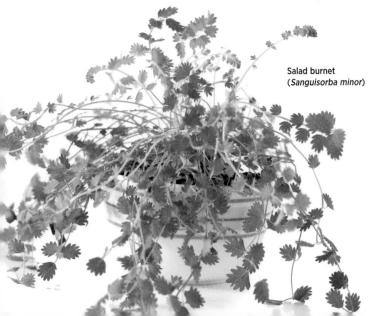

Salad burnet
(*Sanguisorba minor*)

Herb cocktail

The cucumber taste of salad burnet makes it an excellent accompaniment to alcoholic drinks; according to the Elizabethan herbal writer Gerard, the plants "make the heart merry and glad." For a refreshing cocktail, bruise 6 sprays of salad burnet with a rolling pin or with a mortar and pestle, then place in a large pitcher containing 3 cups (750 ml) sweet white wine, 2 cups (500 ml) sherry and 1 thinly sliced lemon. Mix well; allow to infuse for at least 2 hours. Sweeten to taste. Add 4 cups (1 L) of club soda and serve over crushed ice.

Savory

Latin Name *Satureja* sp. Lamiaceae
Part used **Leaves**

***Satureja* is reputed to have been the source of the mythical satyrs' enormous sexual stamina. Species such as summer savory and winter savory are mainly used to flavor food, while yerba buena and Jamaican mint bush are largely used medicinally.**

Gardening

Summer savory (*S. hortensis*), an annual growing to 1.5 ft. (45 cm), has slender dark green leaves, pink flowers and an aroma of thyme and oregano. Winter savory (*S. montana*) is a perennial subshrub with dark green, narrow-leafed foliage and white flowers. Creeping savory (*S. montana* subsp. *montana* var. *prostata*) is semi-prostrate, very ornamental and resembles white heather when in flower.

Lemon or African savory (*S. biflora* syn. *Micromeria biflora*) is an excellent culinary perennial herb with creeping branches, attractive mauve flowers and bright green, fine leaves that are strongly lemon- and oregano-scented.

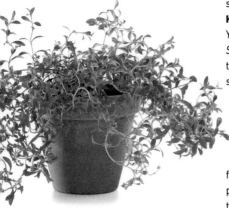

Winter savory (*Satureja montana*) can be used for similar culinary purposes as summer savory.

Thyme-leafed savory or za'atar rumi or savory of Crete or pink savory (*S. thymbra*) is a low-growing, stiffly branched perennial with whorls of small grayish leaves that have an intense oregano and thyme fragrance. Yerba buena (*S. douglasii*) is a perennial herb with trailing branches of fragrant round leaves. Jamaican mint bush (*S. viminea*) is an intensely mint-scented plant with small, oval, glossy bright green foliage.

Position ▶ Except for yerba buena, which grows well in a hanging basket out of direct sunlight, all species should be grown in full sun in well-drained neutral to alkaline soil. In cold areas, give plants winter protection.

Propagation ▶ All species can be propagated by seed sown shallowly in spring. Perennial species are also propagated by cuttings in spring and early autumn.

Maintenance ▶ Plants should be regularly weeded.

Pests and diseases ▶ No significant pest or disease problems.

Harvesting and storing ▶ You can cut down whole plants of *S. hortensis* before flowering and dry them. Harvest the leaves of other species fresh as required, and dry or freeze them in sealed containers.

Cooking

Both summer and winter savory have a similar aroma — fragrant, with a hint of thyme, and a peppery, distinctive taste, although the flavor of summer savory is stronger. The flavor is better before the plant flowers. Savory retains its flavor when dried; in this form it is preferred for cooking.

Savory goes well with lentils and peas, slow-cooked soups, stews, meatloaf and egg dishes. Use it in coatings for delicate meats, such as veal, and for fish. Add to sauces, pâtés and homemade sausages. It is a key herb in herbes de Provence (see below). Use summer savory in marinades, especially for olives. In Croatian cooking, a lemon-scented strain of savory is used with fish and seafood.

Summer savory (Satureja hortensis)

Herbes de Provence

Use this classic herb mix to season vegetables, chicken and red meat.

4 tablespoons dried rosemary leaves
3 tablespoons dried sweet marjoram leaves
2 tablespoons dried thyme leaves
3 tablespoons dried savory leaves
2 tablespoons dried lavender flowers
1 teaspoon dried sage leaves

1. Combine the dried herbs. Place in an airtight jar.
2. Store in a cool, dark place for up to 4 months. If using the mix with fish, add a pinch of fennel seeds.

Scented geranium

Latin Name *Pelargonium* sp. **Geraniaceae**
Parts used **Leaves, roots, flowers**

Scented geraniums are the great mimics of the plant world. At the slightest touch, they release intense true-to-name fragrances, from lemon sherbet and ripe apples to peppermint and red roses, making watering a collection a blissful experience.

Gardening

The species used to create the scented geraniums originated mainly from the Cape of Good Hope area in South Africa. They were introduced into England as a curiosity in the 1630s, but by the 1840s the French realized their potential as an essential oil source.

Steam distillation of rose geranium (*P. graveolens*) yields an essential oil with an enlivening true rose fragrance that is added to perfumes and toiletries. It is produced on the island of Réunion and also in Algeria, China, Egypt, India and Morocco.

The scented geraniums are soft to semi-hard wooded shrubs or subshrubs with a very wide range of leaf shapes. *P. graveolens* is an upright multi-stemmed small shrub to 3 ft. (90 cm), with bright green, much indented leaves that create a lacy shape. The small flowers are mid-pink rouged with bright ruby on the upper petals, and are borne in terminal umbels. The seed head somewhat resembles that of a stork's head.

Other rose-scented species distilled for oil are *P. capitatum* and its variety 'Attar of Roses,' together with *P. radens*. The oil is valued in aromatherapy, and is used in massage oils to relieve tension and soothe the symptoms of dermatitis and eczema. Antifungal and antibacterial in activity, the oil is currently used in the United States as a tick repellent for dogs, and is considered both mosquito- and lice-repellent. The oil of apple geranium (*P. odoratissimum*) is astringent and antiseptic, and repels insects. Hybridization led to a proliferation of varieties, and scented geraniums became great favorites with 19th-century gardeners, particularly as they proved adaptable to cultivation in greenhouses and on sunny kitchen windowsills during the winter months. They are fashionable once again, but fewer than 100 varieties have survived.

Rose geranium
(*Pelargonium graveolens*)

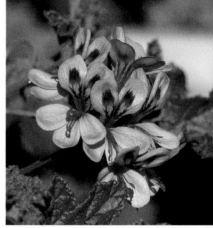

Pelargonium quercifolium 'Fair Ellen'

Those suited to cultivation in pots include the following plants:
- 'Nutmeg' and its variegated form, together with 'Old Spice,' 'Apple Cider' syn. 'Cody' and 'Tutti Frutti' (all derived from *P.* x *fragrans*)
- *P. odoratissimum* 'Apple'
- *P. nervosum* 'Lime' and its hybrid 'Ginger' syn. 'Toronto'
- varieties of *P. crispum* such as 'Fingerbowl,' 'Prince Rupert' and 'French Lace' (all with an intense lemon fragrance)
- cream-variegated *P.* x *asperum* 'Lady Plymouth'
- *P.* x *citronellum* 'Lemon Tart'
- carrot-scented 'Scarlet Pet' syn. 'Moore's Victory'

Natural beauty

Rose geranium (*Pelargonium graveolens*) is the classic beauty pick-me-up. Its toning effect revives tired skin and the fresh, pungent smell revives body and mind. Its toning and balancing properties leave hair and scalp clean and fresh. It is a mild anti-irritant, making it helpful for any inflammation, including minor wounds and insect bites. It also helps control stress-triggered oil production, which can result in pimple breakouts.

- hazelnut-scented *P.* x *concolor* 'Concolor Lace' and 'Strawberry' syn. 'Countess of Scarborough'
- *P.* x *scarboroviae* 'Gooseberry' (lemon-, clove- and mint-scented)
- Plants better suited to large pots or garden beds include these pelargoniums:
- the darkly handsome, velvety-leafed, semi-prostrate *P. tomentosum* 'Peppermint' and its hybrid 'Dark Lady'
- white-speckled 'Snowflake'
- *P.* x *graveolens* 'Robert's Lemon Rose'
- *P.* x *capitatum* 'Dr Livingstone' syn. 'Skeleton Rose'
- *P.* x *asperum* 'Mint Rose'
- *P. graveolens* var. 'Camphor Rose'
- *P.* x *asperum*, the 18th-century 'M. Ninon' (apricot)
- *P.* x *scabrum* 'Mabel Gray' (intense lemon sherbet)
- the pungently woodsy-scented hybrids of *P. quercifolium,* such as 'Staghorn Oak,' 'Clorinda,' 'Chocolate Mint,' 'Fair Ellen,' 'Endsleigh' and 'Pretty Polly'
- *P. citrosum* 'True Lemon'
- the reputedly insect-repelling 'Citronella' syn. 'Citrosa,' a derivative of *P.* x *asperum*

Position ▶ Pelargoniums are drought-resistant, and where space is limited, a collection can be kept in well-drained pots in a sunny position.

Propagation ▶ Propagate scented geraniums from 4-in. (10-cm) cuttings taken in late summer and inserted into a sterilized mix. Make sure to protect them from frost.

Maintenance ▶ Regular harvesting restricts the size of larger specimens. They should be only lightly fertilized, preferably in spring. Water thoroughly when the upper soil dries out.

Pests and diseases ▶ They cannot tolerate poorly drained soil and will suffer root rot and death from soil fungi, such as *Pythium, Verticillium* and *Fusarium.*

Harvesting and storing ▶ Harvest and dry leaves at any time for potpourri and for sleep pillows. Harvesting for distillation occurs around midsummer.

Herbal medicine

Pelargonium sidoides, P. reniforme. Part used: root. In their native South Africa, where these two *Pelargonium* species have been used medicinally for centuries, a preparation of their

Peppermint geranium leaves make an instant poultice for sprains and bruises.

roots is called umckaloabo. It is traditionally prescribed for digestive complaints, such as diarrhea and dysentery, and for infections of the respiratory tract, including colds, coughs and tuberculosis. The name is derived from Zulu words meaning "symptoms of lung disease" and "breast pain."

Umckaloabo is widely used today by traditional healers in Southern Africa for treating tuberculosis; in the early 1900s, it enjoyed a rather controversial success as a remedy for this condition in Europe.

In more recent times, it has become popular in Europe for treating acute bronchitis, tonsillitis and sore throat; a number of clinical trials have shown that *P. sidoides* reduces symptoms of acute bronchitis by the seventh day of treatment. Laboratory studies suggest that compounds

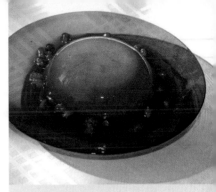

Cooking with scented geraniums

Scented geraniums, with their attractive leaves in a wide range of heavenly scents, are a culinary treat. Try using them in the following ways.

- Add dried leaves of rose or lemon varieties to the tea caddy.
- Finely chop fresh leaves. Infuse in warmed liquid such as cream or milk. Strain, and use liquid to make ice creams, sweet custards and sauces for desserts.
- Infuse red wine vinegar with rose geranium and fresh raspberries. Strain after a week for a summer salad vinegar.
- Place a cake still warm from the oven on top of leaves to absorb the fragrance. Try rose geranium with vanilla pound cake or peppermint geranium with a chocolate sponge. Remove the leaves when the cake has cooled.
- Line Jell-o molds with leaves (above) and pour a gelatine on top to set.

contained in the root may reduce the ability of bacteria to adhere to the lining of the respiratory tract and thus prevent infection as well as improve immune function.

For the safe and appropriate use of these herbs, consult your healthcare professional. Do not use these herbs if you are pregnant or breastfeeding.

Sorrel

Latin Name *Rumex acetosa, R. scutatus, R. acetosella* Polygonaceae
Parts used **Leaves (sorrel); roots (yellow dock)**

Gardening

Three species of sorrel are commonly grown for culinary purposes — broad leaf, garden or sheep's sorrel, or sour grass (*R. acetosa*); French or buckler-leaf sorrel (*R. scutatus*); and sheep's sorrel (*R. acetosella*).

Broad-leaf sorrel is a perennial forming a basal rosette of leaves up to 6 in. (15 cm) long. In early summer the slender flowering stems, to about 4 ft. (1.2 m), produce spikes of tiny reddish flowers, followed by hard nutlets. French sorrel has smaller ovate to hastate leaves, tiny green flowers and grows to about 1 ft. (30 cm).

Varieties ▶ *R. acetosa* 'Blond de Lyon,' with large succulent leaves, is used for classic sorrel soup and to produce blue and green dyes. A pretty silver-leafed variety of *R. scutatus* is 'Silver Shield.'

Position ▶ Sorrel requires a rich, moist soil and a sunny to partly shaded position.

Propagation ▶ Sow sorrel seed in situ when the soil has warmed in spring, or start it indoors and transplant it. Seeds germinate within 14 days. Thin plants to 1 ft. (30 cm) apart. Considered weedy, *R. crispus* is under statutory control in Australia.

Maintenance ▶ Regularly trim plants of all three culinary sorrels to keep up the supply of fresh, tender young leaves. Remove the flowering heads whenever they appear.

Pests and diseases ▶ There are none of significance.

Harvesting and storing ▶ Pick sorrel fresh throughout the growing season. It does not dry well, but like spinach, it can be frozen. Lift the roots in autumn and dry them for herbal preparations.

Cooking

This spinachlike leaf is quite delicious if picked when young and tender. Cook it briefly to retain the flavor; do not use aluminium or iron pots or utensils, because they will make sorrel go black and cause a disagreeable metallic taste. If using raw, select the young, tender leaves. A purée of cooked sorrel is a good accompaniment to fish, eggs, pork and veal. Sorrel's acidity also acts as a meat tenderizer.

Sorrel sauce is a French classic that goes well with poached fish.

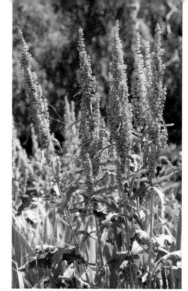

French sorrel (*Rumex scutatus*)

Sorrel (*Rumex acetosa*)

Sweet cicely

Latin Name *Myrrhis odorata* Apiaceae
Another common name **English myrrh**
Parts used **Young leaves and stalks, young roots**

This delightfully ornamental herb has leaves with a sugary anise scent. It is one of the important ingredients in Chartreuse liqueur, and is also included in Scandinavian aquavit, which is used as a digestive and an aperitif.

Gardening

Native to cool, moist mountainous areas of Europe, sweet cicely is the lone species in its genus. It is a fully hardy perennial, forming a clump of delicate, fernlike and very sweet-tasting leaves. The large, handsome umbelliferous heads of white flowers are followed by slender, 1-in. (2.5-cm) seeds, which are technically fruits. They are aromatic and deliciously nutty when eaten raw and green. Both the leaves and green fruits are very high in anethole, which gives them their sweet anise scent. Mature seed are a shiny dark brown.

If you're gathering sweet cicely in the wild, do not to mistake *Myrrhis* for highly toxic hemlock (Conium maculatum), which has dark stems spotted red-purple.

Position ▶ It requires a humus-rich moist soil, a cool climate and a shady location.

Propagation ▶ Allow the seed to fall around the parent plants, where they will germinate in spring. Alternatively, stratify the seed by placing it in moist, sterile sand or vermiculite inside a sealed plastic bag, and store in the refrigerator crisper tray for 8 weeks before sowing in spring (see box *page 40*).

Maintenance ▶ Remove flowering stalks to prolong leaf production.

Pests and diseases ▶ None of any significance.

Harvesting and storing ▶
Harvest young leaves for fresh use. They retain little fragrance after drying. Pickle the unripe seeds, and clean and store the young roots in brandy.

The cooked young roots are considered beneficial for those who are "dull and without courage."

American sweet cicely

Osmorhiza longistylis, a native North American species of Apiaceae, also known as sweet cicely (or aniseroot, licoriceroot or longstyle sweetroot), is a perennial with small, white umbelliferous inflorescences and coarse, rather celery-like leaves. It is found in rich woodland in eastern North America. The sweet-tasting root, with its strong anise scent, was used by Native Americans as a digestive and antiseptic.

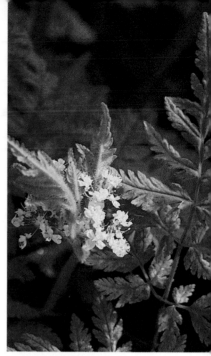
Sweet cicely (*Myrrhis odorata*)

Cooking

Boil the roots as a vegetable; they can also be candied like angelica and used as a decoration for desserts. Use the crisp, celery-tasting stems in salads.

The leaves of sweet cicely have a warm, anise aroma and a pleasantly sweet taste. Use them fresh in salads or add them when cooking sharp fruits such as gooseberries and rhubarb and some varieties of apples, because their natural sweetness will counteract the tartness. They are a safe sweetener for diabetics. The green seeds can be used for the same purpose.

Sweet cicely leaves add a lovely flavor to cream, yogurt, rice pudding, fruit and wine, soups, stews and dressings. Use leaves in omelettes, too. They also make a very pretty garnish.

Sweet myrtle

Latin Name **Myrtus communis** Myrtaceae
Other common name **Greek myrtle**
Parts used **Leaves, buds, flowers, fruits**

Myrtle was sacred to Venus in ancient times, and groves of fragrant myrtles were grown around her temples. Myrtle also symbolized honorable victory and was woven into bay wreaths at the early Olympic Games. Brides still tuck sprigs of myrtle into their bouquets.

Gardening

Sweet myrtle is native to the south-eastern Mediterranean. The sweetly spicy essential oil, also known as *eau d'anges* (angel's water), is used in perfumes and for medicinal purposes. The plant varies from a shrub to a small tree with oval, shiny, fragrant green leaves and small white flowers with a central "powder puff" of stamens.

Varieties ▶ Varieties of myrtle include the double-flowered 'Flore Plena'; the box-leafed myrtle, 'Tarentina,' which is useful for topiary; 'Variegata,' a variety with white-edged leaves; a white-fruited variety called 'Leucocarpa'; and the broad-leafed or Roman myrtle, 'Romana.'

Position ▶ Sweet myrtle requires sunshine and good drainage.

Propagation ▶ You can propagate myrtle by seed, although the resulting plants can be quite variable. Propagate named varieties by tip cuttings in mid- to late summer.

Maintenance ▶ In frost-prone areas, grow sweet myrtle in pots and bring it under cover in winter.

Pests and diseases ▶ There are none of significance.

Harvesting and storing ▶ You can air-dry the buds, flowers, fruits and leaves.

Lay sprigs over barbecued or roast meats toward the end of cooking to add a spicy flavor.

Cooking

Although of limited culinary use, the leaves, flower buds and fruits of sweet myrtle feature in Mediterranean cooking, especially Corsican and Sardinian recipes, to flavor pork, lamb and small game birds. They are also used in sauces and some liqueurs. The berries have a mild juniper flavor, and both the dried flowers and dried fruits are ground into a spice that has the same flavor. The infused oil is used in teas, salad dressings, fish and chicken dishes, desserts and bakery items.

Other myrtles

Lemon myrtle (*Backhousia citriodora*), anise myrtle (B. anisata) and cinnamon myrtle (*B. myrtifolia*) are rain forest trees from eastern Australia that are rapidly gaining prominence for their culinary and perfumery uses; they are now plantation grown. Lemon myrtle is a broad-leafed evergreen tree with panicles of small, scented white flowers. The leaves have an intensely fresh lemon fragrance, and the essential oil is typically very high in citral. Anise myrtle (see Anise, *page 10*) is used in teas and also as a culinary flavoring. Cinnamon myrtle or carrol forms a shrub with spicy cinnamon-scented ovate leaves that can be used in cooking. Bog myrtle or sweet gale *(Myrica gale)* of the family Myricaeae has sweetly resinous leaves that repel insects. They are used in perfumery, as a condiment, and also in treating skin problems.

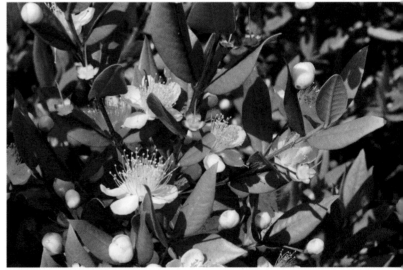

Sweet myrtle (*Myrtus communis*)

Sweet violet

Latin Name *Viola odorata* Violaceae
Parts used **Leaves, flowers**

The sweet fragrance of violets is often detected on early spring breezes long before the flowers are seen, leading inevitably to sayings such as "shy violet" and "modest as a violet." But sweet violets hold a proud place in history, associating freely with gods, kings, and emperors.

Gardening

Of the 250 or so species of *Viola*, two are used medicinally: *V. odorata* (sweet violet) and *V. tricolor* (Heartsease, page 58). There are single, semi-double and fully double forms of V. odorata occurring naturally in a number of different colors.

Among recommended garden varieties of sweet violets are 'Victoria,' which is the foundation of the French Riviera industry; 'Princess of Wales' (grown commercially in Australia); sky-blue 'John

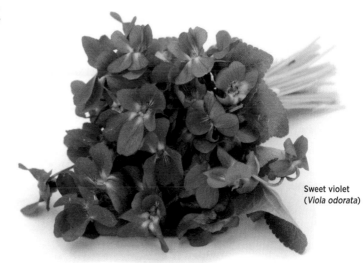

Sweet violet
(*Viola odorata*)

"Forgiveness is the fragrance that violet sheds on the heel that has crushed it."

Mark Twain, American writer 1835–1910

Raddenbury'; red-purple 'Admiral Avellan'; pink 'Rosina'; the richly colored 'Queen of Burgundy'; white 'Alba'; apricot-colored 'Crépuscule'; and the large purple- and white-striped 'King of the Doubles.'

The very double Parma violets have shiny heart-shaped leaves and profuse, large, intensely fragrant flowers that resemble rosebuds. Excellent varieties include white 'Comte de Brazza,' deep lavender 'D'Udine,' pale lavender 'Neapolitan' and 'Parme de Toulouse.'

Position ▶ Sweet violets thrive in a well-composted, moist soil. Flowering is reduced in shaded locations, so a position under deciduous trees is ideal. Mulching ensures good summer growth.

Propagation ▶ Propagate plants by runners formed in autumn.

Maintenance ▶ Remove old plants when they become woody. Apply a liquid seaweed fertilizer once or twice annually; overfeeding

encourages foliage rather than flowers.

Pests and diseases ▶ Check for red spider mite, which thrives under dry conditions. Water under foliage and spray with a seaweed solution.

Harvesting and storing ▶ During the blooming season, gather flowers and leaves before they wilt. Deadheading prolongs the flowering season as long as possible.

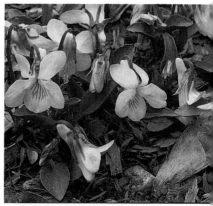

Sweet violets grow well in dappled shade beneath deciduous trees.

Napoléon and Josephine

In the 19th century, when violets were very fashionable, entire districts were devoted to their production. Victorian women pinned sweet-scented corsages to their gowns, and the fragrance was captured in many products, from perfumes to toiletries, prepared from the essential oil, which is distilled from the leaves. Josephine, wife of the French emperor Napoléon, loved the scent of violets. After his death, sweet violets and a lock of her hair were found in a locket he had kept.

Sweet violet *Continued*

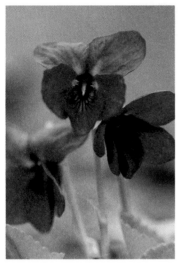

Sweet violet (*Viola odorata*)

Herbal medicine

Viola odorata. Parts used: leaves, flowers. The medicinal properties of sweet violet closely resemble those attributed to its relative, heartsease (*V. tricolor*). Sweet violet is used for skin conditions such as eczema and psoriasis as well as catarrhal conditions of the respiratory tract, where it can help remove mucus from the lungs.

In traditional herbal practice, sweet violet has a longstanding reputation as an adjunctive remedy in the treatment of certain types of cancer, including those of the breast and lung. Laboratory studies have elucidated the presence of specific compounds in the plant that show an inhibitory effect on tumor growth; further investigations need to be undertaken before this traditional use can be substantiated.

For the safe and appropriate use of sweet violet, consult your healthcare professional. Do not use sweet violet if you are pregnant or breastfeeding.

Cooking

The flowers of sweet violet are edible and, from the time of the ancient Romans, who used the fragrant blooms to sweeten their wine, have a long history of culinary use. In Victorian times, fresh flowers were used to create herbal jellies, syrups, pastilles, liqueurs and chocolates.

You can use freshly picked flowers to garnish and add flavor to desserts and fruit salads. Like heartsease, sweet violets can be crystallized for cake decoration.

The flowers and young leaves can be scattered through salads and the flowers can be made into tea or steeped in vinegar to add both flavor and a delicate mauve tint.

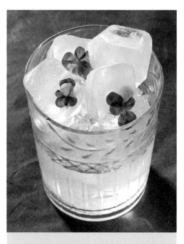

Cool and pretty

To add a splash of color to summer drinks, freeze sweet violet and heartsease flowers in water in ice-cube trays and then pop a few cubes into a jug of lemonade or mix them in with cake batter or cookie dough to give the flavor an extra kick.

Crystallized flowers

Crystallized flowers are available from shops that sell cake-decorating supplies. Alternatively, it's easy to make your own. Cupcakes provide an ideal platform for your creative skills.

12–24 violets, or other edible
   flowers or petals
1 egg white, at room temperature
1 cup (230 g) caster sugar

1. Combine egg white in a small dish with a few drops of water. Using a fork, beat lightly until the white just shows bubbles. Place sugar in shallow dish.

2. Hold a flower or petal in one hand; with other hand, dip a small paintbrush into egg white and gently paint flower or petal, covering it completely but not excessively.

3. Gently sprinkle sugar over flower or petal. Place on wire rack covered with baking paper to dry. Repeat with remaining flowers or petals.

4. Allow flowers or petals to dry completely before use (about 12 to 36 hours, depending on humidity). Store crystallized flowers or petals in an airtight container until required.

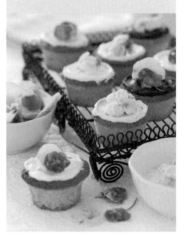

Sweet woodruff

Latin Name *Galium odoratum* syn. *Asperula odorata* Rubiaceae
Parts used Leaves (*G. odoratum, G. verum*), flowers (*G. odoratum*),
roots (*Rubia tinctorium*), whole plant (*G. aparine*)

Sweet woodruff and its close relatives, ladies' bedstraw, madder and cleavers, have all been used since medieval times. Known in Germany as master of the woods for its groundcovering habit, sweet woodruff is used to flavor May wine.

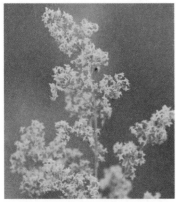

Ladies' bedstraw (*Galium verum*) produces panicles of honey-scented flowers in summer.

Gardening

Sweet woodruff (*G. odoratum*) is a stoloniferous perennial growing to about 9 in. (23 cm). The ascending stems have whorls of 6 to 8 shiny leaves borne at each node, while the starry white flowers are borne in loose clusters. In 1954, the U.S. Food and Drug Administration banned the use of sweet woodruff in food and non-alcoholic drinks as a suspected carcinogen. The ban remains in place but it is controversial because the evidence is contradictory.

Ladies' bedstraw (*G. verum*), also known as yellow bedstraw and Our Lady's bedstraw, resembles a slender form of sweet woodruff. 'Bedstraw' refers to the plant's former use as mattress stuffing.

Cleavers or goosegrass (G. aparine), an annual resembling a coarse version of sweet woodruff, has white flowers and stems and leaves that are covered with hooked bristles. Cleavers has been used as a potted herb, and its seed roasted as a good coffee substitute.

Madder (*Rubia tinctorium*), a scrambling perennial with starry yellow flowers, resembles a larger and coarser version of sweet woodruff. The roots can reach 3.5 ft. (1 m) long and are the source of a valuable pigment, red madder, which is used to make fabric dye, inks and paints.

Position ▶ Sweet woodruff and its close relatives all prefer a moist, compost-enriched soil. Woodruff and cleavers prefer a partly shaded position, while bedstraw requires full sun.

Propagation ▶ Grow sweet woodruff, ladies' bedstraw and madder by seed or by division; grow cleavers by seed.

Maintenance ▶ Weed as required.

Pests and diseases ▶ None of any significance.

Harvesting and storing ▶
Harvest sweet woodruff and bedstraw, then air-dry as required. Once dried, sweet woodruff develops a pleasing scent of fresh-mown hay. When madder roots are 2 years old, strip them of bark and dry them. They are used to make dye.

Herbal medicine

Galium aparine. Parts used: whole plant. Cleavers is an important medicinal herb in the Western herbal

Sweet woodruff (*Galium odoratum*)

tradition. Essentially, it is regarded as an exceptional lymphatic-system cleanser, helping to remove toxins from the body. It is a valuable remedy for chronic skin conditions such as eczema and psoriasis and, due to its diuretic and detoxifying effect, can also be of use for fluid retention. In addition, it is prescribed for conditions presenting with swollen lymph nodes, including tonsillitis.

For the safe and appropriate use of cleavers, see Detox, *page 183*. Do not use cleavers if you are pregnant or breastfeeding.

Traditional uses

Woodruff was once used as a strewing herb because it produces a fresh hay-like scent as it dries. Traditionally, it was used as a flavoring for jellies, jams and ice-creams as well as beer and sausages in Germany, where it is now replaced with synthetic flavorings and aromas. Woodruff is still in use as a flavoring for tobacco.

Ladies' bedstraw (pictured) has long been used to curdle milk for making cheeses, especially vegetarian types, while its roots were used to dye tartans in Scotland until 1695, when the erosion of native grasslands resulted in the practice being banned.

Tansy

Latin Name *Tanacetum vulgare* syn. *Chrysanthemum vulgare* Asteraceae
Another common name **Golden buttons**
Parts used **Aerial parts**

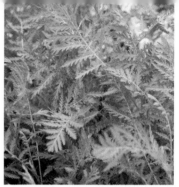

Plant tansy with potato crops to deter the highly destructive Colorado beetle.

A bitter herb included in liqueurs, in medieval times tansy was eaten in dishes as a penance at Eastertide. The name is derived from the Greek word for "immortality," reflecting the fact that tansy stays in flower for a long period. The plant produces a yellow dye.

Gardening

A very hardy rhizomatous perennial herb, tansy grows to about 4 ft. (1.2 m), with pinnate leaves, which typically have a camphor scent. There are a number of chemotypes, with the scent of rosemary, artemisia, chrysanthemum or eucalyptus. Tansy bears flat-topped ornamental inflorescences of golden button flowers that dry well.

Crisp-leafed or fern-leafed or curly tansy is a more compact ornamental form with ferny leaves. Costmary or alecost or bible leaf (*T. balsamita*) is a rhizomatous perennial with clusters of white daisy flowers and silvery green, sweetly mint-scented leaves.

Camphor plant (*T. balsamita* subsp. *tomentosum*) has camphor-scented foliage and is used in moth-repellent herb mixtures. *T. cinerariifolium* syn. Pyrethrum cinerariifolium is an aromatic, white daisy-flowered perennial, the source of Dalmatian insect powder. The pink-flowered *T. coccineum* is the source of the less-effective Persian insect powder.
Varieties ▶ 'Silver Lace' is a variegated variety of *T. vulgare*.
Position ▶ All *Tanacetum* species listed prefer a well-drained, sunny position.
Propagation ▶ Propagate the species and its varieties by seed, root division in spring or semi-ripe tip cuttings in summer.
Maintenance ▶ Tansy can become invasive, so in garden beds take care to keep the rhizomes under control.
Pests and diseases ▶ There are none of significance.
Harvesting and storing ▶ Harvest tansy foliage during flowering for drying or oil extraction. Harvest the leaves of costmary and camphor plant as required, and the flowers of pyrethrum when they open, then dry and grind them.

Herbal medicine

Tanacetum vulgare. Parts used: aerial parts. Tansy was once used as a short-term remedy for the treatment of worm infestations of the gut. Today this herb is no longer used medicinally, because we now know that thujone, a component of the essential oil of the plant, is associated with significant toxic effects.

Thujone also has a strongly stimulating effect on the uterus and can have serious negative side effects in pregnant women or those attempting to become pregnant. Do not use tansy or its essential oil, and take extra care with this plant if you are pregnant or breastfeeding.

Around the home

A natural insect repellent, tansy can be grown outside in pots around outdoor entertaining areas to deter flies and mosquitoes. Indoors, use dried tansy to deter ants, clothes moths or fleas in your pet's bedding. A strong tansy tea can be spritzed over the carpet to keep flea populations under control, but do not spray it directly onto your pet or its bedding. Also, do not use it if you are pregnant or breastfeeding.

Bible leaf

Costmary (*Tanacetum balsamita*), once had the common name of bible leaf, in reference to its use as a Bible bookmark — its mintlike scent was perfect for reviving the faint-hearted during interminable Sunday sermons. The word *tanacetum* is from *athanasia*, Greek for "immortality," and in ancient Greece, corpses were packed with tansy leaves to preserve them and ward off insects until burial took place.

Tansy (*Tanacetum vulgare*)

Tarragon

Latin Name *Artemisia dracunculus, A. dracunculoides* Asteraceae
Part used **Leaves**

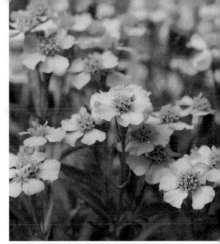

Dracunculus is Latin for "little dragon," and once tarragon was reputed to cure the bites of not only diminutive dragons but also all serpents. Today its unique, delicious and piquant flavor is indispensable to the classic cuisine of France.

Gardening

French tarragon (*A. dracunculus*) is a selected form of exceptional flavor. It rarely sets seed, especially in cool climates, although it may produce tiny, greenish, ball-shaped inflorescences. Its slender linear leaves are warmly aromatic, with a complex fragrance and taste that blends sweet anise, basil and resinous undertones.

Russian tarragon (*A. dracunculoides*) regularly flowers and sets viable seeds. It often improves in flavor the longer it is grown, but seed-grown Russian tarragon has an earthy balsamic scent.

Winter tarragon, or Mexican mint marigold or Mexican tarragon or sweet mace (*Tagetes lucida*), is a true mimic of French tarragon. A half-hardy perennial with finely toothed, linear, deep green aromatic leaves, it produces a lavish display of small, bright golden flowers, borne in clusters in autumn to 2.5 ft. (74 cm).

Position ▶ Winter tarragon thrives in hot, humid climates. French tarragon is cold-hardy and drought-resistant, and can grow in high summer temperatures. It is, however, very susceptible to high humidity and easily infected with fungal diseases. Avoid overhead watering.

Propagation ▶ Propagate French tarragon by tip cuttings in spring and early autumn, or by root division.

Maintenance ▶ Regularly thin plants of French tarragon by harvesting. Remove any diseased branches.

Pests and diseases ▶ Tarragon is susceptible to nematodes (eel worms) and leaf fungal diseases, particularly rust.

Harvesting and storing ▶ Harvest foliage until mid-autumn.

Herbal medicine

Artemisia dracunculus, A. dracunculoides. Part used: leaves. These days, tarragon is more likely to be used for culinary than therapeutic purposes. Tarragon contains an essential oil component that is reputed to have similar properties to that of anise, which is often used to treat digestive symptoms. Russian tarragon has been used for stimulating the appetite.

In some countries, tarragon is traditionally used to treat the symptoms of diabetes; recent scientific research appears to support this. Preliminary studies in diabetic animals found that an alcoholic extract of French tarragon lowered the levels of both insulin and sugar in the blood.

For the safe and appropriate medicinal use of tarragon, consult your healthcare professional. Do not use tarragon in greater than culinary quantities if you are pregnant or breastfeeding.

Winter tarragon (*Tagetes lucida*). The leaves have a tarragon-like flavor, with hints of anise.

Tarragon's unique and piquant flavor is indispensable to the classic cuisine of France.

Cooking

French tarragon's flavor diffuses rapidly through cooked dishes, so use it carefully. Use it fresh with fish and shellfish, turkey, chicken, game, veal and egg dishes. Use chopped leaves in salad dressings, fines herbes, mustard, ravigote and béchamel sauces, sauce verte and mayonnaise.

Oil of tarragon is used in commercial salad dressings, beverages, confections, perfumes and mustards.

French tarragon
(*Artemisia dracunculus*)

Tea

Latin Name *Camellia sinensis* syn. *Thea sinensis* Theaceae
Parts used **Leaf tips, leaves, seeds**

Tea has been the favored beverage of China for 3,000 years. While Western palates favored the more robust flavor of black tea, green tea has been shown to be richer in antioxidants and is credited with a number of uses in traditional medicine.

Gardening

There are some 350 varieties of *Camellia sinensis*, and they vary considerably in form. The smooth, leathery leaves are oval, pointed and faintly scented. The small white flowers are single, with a boss of gold stamens, and are borne in the leaf axils.

Tea contains polyphenol antioxidants, the levels being higher in green tea, which has undergone minimal oxidation. An essential oil is distilled from the mature leaves, which is used both in perfumery and as a commercial flavoring. The seeds are pressed for a fixed oil that is processed to remove saponins. Other species that are used for oil production include *C. crapnelliana*, *C. oleifera*, *C. octapetala* and *C. sasanqua*.

Position ▶ *Camellia sinensis* is frost-hardy and requires full sun to partial shade, and a rich, moist but well-drained soil.

Propagation ▶ It is propagated from freshly harvested seed, and by semi-ripe wood cuttings for named varieties.

Maintenance ▶ Maintain bushes to a height of about 3⅓ ft. (1 m).

Pests and diseases ▶ There are none of significance.

Harvesting and storing ▶ Harvest leaf tips for tea once bushes are 3 years old.

Herbal medicine

Camellia sinensis. Part used: leaves. Leaves picked from the tea plant are subjected to various processing methods to produce green, black, white and oolong varieties of tea: For instance, leaves are fermented and dried for black tea, but steamed and dried for green tea. Each type of tea contains different levels of important compounds, known as polyphenols, which are primarily responsible for the plant's medicinal properties. Green tea contains the highest levels of polyphenols and is regarded as having the greatest therapeutic activity of all these teas.

Green tea polyphenols possess a potent antioxidant capacity that is far greater than that of vitamin C or E, and which may help in the prevention and treatment of numerous chronic diseases of our time. Studies of large populations of regular green-tea drinkers report lower rates of some cancers and reduced risk of cardio-vascular disease.

Further human trials have reported a protective effect of green tea against sunburn when applied topically, and regular consumption of chewable green-tea tablets has been shown to reduce gum inflammation and plaque formation.

Due to its caffeine content, green tea continues to be a popular aid for improving mental alertness and concentration, and it has also been investigated for its use as a potential weight-loss agent. Some studies also suggest a potential role for green tea in the treatment of diabetes as a result of a blood sugar-lowering effect in addition to its antioxidant properties.

For the safe and appropriate medicinal use of green tea, consult your healthcare professional. Do not use green tea in greater than culinary quantities if you are pregnant or breastfeeding. Caffeine intake should be monitored during these times.

Tea (*Camellia sinensis*)

Rooibos tea

In South Africa, the leaves of the rooibos (pronounced roy-boss) plant (*Aspalathus linearis*) have been brewed as a refreshing beverage for centuries. Now, rooibos tea is becoming a popular drink all over the world as a result of its pleasant taste, caffeine-free content and, more important, the discovery of its remarkable antioxidant capacity; therefore, it may have the potential to improve general health and well-being as well as help in the treatment of many serious illnesses.

Opposite page: Hand harvesting of Camellia sinensis leaves for tea, one of the world's most popular beverages.

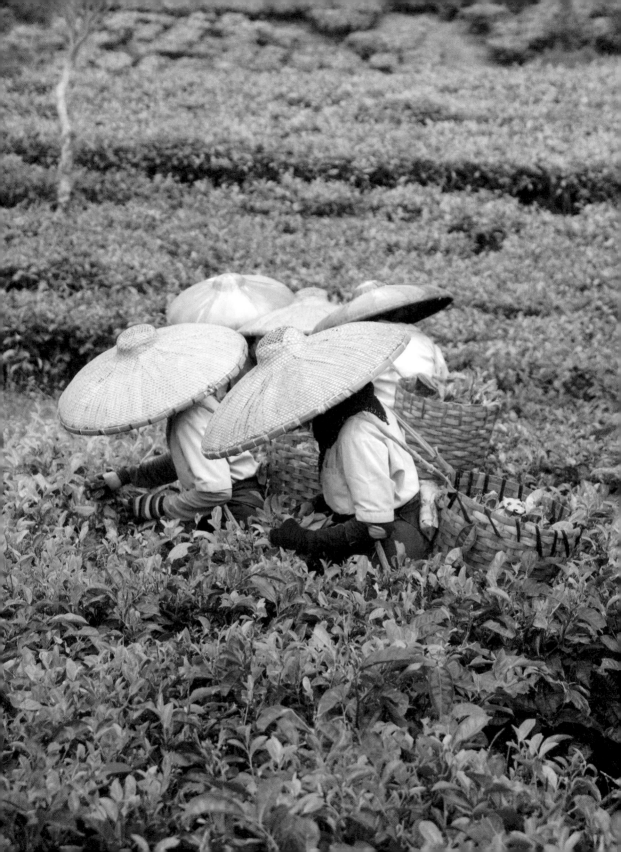

Tea tree

Latin Name *Melaleuca* sp. Myrtaceae
Parts used **Leaves, branches**

In the 18th century, Aboriginal Australians taught Captain James Cook and his crew how to make poultices from crushed tea tree leaves to treat cuts and skin infections.

Gardening

"Tea tree" is a misnomer, because that term also applies to *Leptospermum* species, while *Melaleuca* species are actually paperbarks. This has caused confusion and the widely held belief that the tea trialed by the Cook expedition was prepared from *Melaleuca*, which is not recommended.

Tea tree (*M. alternifolia*) is plantation-grown in Australia for high-quality essential oil. The species grows to about 23 ft. (7 m) and occurs naturally on the warm east coast of Australia, where it is often associated with swampy conditions.

M. leucadendron, a tall species, is the source of cajeput oil. Both *M. viridiflora* and *M. quinquenervia* are sources of niaouli oil, used in perfumery and as an antiseptic. All four species have whitish, layered, papery bark, stiff pointed

narrow linear (*M. alternifolia*) or oval smooth leaves, and profuse, intensely honey-scented bottlebrush inflorescences, which are white, except in *M. iridiflora* where they are greenish white or, rarely, pink to red. Trees may literally drip nectar.

Position ▶ The species of *Melaleuca* described require an acid, very moist soil, full sun and warm conditions.

Propagation ▶ All species can be grown by seed, but trees with desirable chemotypes are raised by seed from selected trees or cuttings.

Maintenance ▶ Irrigation is important.

Pests and diseases ▶ None of note.

Harvesting and storing ▶ Trees are cut for foliage, which is water- or steam-distilled and cured for 6 weeks.

Herbal medicine

Melaleuca alternifolia. Parts used: essential oil from leaves and branches. Scientific research has confirmed that the essential oil of the tea-tree plant possesses potent antimicrobial actions against many common bacterial, viral and fungal disease-causing organisms.

These days, tea-tree essential oil continues to be used extensively for its topical antiseptic actions. It is used to treat acne, gum infections and fungal infections of the foot, and clinical trials have shown that its effectiveness is comparable to some conventional treatments.

For the safe and appropriate external use of tea-tree oil, see First aid, *page 194;* Acne, *page 190;* and Athlete's foot, *page 192.* Tea-tree oil should not be used internally.

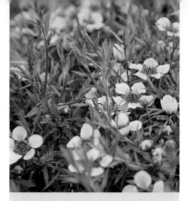

New Zealand tea tree

The essential oil of the New Zealand tea tree or manuka (*Leptospermum scoparium*) is strongly antimicrobial and can be diluted and used to disinfect wounds.

A particularly important remedy is honey from bees that graze on manuka, which contains a compound called Unique Manuka Factor (UMF), which supercharges its ability to heal infections. High-UMF honey is labeled as 'active manuka' honey. Other manuka honeys without the 'active' label (or a UMF rating of at least 10) are not likely to be as potent.

Do not use tea-tree oil if you are pregnant or breastfeeding.

Around the home

Tea-tree oil is powerfully antiseptic, with antimicrobial and antibacterial properties.

● Wipe down surfaces with a disinfectant solution – mix tea-tree oil with either water or vinegar.

● Disinfect a shower and remove mold by mixing ¼ cup (60 g) borax, 2 cups (473 g) very hot water and ¼ teaspoon tea-tree oil. Shake in a spray bottle until borax dissolves. Spray on surfaces, leave overnight, then rinse.

● Deodorize and disinfect garbage bins — wipe them out with a solution of ½ teaspoon tea-tree oil and a little detergent in hot water.

Tea tree
(*M. alternifolia*)

Thyme

Latin Name *Thymus* sp. Lamiaceae
Part used **Leaves**

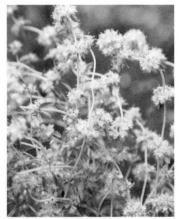

Common thyme
(*Thymus vulgaris*)

There are an astonishing number of aromatic thyme species with a wide variety of fragrances, flavors and uses, from culinary and medicinal to mystical and magical. No wonder the highest praise in ancient Greece was the expression "To smell of thyme."

Gardening

There are some 350 species of thyme. They share much in common, most being sun-loving, perennial woody subshrubs or creeping woody plants with a neat habit that are high in fragrant essential oils.

Garden or common thyme
(*T. vulgaris)* is the principal culinary thyme. The leaves of all forms are tiny, narrow, elliptic, gray-green and aromatic. The tiny white or lavender flowers are borne terminally in many-layered whorls.

Selected forms include 'Silver Posie,' with soft green and white variegated foliage; 'German Winter,' a very hardy spreading form; 'Provence,' a selected high-quality culinary variety from France; a hybrid called 'Fragrantissimus,' or orange thyme, with very fine, erect, thyme- and citrus-scented gray foliage; and 'Erectus,' with strong vertical growth.

Caraway or seedcake thyme
(*T. herba-barona)* is a wiry carpeting thyme with a delicious caraway scent and lavender flowers. The neat foliage is deep green and the loose flower heads are mauve. Varieties include 'Lemon Caraway' and 'Nutmeg.'

Conehead thyme (*T. capitatus* syn. *Coridothymus capitatus*) is another very popular cooking thyme. It is an intensely scented, compact spreading subshrub with distinctive terminal conical clusters of deep pink flowers.

Spanish thyme (*T. mastichina*) forms a neat gray, upright subshrub. The scent is predominantly of common thyme with an element of eucalyptus leaf. This thyme is excellent for barbecues.

Lemon thyme (*T. x citrodorus*) has neat, bushy, fresh green-leafed plants that are redolent of lemon and thyme, making them ideal for fish and chicken dishes. The plants have somewhat sparse heads of lilac flowers. 'Silver Queen,' also known as 'Silver Strike,' is a white-variegated form, and golden-variegated thyme was the old Elizabethan 'embroidered thyme.' 'Lime' is a low-growing fresh green variety with a tangy lime scent.

Broad-leafed thyme has broadly elliptical leaves with the true thyme fragrance and interrupted inflorescences with whorls of mauve flowers. Varieties include 'Oregano' or 'Pizza' thyme, which is often listed as *T. nummularium*; 'Pennsylvania Tea,' with broad leaves and a gentle flavor that's ideal for tisanes; and 'Bertram Anderson' syn. 'Archer's Gold,' with pink flowers and bright golden foliage in summer.

Winter-flowering thyme
(*T. hyemalis*) forms a small, densely clothed gray bush and is harvested for commercial dried thyme and essential oil.

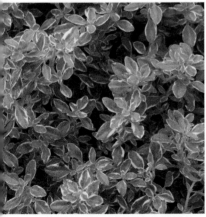

'Bush BBQ' thyme is very aromatic, perfect for adding flavor to barbecued meat.

A number of thymes are popular as much for their profuse flowering and dense matting habit as for their fragrance.

Azores or orange peel thyme
(*T. micans* and *T. caespititius* syn. *T. azoricus*) resembles a dense, bitter orange-scented, mosslike carpet. The flowers are white or lavender.

Thymus vulgaris 'Silver Posie' bears pink-purple flowers in late spring to early summer.

Thyme *Continued*

Mother of thyme (*T. serpyllum*) has been divided taxonomically into two species, previously classified as subspecies — *T. serpyllum* and *T. quinquecostatus*, with reddish stems. Many popular varieties of carpeting thymes have been developed from the latter, including red-flowered 'Coccineus,' 'Minimus,' 'Pink Chintz,' 'Russetings' and 'Snowdrift.'

Woolly thyme (*T. pseudolanuginosis*) has soft, gray, dense foliage. Hybrid carpeting varieties also include 'Coconut' and gold-speckled, lemon-scented 'Doone Valley.' 'Porlock' and 'Westmoreland' (Turkey) thyme are both robust culinary varieties.

Position ▶ Thymes require good drainage and a sunny position.

Propagation ▶ Raise thyme from seed in spring, but propagate varieties by cuttings and by division.

Maintenance ▶ Weed the carpeting thymes regularly.

Pests and diseases ▶ There are none of significance if grown in full sun. Substances leached from the leaves of thyme inhibit surrounding

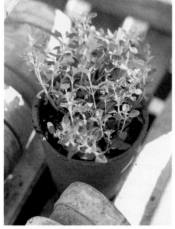

Grow common thyme (*Thymus vulgaris*) in pots or as a border plant in the garden.

plant growth, reducing weed and grass competition.

Harvesting and storing ▶ Thyme is low in moisture and easily air-dried out of direct sunlight. It retains its flavor.

Herbal medicine

Thymus vulgaris. Parts used: leaves, flowering tops. Thyme has potent anti-microbial properties, attributed to the high content of essential oil found in the plant. Thyme also possesses a muscle-relaxant effect and an ability to thin mucus in the lungs, making it easier to expel. These combined effects make thyme a formidable remedy when it comes to treating respiratory conditions, such as colds and flus. Thyme can also be used as a gargle for sore throats and tonsillitis.

Thyme alleviates the symptoms of indigestion, such as gas, bloating and cramps, and its antimicrobial action can also be helpful in treating gastrointestinal infections.

For the safe and appropriate medicinal use of thyme, see Sore throats, colds & flu, *page 174*. Do not use thyme in greater than culinary quantities and do not use the essential oil if you are pregnant or breastfeeding.

Around the home

Thyme essential oil is a great addition to cleaning products and disinfectant sprays. For a powerful and fresh-smelling bathroom cleaning spray, mix ¼ teaspoon each of lemon, bergamot, pine, thyme, citronella and tea-tree essential oils with 2 teaspoons vinegar, 1 tablespoon cloudy ammonia and 4 cups (1 L) water. Then, to this

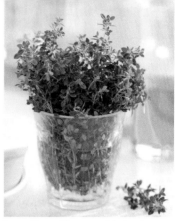

Lemon thyme (*Thymus x citriodorus*)

According to folklore, a garden full of thyme will attract fairies.

solution add 2 tablespoons club soda and shake until well combined.

Use thyme essential oil in an oil diffuser in a sick room for its antibacterial qualities and soothing aroma.

Cooking

Various types — including lemon thyme and caraway thyme — have the flavor suggested by their names. Lemon thyme and common thyme, with their warm, pleasant aromas, are the ones commonly used in cooking, but it's well worth trying other varieties.

Thyme is a major culinary herb in Europe, where it shines in slow-cooked casseroles and dishes containing meat, poultry or game. It can be assertive and dominate other milder flavors, so robust companions, such as onions, red wine and garlic work well. Use thyme in terrines, pâtés, meat pies, marinades (especially for olives), eggplant and tomato dishes and thick vegetable-based soups. Dried thyme is often used in the jambalayas and gumbos of Creole and Cajun cooking.

Turmeric

Latin Name *Curcuma longa* Zingiberaceae
Part used **Leaves**

Turmeric is a member of the ginger family and its rhizomes add a golden color to curries. It has long had medicinal herbal use, particularly in Ayurvedic medicine, and a rhizome constituent, curcumin, is currently exciting scientific interest for its potential in treating a range of diseases.

Gardening

Turmeric is an herbaceous perennial native to tropical Southeast Asia. It forms a dense clump of aromatic foliage to about 3.5 ft. (1 m), spreading by rhizomes that are brown with bright yellow flesh. The flowers are borne in dense spikes with yellow and white to orange tubular flowers. The leaves are simple and the lamina extends to the base of the stems. There are ornamental forms of *C. longa*, including 'Bright White,' 'Jamaican Red' and 'Vietnamese Orange.'

Position ▶ Turmeric requires a rich, moist soil and consistently warm temperatures in order to flourish. Plants die back underground each winter and will survive some frosts.

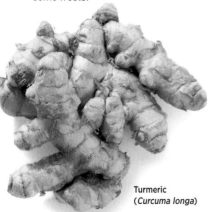

Turmeric
(*Curcuma longa*)

Propagation ▶ Propagate from sections of rhizome.
Maintenance ▶ Divide each year.
Pests and diseases ▶ It repels ants.
Harvesting and storing ▶ Boil the rhizomes for several hours before drying and powdering.

Herbal medicine

Curcuma longa. Part used: rhizome. Turmeric has a long history of use in both Ayurvedic and Chinese traditional medicinal systems, where it is regarded as an excellent tonic and blood purifier and an effective remedy for inflammatory conditions such as arthritis, skin conditions, including psoriasis, and digestive and liver disorders. Extensive scientific research and clinical trials are providing supportive evidence for its therapeutic effects.

Turmeric contains a compound called curcumin, which is responsible for the vivid yellow color and has also been shown to be involved in many of turmeric's medicinal effects. Potent antioxidant and anti-inflammatory properties have been identified, as well as a protective effect on the liver and an ability to increase bile secretion. Turmeric has also been shown to reduce harmful cholesterol levels in the blood and reduce the development of hardened and blocked arteries. Recent research has also led to the discovery of a remarkable range of potential anti-cancer effects.

Clinical trials have shown that turmeric is effective in reducing the symptoms of rheumatoid arthritis and post-operative inflammation. It

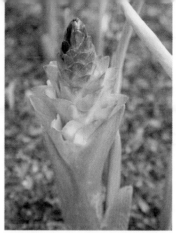

The flowers are accompanied by pale green lower bracts and pink to purple upper bracts.

has also been shown to be effective in the treatment of indigestion, stomach ulcers and inflammatory bowel conditions, such as Crohn's disease and ulcerative colitis.

In addition, studies on large populations have shown that the consumption of large quantities of turmeric is associated with a reduced risk of developing certain cancers.

For the safe and appropriate medicinal use of turmeric, see Liver support, *page 182;* High blood pressure & cholesterol, *page 202;* and Psoriasis, *page 191.* Do not use turmeric in doses greater than culinary quantities if you are pregnant or breastfeeding.

Cooking

Buy plump, firm, clean rhizomes. They should have a warm, mild aroma and an earthy, musky flavor. Turmeric can be used fresh or dried and ground, and adds a brilliant yellow color to foods. It is used in curry powders and pastes, pickles and chutneys, vegetable, rice and lentil dishes (especially in India, where it often partners potatoes and cauliflower), and with poultry, fish and shellfish. It is also an ingredient in the Moroccan spice blend chermoula.

Valerian

Latin Name *Valeriana officinalis* Valerianaceae
Part used **Root**

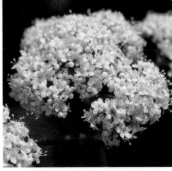

Valerian (*Valeriana officinalis*) bears clusters of white flowers, followed by tiny seeds.

Valerian root is believed to be the attractant used by the Pied Piper in the medieval German milling town of Hamelin in 1284. It certainly proved to be profitable knowledge for the rat catcher, at a time when the mayor was desperate to save the town's food supplies.

Gardening

Once praised by Arab physicians, valerian (*V. officinalis*) is an herbaceous perennial forming a large basal rosette of compound, fernlike leaves. The tall flowering stem bears large, dense pale pink to pure white heads of sweetly scented flowers. The essential oil is used commercially for such purposes as flavoring tobacco and beer.

Chinese medicine has employed several additional species, such as *V. coreana*, *V. fauriei*, *V. amurensis* and *V. stubendorfi* for indications similar to those used in the West. Note that red valerian or kiss-me-quick is *Centranthus ruber*, which is of no value medicinally.

Position ▶ Native to Western Europe, valerian prefers a cool root run, a sunny to lightly shaded position, and a moist, well-composted, well-drained loam.

Propagation ▶ Valerian is propagated by seed sown in spring, scattered over the propagation mix and gently pressed down, because the seed requires light to germinate. Transplant 2 ft. to 2.5 ft. (60 cm to 74 cm) apart.

Maintenance ▶ Divide mature plants in autumn or early spring. Cats are as enchanted by valerian roots as rats, so you may need to provide protection for young plants.

Pests and diseases ▶ There are none of significance.

Harvesting and storing ▶ Lift the rhizomes in early spring, then rinse gently and dry them in a cool 200°F (100°C) fan-forced oven with the oven door left ajar. Grind if desired.

Herbal medicine

Valeriana officinalis. Part used: root. Valerian has been used medicinally as a remedy for aiding sleep and relaxation for hundreds of years. Pharmacological studies on the plant have confirmed its sedative effects on the nervous system as well as its relaxant action on muscles.

A number of clinical trials have assessed the efficacy of valerian on its own or in combination with other relaxing herbs for insomnia, when there is difficulty falling asleep and/or sleep that is easily disturbed. The results of these trials are mixed and may be the result of large variations in the dose and preparation of valerian used as well as the length of time it was taken; however, they are strongly suggestive of positive effects on sleep, particularly if taken consistently for more than 2 weeks.

A small number of human trials have also shown a beneficial effect of valerian in alleviating the symptoms of anxiety and mental stress.

Valerian's calming effect on nerves and muscles explains the traditional use of the herb for gastrointestinal cramps, period pains and headaches as well, particularly when they are related to nervousness and tension.

For the safe and appropriate use of valerian, see Insomnia, *page 188*. Do not use valerian if you are pregnant or breastfeeding.

Shell shock

The name "valerian" is derived from the Latin *valere*, "to be strong" or "to be well." The herb was used by ancient Greek physicians such as Hippocrates and, in the Dark Ages, it was recommended in Anglo-Saxon herbals for treating shock. During World War I, it was used in a tincture to treat soldiers who were suffering from shell shock, which is now better known as post-traumatic stress disorder, or PTSD.

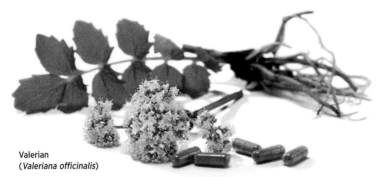

Valerian
(*Valeriana officinalis*)

Vervain

Latin Name *Verbena officinalis* Verbenaceae

Other common names **Devils' bane, enchanter's plant, herb of grace, herb of the cross, herb Venus, holy herb, pidgeonweed (it is a bird attractant), simpler's joy, tears of Isis**

Parts used **Aerial parts**

Despite its lack of looks and scent, vervain was once considered the most magical of all herbs in Europe, the Middle East and China, and was used for purifying sacred spaces and in spells and potions for divination, immortality, crop fertility, prosperity, love and for protection from evil forces and lightning.

Gardening

Vervain is native to Europe, Asia and Africa and is naturalized in North America. A slender erect herbaceous perennial growing to 4 ft. (1.2 m), it is found on dry, stony ground such as roadsides. The leaves are coarsely and irregularly toothed, and the slender, branched, terminal flowering spikes bear small tubular lavender flowers. Blue vervain (*V. hastate*) finds similar uses. Pineapple verbena (*Nashia inaguensis*, family Verbenaceae) is used as an herbal tea.

Position ▶ Grow plants 1 ft. (30 cm) apart, in full sun, in well-drained soil.

Propagation ▶ Grow vervain from seed in spring. Germination is erratic and can take 4 weeks.

Maintenance ▶ Keep plants weed-free.

Pests and diseases ▶ Knotlike galls caused by insects can form in the stem.

Harvesting and storing ▶ Harvest the green tops just before the flowers open, then air-dry them. Store under airtight conditions.

Vervain tea was once used to protect people from vampires.

Herbal medicine

Verbena officinalis. Parts used: aerial parts. Vervain has both calming and restorative effects on the nervous system and an uplifting effect on mood. It can help to relieve nervous exhaustion and depression, and act as a supportive remedy during times of tension and stress. Vervain is particularly effective for those who feel miserable and fatigued during recovery from feverish illnesses such as flu. The plant's relaxing effects are also of benefit for any muscular tension in the body, reducing intestinal cramps and easing the discomfort of period pains.

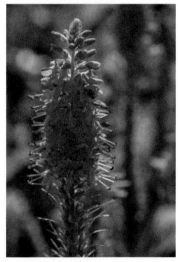

Vervain (*Verbena hastata*)

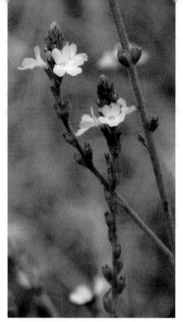

Vervain (*Verbena officinalis*)

Vervain is also traditionally prescribed during the early stages of fever. Further, it is regarded as a liver remedy and can be used to treat some conditions associated with this organ.

For the safe and appropriate use of vervain, consult your healthcare professional. Do not use vervain if you are pregnant or breastfeeding.

Devil's bane

Derived from the Celtic *ferfaen*, from *fer*, "to drive away" and *faen*, "a stone," vervain has a multitude of religious, cultural and magical associations. For instance, the names herb of the cross, holy herb and devil's bane derive from vervain's reputation for staunching Christ's wounds on the cross, and it was also used in sacrifice and purification ceremonies by the ancient Romans and Druids. In more recent times, the Iroquois people of North America used a concoction of smashed blue vervain (*Verbena hastate*) leaves to make an obnoxious person go away.

Viburnum

Latin Name *Viburnum opulus, V. prunifolium* Caprifoliaceae
Other common names **Cramp bark, European cranberry bush, guelder rose**
(*V. opulus*); **American sloe, black haw, stagbush** (*V. prunifolium*)
Parts used **Stem bark** (*V. opulus*); **stem and root bark** (*V. prunifolium*)

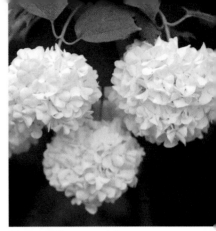

Viburnum (*Viburnum opulus*)

Viburnum species are shrubs grown for their outstanding spring displays of usually fragrant flowers, colorful autumn leaves and berries. But the bark of two species has also found herbal use as a muscle relaxant in treating cramps, especially those associated with menstruation.

Gardening

Cramp bark (Viburnum opulus) is a widely distributed deciduous shrub, with vine-shaped leaves that turn red in autumn and large lacy heads of white flowers borne in late spring.

Black haw (V. prunifolium) forms a spreading deciduous shrub to small tree that reaches to 16 ft. (5 m). It has fine and sharply toothed, rounded leaves and flat-topped lacy heads of reddish buds opening to white flowers in spring, followed by lime green berries that ripen black in autumn. Do not eat the berries of either species.

Another species sometimes used is American highbush cranberry (*V. trilobum* syn. *V. americanum*).

Varieties ▶ *V. opulus* varieties include 'Sterile' (the snowball tree); 'Notcutt's Variety,' with excellent autumn foliage and large red fruits; and 'Xanthocarpum,' with translucent golden berries.

Position ▶ The species described above are all deciduous shrubs for cool to mild climates, and prefer an open position and well-drained soil. Once established, they have modest drought resistance.

Propagation ▶ The species above are easy to grow from seed, while the varieties can be propagated by semi-hardwood cuttings.

Maintenance ▶ Prune after flowering, if required.

Pests and diseases ▶ There are none of significance.

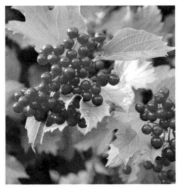

The shiny red berries of cramp bark (*Viburnum opulus*) are ornamental, but toxic.

Poisonous plants

The berries of *Viburnum opulus* are poisonous, while those of European cranberry bush can cause vomiting and diarrhea. And there are other species in the plant world that should not be grown in a garden that young children can access. Poisonous foxgloves (*Digitalis* sp.), for instance, produce tall spires of flowers that fit neatly over the fingers, tempting children to play with them. Monkshood (*Aconitum* sp.), which has a similar flowering habit, contains an extremely toxic compound that was once used to poison arrow tips. According to Greek mythology, aconite was created by the goddess of the Underworld, Hecate, from the mouths of Cerberus, a three-headed dog that guarded the gates of Hades.

Harvesting and storing ▶ Peel off the outer bark in strips and dry it.

Herbal medicine

Viburnum opulus. Part used: bark. As its name suggests, cramp bark is effective for most types of muscular tension and can help to relax the muscles of the body after strenuous or ongoing physical activity. Cramp bark is also prescribed for tension and cramping in the digestive system, and it will ease the symptoms of indigestion, colic and gut cramps, including those brought on by nervous tension.

The medicinal properties of cramp bark are particularly useful in treating menstrual and menopausal symptoms. Its muscle relaxant properties help to ease the spasm and discomfort of period pains and, due to a slightly astringent or drying effect, cramp bark can reduce heavy bleeding during menstruation as well as irregular bleeding that can occur during menopause. Black haw (*V. prunifolium*) is used for similar indications.

For the safe and appropriate use of cramp bark, see Sports injuries, *page 196.* Do not use cramp bark if you are pregnant or breastfeeding, except under professional supervision.

Watercress & nasturtium

Latin Name *Nasturtium officinale, Tropaeolum majus* Brassicaceae
Parts used **Leaves, young stems (watercress); aerial parts (nasturtium)**

Watercress is cultivated for its attractiveness as a garnish as well as the bite it gives to soups, pesto, trout, salads, sandwiches and vegetable juices. It is high in vitamin C, folic acid, beta-carotene and minerals, including potassium.

Gardening

Watercress is a semi-aquatic perennial herb found wild in streams passing through chalk soils. The cultivated form, now usually grown hydroponically, is preferred, because wild watercress is often a refuge for liver flukes (*Fasciola hepatica*) in areas where sheep graze. The plant has compound green leaves, a hollow stem and insignificant white flowers. The plant is notably more bitter when flowering.

Nasturtium, or Indian cress (*Tropaeolum majus*), has large, shield-shaped, peppery leaves and cheerful, helmet-shaped flowers in yellow, orange and red.

Position ▶ You can grow watercress in pots in a partially shaded position. It prefers a well-limed soil. The large seeds of nasturtium germinate easily in spring, either planted directly into moist soil or germinated in pots and transplanted into a sunny position.

Propagation ▶ To propagate, use tip cuttings grown in regularly changed water, rooted runners or seeds. Grow all other cresses by seed.

Maintenance ▶ Water regularly.

Pests and diseases ▶ None of note.

Harvesting and storing ▶ Harvest watercress fresh and only use before flowering. Store it at room temperature with its roots in water.

Herbal medicine

Tropaeolum majus. Parts used: aerial parts. Nasturtium and watercress belong to the same family as horseradish and, like their relative, contain pungent compounds known as mustard oil glycosides, which are responsible for the major medicinal effects of nasturtium. These compounds possess potent antibacterial and anti-fungal properties that have particular application in the treatment of infectious conditions of the respiratory and urinary tracts. They can help the body fight off colds, flus and other infections of the lungs as well as cystitis.

The fresh form of the herb is reputed to have a higher antimicrobial effect than the dried form, and is commonly prepared as an infusion. Applied externally as a poultice or compress, the fresh herb is also used as a local antibacterial agent for cuts and wounds. Interestingly, fresh nasturtium juice

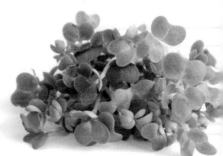

Watercress (*Nasturtium officinale*)

rubbed onto the scalp is said to stimulate hair growth.

For the safe and appropriate use of nasturtium, consult your healthcare professional. Do not use nasturtium if you are pregnant or breastfeeding.

Cooking

The sharp, peppery taste of watercress makes it a good salad green. It goes well with a citrus dressing. Use watercress in soups, sandwiches and sauces for fish. Nasturtium flowers make an attractive edible garnish.

Other cresses

A number of other species share the hot peppery flavor of watercress and find similar culinary uses. Upland or winter cress (*Barbarea verna*) is a cold-hardy dry-land cress. The cress sold in trays to be clipped for salads is garden cress (*Lepidium sativum*). The cucumber-flavored Lebanese cress (*Apium nodiflorum*) resembles watercress but is, in fact, a land plant that's related to celery.

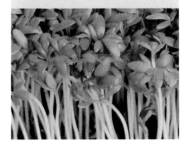

Nasturtium
(*Tropaeolum majus*)

White horehound

Latin Name *Marrubium vulgare* Lamiaceae
Parts used **Leaves, flowering tops**

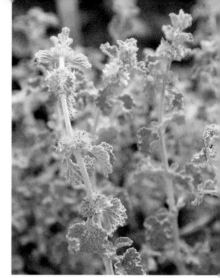

White horehound (*Marrubium vulgare*)

Used as a cough and bronchitis medicine since Egyptian times, horehound is a member of the mint family and has attractive white furry foliage. It is also used in making horehound ale and flavoring liqueurs, and attracts bees to gardens.

Gardening

White horehound is a perennial with attractive crinkled, downy, gray-white, toothed foliage. The small white flowers, borne in summer, are densely clustered in successive upper leaf axils. The plant yields an aromatic bitter juice with a distinctive and not unpleasant smell.

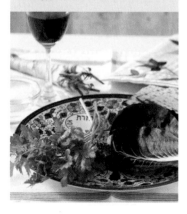

Passover plate

In late March or in April each year, Jews celebrate Passover with a meal that symbolizes the flight of the Jews from Egypt. Each of the six items on the plate, or *seder*, represents part of the story of their escape: Along with romaine lettuce or grated horseradish, white horehound is one of the bitter herbs eaten to symbolize the harshness of living as a slave in Egypt.

Black horehound (*Ballota nigra*), a member of the same family, was also used medicinally, but this use has largely fallen away now. Native to Mediterranean Europe and Asia, black horehound is a fully hardy perennial herb that is still widely grown in herb gardens.

Variety ▶ A very attractive, heavily white-variegated form of *B. nigra*, 'Archer's Variety,' has deep green, toothed leaves and small, hairy, tubular lilac (rarely white) flowers borne in whorls in the upper stem axils. The scent is rather disagreeable.

Position ▶ Grow white horehound in a sunny, well-drained position, and black horehound in well-drained soil in sun to partial shade.

Propagation ▶ Propagate both white and black horehound by seed. The latter's variegated form can only be reliably propagated by cuttings.

Maintenance ▶ Both forms are hardy plants needing little care.

Pests and diseases ▶ There are none of significance. White horehound has been used as a grasshopper repellent on various crops.

Harvesting and storing ▶ Cut down the whole plant just as flowering begins and dry it for herbal use.

Herbal medicine

Marrubium vulgare. Parts used: leaves, flowering tops. Not to be confused with black horehound, which is used for quite different purposes, white horehound is best known as a remedy for respiratory conditions such as colds and bronchitis — especially when there is mucus that is difficult to expel by coughing. White horehound relaxes the bronchial muscles while at the same time encouraging easier removal of mucus from the lungs.

As a result of its pronounced bitter taste, due to the presence of specific compounds, white horehound has an appreciable and somewhat stimulating effect on the digestive system. It can improve a poor appetite as well as ease symptoms of indigestion, particularly when there is gas and bloating.

It also has a positive effect on liver function and increases the secretion of bile, which can aid the digestive process as a whole.

For the safe and appropriate use of white horehound, see Sore throats, colds & flu, *page 174*. Do not use white or black horehound if you are pregnant or breastfeeding.

Fresh white horehound can be used to make syrup and candy to ease sore throats and coughs.

Yarrow

Latin Name *Achillea millefolium* Asteraceae

Other common names **Achillea, allheal, bloodwort, carpenter's herb, milfoil**

Parts used **Leaves, flowers**

Yarrow is one of our oldest herbs. In China, stripped and dried yarrow stalks were tossed to consult the *I Ching*, the *Book of Changes*, and, in the West, it has been widely used as an herb of powerful but neutral magic.

Gardening

Yarrow is a tough, fully hardy perennial forming a rosette of very finely divided feathery leaves with a pungent, refreshing scent that is strangely uplifting to the senses. It multiplies via underground rhizomes. The small white flowers form dense, flat-headed, large inflorescences borne on wiry stems to about 2.5 ft. (74 cm).

There are some 85 species of *Achillea*, and many hybrids. Yarrows are among the toughest and prettiest modern ornamental perennials; many have been bred from *A. millefolium*.

Varieties ▶ Some beautiful varieties include 'Lemon Queen,' 'Paprika,' 'Cerise Queen,' 'Appleblossom,' cream-flowered 'Credo,' blackcurrant-colored 'Cassis,' Damask rose-scented 'Fawncett Beauty,' 'Lilac Beauty' and coppery 'Colorado.'

Other widely cultivated species include feathery, woolly yarrow (*A. omentosa*); fern-leaf yarrow (*A. filipendulina*) and its golden-flowered hybrid 'Coronation Gold'; sneezewort (*A. ptarmica*); and *A. taygetea* and its famous hybrid 'Moonshine.'

Position ▶ The yarrows described above all require a sunny, well-drained position. They are frost-hardy and have good drought resistance.

Propagation ▶ Raise species by seed sown in pots and transplant about 6 to 8 weeks later. Propagate named varieties by division.

Maintenance ▶ Divide clumps every 3 to 4 years in late autumn or, in cooler climates, early spring.

Pests and diseases ▶ There are no pests or diseases of any consequence. Cold, wet winters may cause rotting if plants are poorly drained.

Harvesting and storing ▶ Harvest the flowering stalks just as they fully open, and dry in small bunches hung upside down out of direct sunlight. Harvest leaves at any time.

Herbal medicine

Achillea millefolium. Parts used: aerial parts. Yarrow has been used since ancient times for its healing effects on wounds, quickly stopping bleeding and reducing inflammation. It is also well known for its application in any feverish condition where it encourages

perspiration and reduces body temperature; for this purpose it is commonly taken with elderflowers.

Yarrow is a valuable digestive remedy, alleviating colic and indigestion and improving appetite while also having a stimulatory effect on bile flow and liver function. Traditionally regarded as a women's herb, yarrow was commonly used to treat menstrual complaints associated with particularly heavy and painful bleeding.

For the safe and appropriate use of yarrow, *see* Sore throats, colds & flu, *page 174*. Do not use yarrow if you are pregnant or breastfeeding.

Yarrow
(*Achillea millefolium*)

Spices

Bark, resin, seeds, seed pods, fruit, flower buds, even stigmas — various parts of these plants are used as culinary spices as well as in herbal medicinal preparations.

1 Asafetida *Ferula asafetida*
The resin is used as a remedy for flatulence, so it's worth adding it to dishes based on legumes and pulses that tend to cause wind.

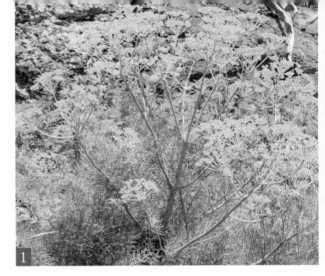

2 Fenugreek *Trigonella foenum-graecum*
Fenugreek is used under professional supervision to help manage blood sugar in patients with diabetes, and to lower cholesterol.

3 Cinnamon *Cinnamomum verum, C. cassia*
The volatile essential oils of both cinnamon and cassia contain high quantities of a compound called cinnamaldehyde, which is believed responsible for most of the plants' medicinal activity.

4 Cumin *Cuminum cyminum*
A popular cooking spice, medicinally cumin can be used to reduce flatulence and colic; it has a reputation as an appetite tonic.

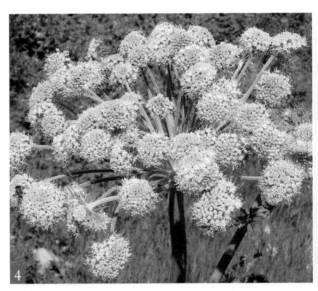

5 Cloves *Syzygium aromaticum*
The essential oil in the flower buds contains eugenol, responsible for its use as a local anesthetic, antiseptic and anti-inflammatory.

6 Saffron *Crocus sativus*
Saffron threads with a vibrant orange-red color contain the highest concentrations of the carotenoid crocin, which may have the potential to help treat cancer.

7 Black pepper *Piper nigrum*
Black, green, white, pink and red peppercorns all come from Piper nigrum. The different appearance and taste characteristics of each type are created by different processing methods.

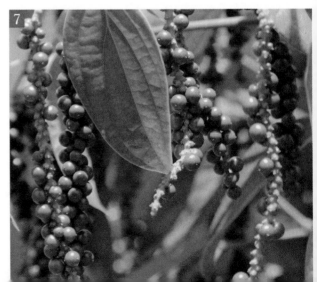

8 Nigella *Nigella sativa*
The peppery flavor of nigella seed is used in cooking and in Ayurvedic medicine to treat a variety of digestive problems.

9 Tamarind *Tamarindus indica*
The fruit is used widely in cooking, and various parts of the plant also have traditional medicinal uses. For example, in India the fruit is used as a laxative and also taken for nausea in pregnancy.

Caution
● Do not use any of these herbs if you are pregnant or breastfeeding, except under the advice of a healthcare professional.

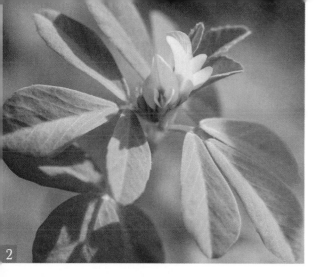

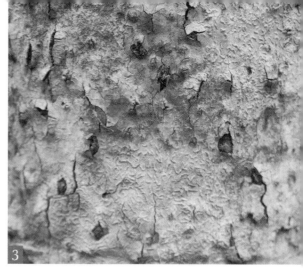

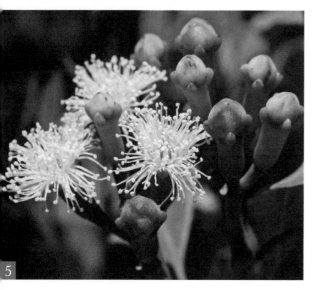

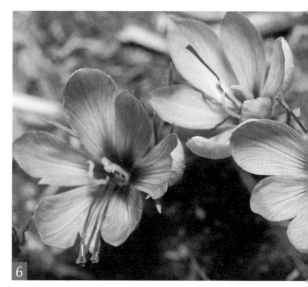

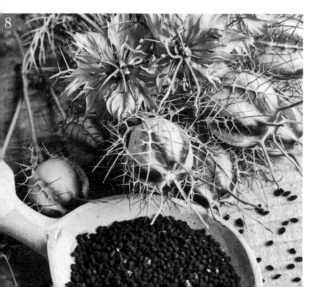

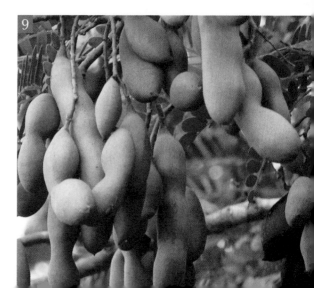

Berries

While some of these berries are delicious and safe to eat, either fresh or cooked, others are strictly for medicinal use only and should always be taken under the supervision of a professional herbalist.

1 Bilberry *Vaccinium myrtillus*
Compounds in bilberries called anthocyanosides have potent antioxidant properties, which contribute to the herb's many benefits, particularly for vision and eye health.

2 Saw palmetto *Serenoa repens*
The berry contains an oily extract that has been clinically proven to reduce symptoms of benign prostatic hyperplasia (BPH).

3 Chaste tree *Vitex agnus-castus*
Chaste tree helps to regulate the menstrual cycle and is used to treat a range of hormonal imbalances, including PMS symptoms.

4 Cranberry *Vaccinium macrocarpon*
Rich in antioxidants, including vitamin C, cranberries are an important remedy for preventing and treating cystitis.

5 Schisandra *Schisandra chinensis*
These berries are prescribed for a wide range of symptoms and conditions, including asthma, cough, insomnia and liver disorders.

6 Juniper *Juniperus communis*
Often taken in combination with other diuretic herbs, an infusion of berries is a traditional remedy for arthritis, gout and rheumatism.

7 Raspberry *Rubus idaeus*
Traditionally used to treat diarrhea, the leaves are also taken during the third trimester to prepare the uterus for childbirth.

8 Wild strawberry *Fragaria vesca*
Rarely used these days, an infusion of the leaves was once taken to relieve mild cases of diarrhea and soothe minor stomach problems.

9 Blackberry *Rubus fruticosus*
Strongly astringent due to large quantities of tannins, blackberry leaves traditionally have been used in the treatment of diarrhea.

Caution
● Except for raspberry leaf, as directed on *pages 210-211*, do not use any of these herbs if you are pregnant or breastfeeding, except under the advice of a healthcare professional.

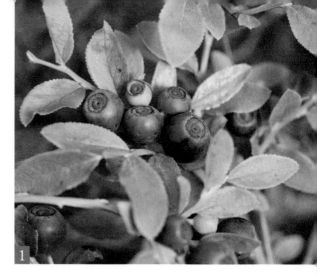

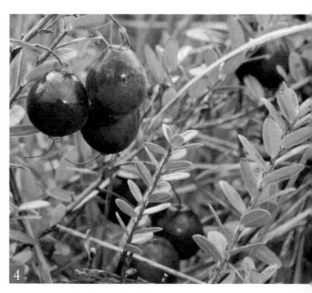

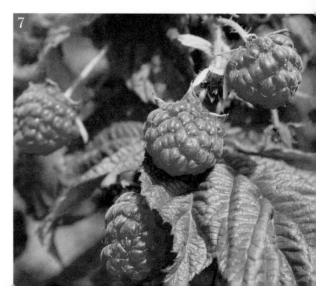

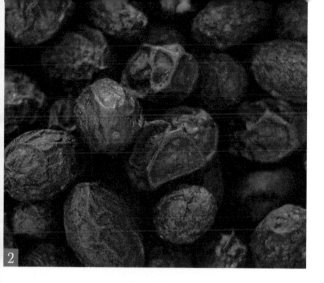

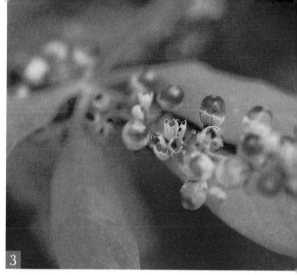

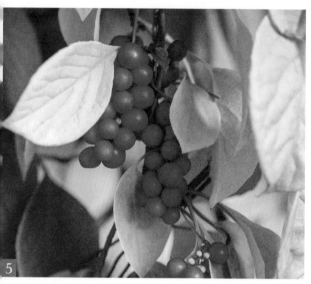

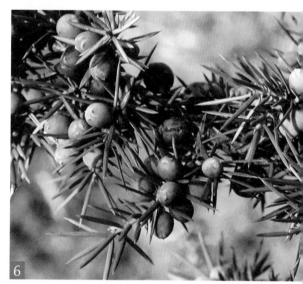

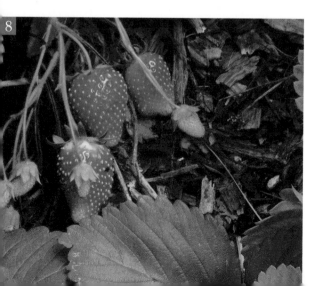

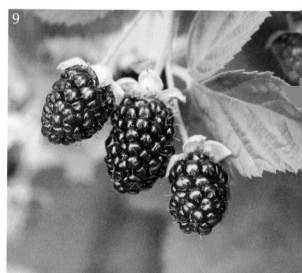

Trees

Admired for their flowers, nuts and fruit, or simply for their form, each of these trees is also the source of medicinal properties that have long been used as herbal remedies.

1 Magnolia *Magnolia officinalis*
Best known as an ornamental tree, the magnolia is a bitter tonic herb used to improve digestion, menstrual and liver problems.

2 Oak *Quercus robur*
Dried oak bark is an astringent herb used to reduce inflammation, control bleeding, and treat diarrhea and various skin conditions.

3 Walnut *Juglans nigra*
Black walnut hulls have traditionally been used for the treatment of worms and intestinal parasites.

4 Hawthorn *Crataegus sp.*
Hawthorn is an aromatic warming herb used to treat circulatory disorders and heart disease in both European and Chinese medicine.

5 White willow *Salix alba*
White willow bark's analgesic and anti-inflammatory properties make it a useful treatment for arthritis, back pain and headaches.

6 Olive *Olea europaea*
Not only does the olive produce wonderful fruit and oil, it is also a blood pressure–lowering herb with antioxidant properties.

7 Horse chestnut *Aesculus hippocastanum*
The seed, or 'conker,' of the horse chestnut tree provides an important circulatory remedy, used to treat varicose veins, leg ulcers and other blood vessel problems.

8 Prickly ash *Zanthoxylum americanum*
This herb is prescribed by herbalists for circulatory problems such as varicose veins and Raynaud's disease.

9 Witch hazel *Hamamelis virginiana*
Soothing and anti-inflammatory, witch hazel is used topically for a range of skin and vascular problems. Its astringent nature means it is also prescribed for diarrhea and heavy menstrual bleeding.

Caution

● With the exception of the topical use of witch hazel, do not use any of these herbs if you are pregnant or breastfeeding, except under the advice of a healthcare professional.

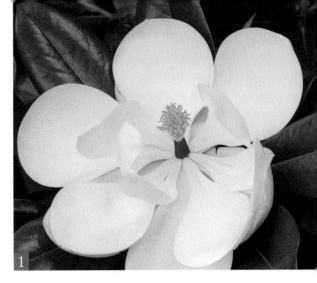

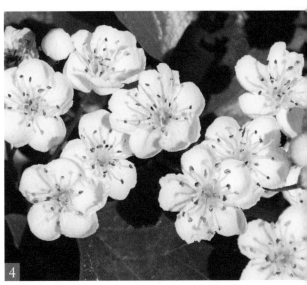

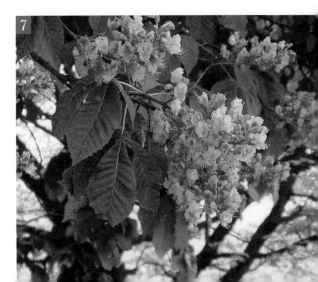

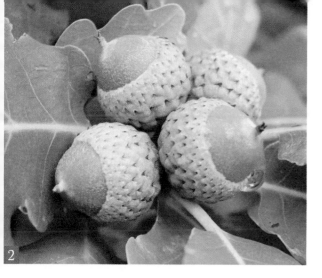

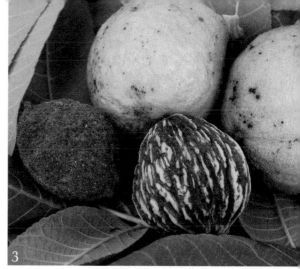

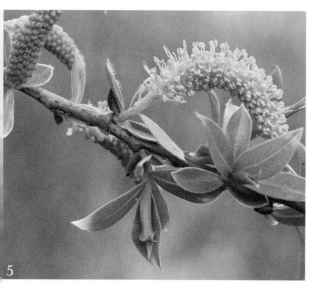

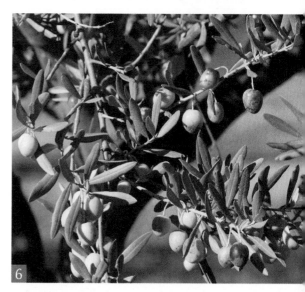

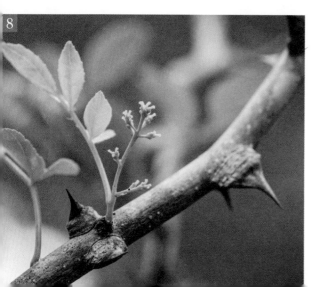

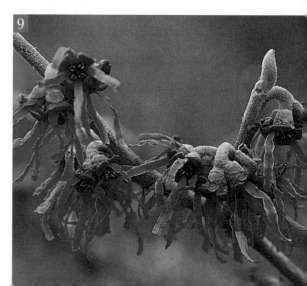

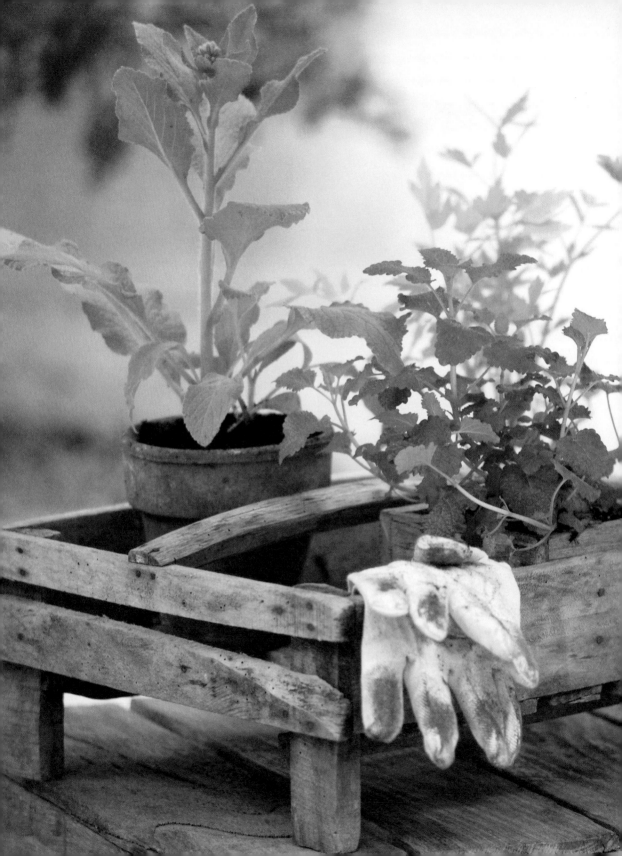

Gardening

Thriving herbs are a beautiful sight. Whether you grow them for health or for cooking and beauty benefits, or simply to enjoy their appearance and aroma.

Soils & organic matter

Good soil is the foundation for growing healthy plants. It provides access to nutrients, water and air, stabilizes roots and assists in plants' natural resistance to pests and diseases. Poor soils that are low in nutrients tend to result in weak, stunted plants, and although some of the tougher, more resilient herbs, such as St. John's wort, thrive in these conditions, you should be aware that this resilience can turn such plants into weeds.

Soil types

There are three main types of soil: sandy, loamy or clay. Sandy soil is easy to dig, but it doesn't hold nutrients or moisture. Heavy clay soils tend to become waterlogged, are difficult to dig into and set hard when dry.

The ideal soil ▶ Loam, on the other hand, is the ideal garden soil, a good balance of clay and sand. A rich brown color, it is slightly moist and crumbly, with a good earthy smell. It holds both air and water and releases the nutrients in the soil to the plant roots.

In a loamy soil, clay particles bind the soil together without making it sticky and impenetrable, while sand particles allow moisture penetration without letting the water run away. If a soil has too much clay, it will hold onto nutrients instead of releasing them.

A large component of loam is decomposed organic matter or humus. Soil microbes, such as bacteria, as well as fungi and earthworms help to break down dead plant material — leaves, branches, twigs, sawdust, kitchen scraps, manure and newspaper — in a process that can occur either naturally or in compost heaps and worm farms.

Improving your soil ▶ Making nutrients available to plant roots is an important aspect of growing healthy plants, so if your soils are too sandy and porous, the best way to improve their structure is to add organic matter in the form of compost or manures.

In addition, to reduce compaction and improve aeration, apply gypsum (calcium sulphate), available from landscape suppliers, nurseries and garden centers, at the rate suggested by the manufacturer.

Sweet or sour soil ▶ To determine the levels of acidity ("sourness") or alkalinity ("sweetness") in your garden soils, use a pH soil-testing kit, available from nurseries and mail-order or online. On a scale of 0 to 14, 7 is neutral, while soils above 7 are alkaline and those below are acidic.

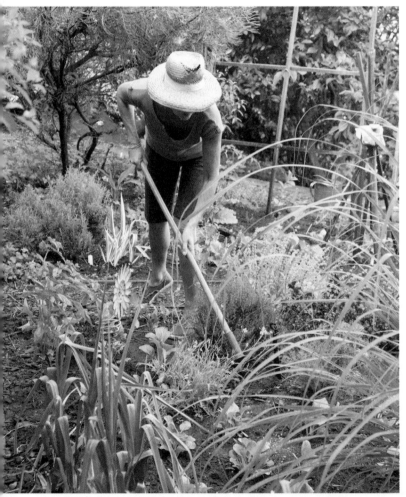

To grow healthy herbs, add plenty of organic matter to the soil, and mulch well.

The acceptable range is between 5 and 7, with most plants enjoying a slightly acidic soil of 6.5. There are exceptions, of course — lavenders, for instance, grow naturally in alkaline, limestone soils while blueberries, rhododendrons and azaleas prefer to be in an acid soil.

Adding organic matter will improve soil and result in healthier plant growth.

Adjusting the pH level ▶ If the pH of the soil is outside its normal range, this can mean the nutrients are either not available to plants or are too readily available. Either way, it can make them toxic. So, if your plants are showing signs of nutrient deficiency, but you know you have applied the correct amount of fertilizer, be sure to check the pH level of your soil.

If your garden soil is too acidic, raise the pH with an application of agricultural lime (calcium carbonate). This will also have a beneficial effect on the structure of clay soils. If your clay soil is also deficient in magnesium, apply dolomite (a combination of magnesium carbonate and calcium carbonate).

Where the soil is too alkaline, and you need to lower the pH level to make it more acidic, add some agricultural sulphur or sulphate of iron. Remember to check the pH again later, because you may need to make annual soil adjustments.

To make a comprehensive analysis, select at least five samples of soil from each garden bed or area.

Testing soil pH

You will need

- pH soil-testing kit
- samples of garden soil

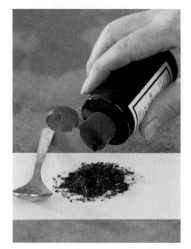

1 Place a level teaspoon of soil onto the test card, and add drops of the indicator liquid. Repeat this process with different areas of the garden.

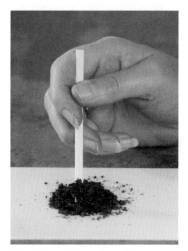

2 Stir the soil sample and keep adding more drops until you can stir it into a thick paste. Use the spoon or a small stick.

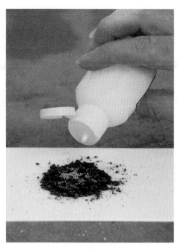

3 Dust the paste with the white powder provided, and wait about 1 minute until it changes color.

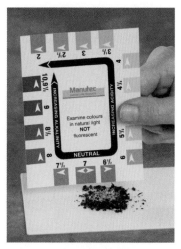

4 To determine if the sample is acidic, alkaline or neutral, match the color of the soil sample with the nearest pH value on the color card. Read the color chart in natural daylight, not fluorescent light. (Alternatively, send your samples to a laboratory for professional analysis.)

Cultivation & propagation

Choosing healthy plants, preparing the soil to suit their needs and giving them the appropriate care and maintenance will result in a thriving herb garden that will supply you with useful plants for medicinal preparations, cooking, natural beauty products, and many uses around the home. Growing plants from seeds is one of the most satisfying aspects of gardeing. Annual herbs are best planted each year from seed, while many perennial herbs are propagated by stem cuttings, layering or division.

When to plant

The best time to plant depends on your climate. In general, planting times are divided into two seasons — warm and cool. The warmer months of spring and summer fall between March and September, while the cooler months of autumn and winter fall between October and February.

From year to year, these times may vary slightly, from a couple of weeks to a month, depending on the weather, with the limiting factor being the temperature — or more specifically, frost. In tropical locations, where many plants can be grown all year round in the hot and humid conditions, the overriding factor is rain. In such climates, the seasons are divided into wet or dry, and the best time for planting is during the wet season.

Plants themselves fall within two groups — frost-tender (including tropical and warm-temperate plants) and frost-hardy (cool-temperate and cold-hardy). If you live in a warm- or cool-temperate climate, you should determine when the first and last frosts are likely to occur and plant accordingly.

Plant frost-tender plants about two weeks after the last cold snap. In frost-prone areas, a good alternative planting method is to start seeds off indoors and then transplant the seedlings into the garden later.

Buying herbs at nurseries

At reputable nurseries and retail garden centers, you'll find large display benches filled with lush, edible herbs of all shapes and sizes. You can select from annual or perennial seedlings in flats, or almost ready-to-eat plants in larger pots. It's good to see what's in season and check out other perennial herbs, shrubs and trees, such as salvias, lavender and bay trees — and companion plants.

You may be tempted to select young plants that look like they're maturing well, perhaps even flowering, but if this is the case, they have probably outgrown their pots. Smaller, immature seedlings will become healthier plants.

Before you buy, check that the herbs have healthy roots and are not pot-bound. Once the roots are tightly compressed, curled around the inside of a container and poking out the bottom, there is no guarantee they will grow well once you plant them in the garden.

For free plants, join a seed-swapping group, or exchange herbs with a friend.

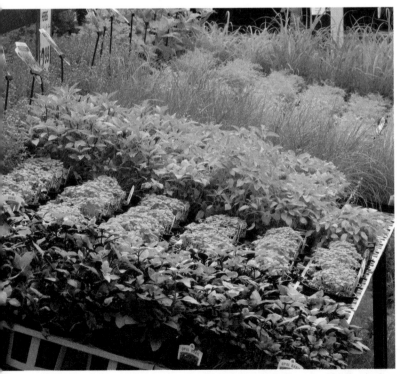

Once you've made your choice at the nursery, check for pests and even growth before buying.

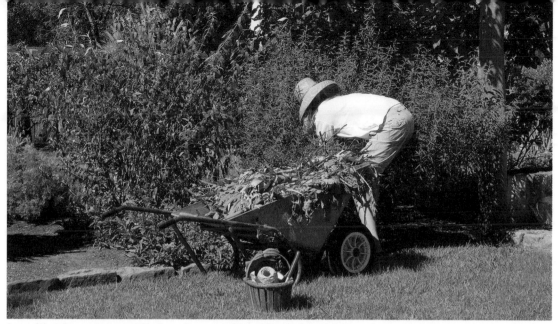

Some of the taller-growing perennial herbs, such as some salvias, require pruning and staking, otherwise they become leggy and look unattractive.

And while you're at the garden center or nursery, ask for advice if you need to. Horticulturalists are employed to share their gardening knowledge with their customers and help them make the best choices, so don't hesitate to ask questions. You'll build a friendly, useful relationship with the staff in the process.

As soon as you get your purchases home, give them a good soak in

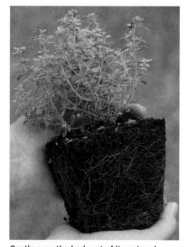

Gently ease the herb out of its pot and check that the root system is healthy, not pot-bound.

a bucket of water for a couple of hours to ensure the rootball gets a thorough watering before planting.

Mail-order plants

Some herbs are hard to find at general nurseries, so you may have to buy them from specialist growers, who usually offer a mail-order service. The Internet is a great place to start your search.

Once you've placed your order, it's exciting to wait for the arrival of your precious package. Plants are packed in various ways, but they will usually be grown beyond seedling stage, but not to maturity, and will be sent in a sturdy cardboard box.

The roots and soil may be encased in plastic wrap or in tube stock pots, and secured with protective material to stop the potting mix from coming loose. Alternatively, you may receive only the roots — as with turmeric and ginger — or the cloves, as with elephant garlic.

They will survive for a day or two, but you'll need to unpack them soon after arrival and place them in a

sheltered area that receives filtered light for several days until they acclimatize to your location.

To minimize transplant shock, water your plants with a weak solution of liquid fertilizer and a seaweed solution.

Preparing garden beds

Before transplanting or buying plants, prepare the areas in which they are going to be grown; these may be existing beds or newly created areas. To achieve the best results, remove any weeds and dig over the soil until it's loose, so the new roots can stretch out and grow unimpeded. It's also a good idea to improve the soil and its water retention and drainage with some organic matter.

Once you've prepared the site, start planting your herbs. Some herbs benefit from added nutrients in the soil, so give them a good start in their new environment by adding a slow-release fertilizer into your beds. Other herbs — such as anise, sweet basil and the various lavenders — like an application of lime.

Sowing Seed

There's something exciting about growing plants from seeds or cuttings and watching them flourish. Annual herbs are best planted each year from seed, while many perennial herbs are propagated by stem cuttings, layering or division.

You will need

- seed tray bag of propagating or seed-raising mix
- various seed packets or collected seed
- piece of dowel or pencil
- plant tag
- pray bottle
- plastic wrap (optional)

1 Fill the seed tray with quality seed-raising or propagating mix. (For best results, use clean sterilized trays and tools that have been washed in a weak solution of bleach.) Gently smooth the surface with a piece of dowel or a small block of wood, but do not compact the mix. Using a pencil or a piece of dowel, create a shallow channel. Gently shake the seeds evenly over the mix or, if they are large enough to handle, drop them one at a time, spacing them according to the packet instructions.

2 Smooth the mix so the seeds are just covered,or use a sieve to add a light covering. Very fine seeds may not need any covering. Select the fine spray setting on the spray bottle and water the tray thoroughly.

3 Place in a warm, dry location with natural indirect light (each plant type will have different light requirements). To retain moisture and humidity, cover trays with plastic wrap or a sheet of glass. Add a tag with the plant name and date of sowing. Remove the cover when the seeds begin to germinate.

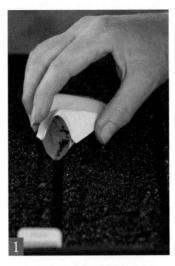

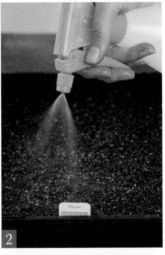

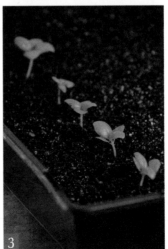

Stem cuttings

You can take soft-stemmed cuttings, such as basil and mint, in spring (after the last frosts) until midsummer, and semi-hardwood cuttings, such as rosemary and myrtle, a bit later, from midsummer to mid-autumn.

Use hormone powder — Cut a piece of soft-stemmed plant about 1.5 in. to 2.5 in. (4 cm to 6 cm) long and remove the lower leaves. Dip the stem into a hormone powder, which will stimulate new root growth. Plant the stem in a small planting hole in a container filled with propagating mix. Using a spray bottle, water thoroughly, then place the cutting in a protected position with natural indirect light.

Use a glass of water — Another method is to place stem cuttings in a glass of water in a position with indirect light, then wait for roots to form within 1 to 2 weeks. Change the water every few days and then transplant the cuttings into individual containers or into the garden. Herbs suitable for this treatment include mint and sage.

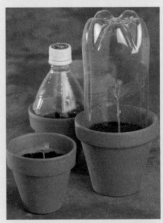

Recycled plastic bottles create an ideal mini greenhouse.

Planting

Once you've prepared your garden beds, it's time for planting. Soak the plant in a bucket of water beforehand, so that it will abosrb moisture more easily. We planted tarragon, a perennial herb that spreads by rhizomes and needs to be replanted every few years. Tarragon likes a well-drained soil that doesn't retain moisture too long; otherwise the rhizomes may rot.

1 Ensure that your soil has plenty of organic matter, such as compost or well-rotted manure, then dig a hole that's larger than the root ball.

2 Tease out the roots and loosen the potting mix so that they will seek out nutrients and moisture from the soil around them.

3 Carefully position the plant in the hole, making sure it sits at the same level in the ground as it did in the pot. Don't cover the crown.

4 Backfill and firm down the soil around the plant. Tarragon can also be propagated by root division in spring.

5 Water the plant well, and then water regularly until established. Prune for culinary use and also to discourage woody stems.

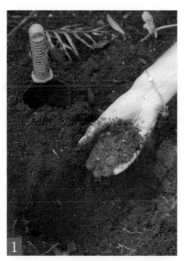

It's easy to forget what you've planted. Write the names on labels and pop them next to each herb.

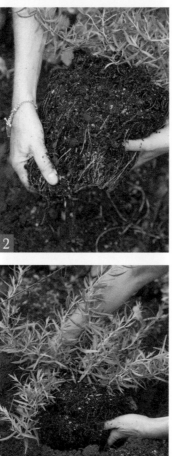

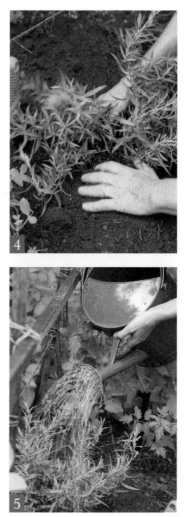

Container gardening

No matter where you live, you can always plant a selection of herbs, whether it's on a balcony, deck or veranda, or in a courtyard — any small garden space where they can thrive in hanging baskets, pots and other containers.

A potted herb garden

Herbs love growing in pots, and some herbs, such as mint and parsley, spread easily and will take over garden beds, so even if you have a huge garden, it's best to contain them. If you put containers in the right sunlit position, use good-quality potting mix and give your herbs the care they need, they will flourish.

The best position ▶ Many herbs, such as marjoram, fennel and thyme, prefer to grow in full sun, while others, such as catmint, chamomile and coriander, are happiest in partial shade.

On the other hand, a few herbs, such as watercress and angelica, actually need the shade. So, determine how much sun your balcony, courtyard or window box will receive throughout the year, and choose your plants accordingly. Alternatively, choose the plants you want to grow and then find the most suitable spot in which to grow them.

In hot climates, it's best to give plants some shade protection, as the heat can be too intense, even if they enjoy full sun in cooler locations. Another important factor is good air circulation; humid conditions can create fungal problems. Also avoid positions open to strong winds; a barrier such as lattice, can diffuse the breeze.

The right pot for the job ▶
Before you buy pots or containers, think about their different shapes, sizes and materials, as these will play an important part in the success of your herbs and the design of your display.

Don't use lots of little pots, particularly in different styles and colors, as these tend to make small spaces look cluttered. You can still grow a variety, but keep it simple: for example, select a single color to pull one area together.

Herbs such as parsley, peppermint and thyme enjoy being contained, and look attractive spilling exuberantly over pot rims, so consider the shape and form of what you're growing and select containers that suit their 'personality.'

Choose containers that complement the location and its surroundings, pick textures and colors to match the area's paintwork, paving or surface, and go for the biggest container that's practical.

Shapes and sizes ▶ Round, square or rectangular, squat or tall, with straight or tapered sides: any of these container types is perfect for growing herbs, as they all allow for good root growth and the display of foliage and flowers. Varying sizes of the same design will give an area a uniform look.

Although they look attractive, urns and 'oil jars' have narrow necks, making it extremely hard to remove plants without damaging them. You could also find yourself with many plant roots and very little foliage. If you favour bell-shaped pots, a cylindrical shape is best because ones that taper in sharply may not provide enough room for roots to space themselves out.

Troughs are generally long and narrow, like window boxes, and are perfect for formal or narrow areas. Team them with a square pot of similar material to create a right angle, then add a round pot to create a point of difference.

Materials ▶ The type of pot material will also affect both the look and the portability of your herb garden. Terracotta pots are popular with gardeners because they're practical, affordable and look attractive in most situations. Limestone and concrete pots, with their lovely pale colorings, are also popular, while alternative materials, such as plastics, are worth exploring.

In fact, the new generation of plastic materials offers a range

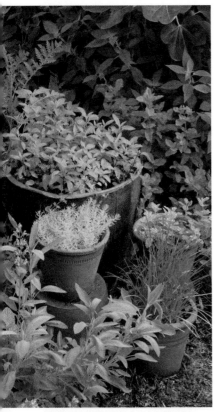

A wide selection of herbs, including sage, chives and apple mint, highlights their different shapes, textures and colors.

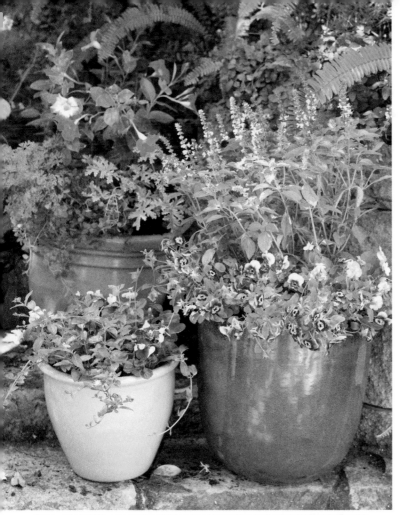

Stagger the heights of complementary pots or containers and underplant tall herbs with trailing plants that will spill over the edge of the pot.

Checklist for success

- **To reduce moisture loss,** apply a seal to porous pots. Or buy glazed ceramic pots, which are not as porous as untreated concrete, terracotta or limestone.

- **If moving pots** is a problem, buy fiberglass or polyethylene ones. They're lightweight and come in many different shapes, sizes and colors.

- **Sit your pots** on saucers to hold any excess water and to stop tile or surface staining. However, make sure you give the roots a chance to dry.

- **To raise pots** and make moving or sweeping easier, use static or movable stands on casters. Make sure pots are secure and won't move around on windy days.

- **Heavy or large containers** are the best choice in areas regularly exposed to strong winds, such as rooftop gardens and balconies.

- **Consider the scale:** A very large pot will look totally out of place squeezed onto a tiny balcony.

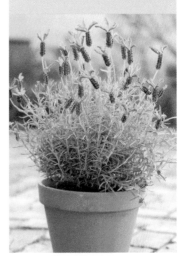

of good-looking, practical choices. Polyethylene and fiberglass (including marine grade) are most commonly used, as they're long-lasting, lightweight, waterproof and available in a wide range of colors. They can also be frost-, UV- and scratch-resistant. And, because these materials are not porous, they'll hold moisture longer than concrete or terracotta.

Experiment with unusual containers, such as old colanders and wicker baskets.

If your chosen pot has no drainage holes (many pots are designed for indoor use and don't have them), just drill a few of them into the base.

Potting mix ▶ One of the most important elements in growing herbs successfully is the right soil or planting mix. Potting mix is better than garden soil, as it's specially designed for container conditions and will provide just the right balance between holding water and providing good drainage. At your local nursery, you'll find various organic mixes that are tailored for different situations, such as hanging baskets.

The best products have a "standards" mark to indicate

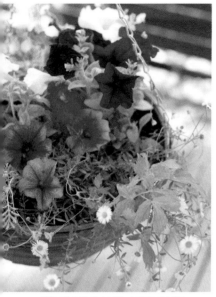

Vibrant petunias add a splash of color to thyme, lovage, chamomile and erigeron.

the potting mix contains extra ingredients, such as a wetting agent to stop it drying out too fast, vermiculite to keep the mix lightweight, and a slow-release fertilizer that gradually feeds the roots. The old adage "You get what you pay for" is true here: it is worth investing in a good quality mix as, over time, you'll have healthier, happier plants.

Feeding tips ▶ There are many fertilizers on the market. A good all-rounder that will suit most herbs is a "balanced" or "all-purpose" one: it will contain all the necessary nutrients to promote strong, healthy roots, flowers and leaves as well as help herbs grow into vigorous, sturdy plants. A soluble fertilizer is ideal for container-grown herbs and also for seedlings, which need to be fertilized regularly so that they will flourish. Always follow the directions on the packet.

If you notice that white 'salt' deposits (fertilizer residues) are appearing on the outside of terracotta pots, you can easily wash them off.

Add a liquid seaweed product to your watering regimen, as this is an excellent tonic. Apply it when you are first planting up pots and containers to help minimize transplant shock.

Watering ▶ While most herbs like to be kept moist, they also need to be allowed to dry out in between waterings so they're not left standing with constantly damp roots.

A good potting mix provides good drainage, while holes in the base of the pots allow the excess moisture to escape. Buy a colorful watering can that's easy to find, fill and carry. Keep it out of direct sun so that it lasts longer.

Hanging gardens ▶ You can also grow herbs in hanging baskets. Those that have a trailing habit, such as heartsease, thyme, mint and pelargonium, are ideal for hanging at eye level where you can easily see your plants maturing and enjoy their fragrance. If you hang baskets higher than eye level, you'll tend to forget about them.

Baskets are commonly made of plastic or wire. Line wire baskets with sphagnum moss, a spongy fibrous material that will hold the potting mix and retain moisture, or use a ready-made basket liner made from coconut fiber. Hanging baskets are prone to drying out in winds, so keep an eye on their moisture levels — another reason to hang them at the right height.

Repotting ▶ About every 12 months or so, give your potted herb garden a boost by repotting or replenishing it.

Discard annual herbs and start again. Remove perennial herbs carefully, compost the old potting mix, and refill the base of the pot with fresh mix. Then trim the roots of the plants if they look congested, and cut off any old stems to give the plant a tidier shape and to promote new growth. Replant them in the container and backfill with fresh mix, gently firming it as you go. Finally, water the herbs thoroughly.

Planting ideas

- **Decide** what you want to use your herbs for — for example, picking — and plant accordingly.

- **Choose** a theme when growing culinary herbs. Select hot and spicy herbs such as chillies and coriander for Mexican or Asian dishes; and dill, lemon balm, horseradish and oregano for fish dishes.

- **Plant** contrasting colors in the same pot. Try "Ruffles," the dark purple-leafed basil, on one side and fine-stemmed chives with mauve flowers on the other.

- **Try** bay trees to create a focal point against a wall or flanking a doorway. They have a lollipop shape that makes them perfect pot specimens.

- **Use** wine barrels for an earthy look. For a classical one, use decorated terracotta.

- **Pot** up culinary herbs, such as chives, rocket, parsley or basil, in a spot near the barbecue, and let your guests snip off their own herbs.

Planting an herbal strawberry pot

It's fun to plant up a strawberry pot with your favorite herbs and flowers.

Buy a few more herbs than you will actually need. Experiment with placement and combinations of herbs to get a look you like. Then get planting.

Always open bags of potting mix in a well-ventilated area. Avoid breathing in the dusty particles, and consider wearing a protective face mask.

You will need

- large terracotta strawberry pot
- selection of trailing herbs (we used variegated and common oregano, thyme and strawberry) and an upright plant (we used fan flower).
- bag of quality potting mix
- potting scoop or trowel
- small bag of coconut fiber (*optional*)

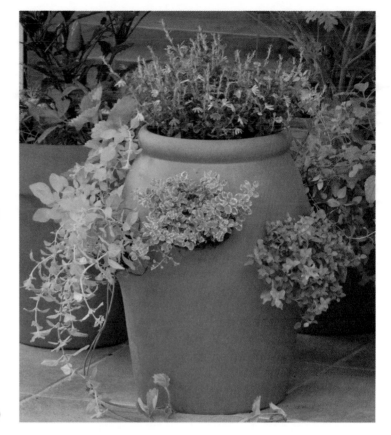

1. Fill the pot with potting mix until it comes to just beneath the level of the first hole.
2. Carefully remove the first herb from its container; tease the roots out so that the surrounding potting mix is loosened. Gently ease the roots into the lowest hole in the pot. Fill pot with more potting mix, gently firming the inside with your hand to ensure that the roots are covered. Add mix until you reach the level of the next hole. Plant until all holes are filled. To stop potting mix falling out the sides of the pot, tuck a small amount of coconut fiber around the edges of each hole.
3. Finish by creating an attractive centerpiece, tucking potting mix around its roots. This final plant doesn't have to be an herb. For a dash of color, you could use a flowering annual or perennial. We selected fan flower (*Scaevola aemula*), but any plant with an upright habit will help to balance the composition of the pot. Place your strawberry pot in a sunny spot, then water well.

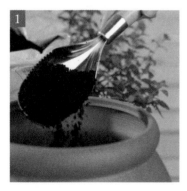

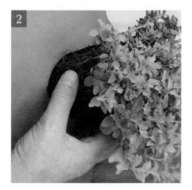

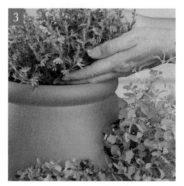

A world of herbs & spices

The extraordinary range of herbs and spices available to us today continues to expand, driven by consumer demand.

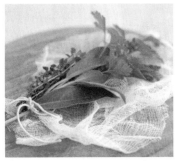

Bouquet garni, an herb mix used in classic French cuisine, includes parsley, bay and thyme.

A multitude of flavors

Can you imagine pasta sauces with no basil, Japanese food without wasabi or Mexican food minus the chilies? Creating authentic dishes from around the world has never been easier.

Asian herbs, in particular, have enjoyed a huge surge in popularity in recent years, and Thai basil, coriander, Vietnamese mint, perilla, kaffir lime leaves, lemongrass and turmeric are becoming easier to source. Also, the seasonings used in Africa, the Middle East, the Caribbean islands and Latin America are more readily available, and in Australia, native plants such as lemon myrtle and other "bush" herbs are being added to the cook's repertoire.

And it's not just the leaves that are used in recipes: flowers, seeds, stems and roots are also often included.

Balancing act

The recipes in this book give measures for the amount of herbs and spices to use, but you can vary them to suit your taste. One of the great bonuses of using herbs is that you'll find you can cut back on the amount of salt you add to your food. The herbs will be flavor enough!

One golden rule is to avoid allowing one flavor to dominate the others. Herb and spice mixes such as garam masala and ras el hanout are a delicate exercise in balancing a wide range of flavors. Even if you like a bit of heat, too much fresh chili can overwhelm the more subtle herbs and spices accompanying it. Very pungent herbs, such as fresh coriander, are not to everyone's taste, so a light hand is recommended.

You can always add more fresh herbs at the table. In Iranian and Vietnamese cooking, a bowl of fresh herbs is a standard appetizer or accompaniment. Similarly, the Lebanese offer a platter of fresh herbs and vegetables as part of a mezze table.

As a general rule, when cooking with herbs, the soft-leafed ones, such as coriander, are best added late in the cooking process to preserve their flavor. The coarser ones, such as rosemary, are ideal for dishes that require long, slow cooking. Dried herbs are usually more concentrated in flavor than fresh ones, so you will need less of them.

Fresh herbs

- Select vibrant, aromatic leaves with no signs of wilting or yellowing.
- Ideally, buy fresh herbs as and when you need them. However well you store them, they quickly deteriorate in flavor and appearance, particularly the soft-leafed varieties such as flat-leaf parsley, coriander and lovage. The coarser herbs, such as thyme and rosemary, are a little hardier.
- Store fresh herbs for no more than 3 or 4 days. Loosely wrap unwashed bunches in damp paper towels and store in an airtight container or sealed plastic bag in a cool place.
- Alternatively, stand the stems in a jug with a little water and loosely

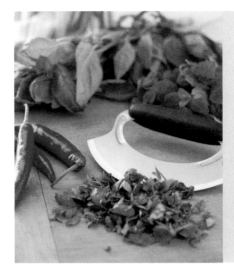

Get chopping!

Chop herbs with a mezzaluna (half-moon-shaped blade), a sharp knife or scissors. You can use a food processor for large bunches, but don't over-process them. Fine-leafed herbs can also be shredded by hand, but coarse herbs, such as rosemary, need fine chopping unless whole sprigs are appropriate for the recipe. Herbs such as basil, coriander and sage discolor if they are chopped too early before use.

cover the leaves with a plastic bag. Store in the refrigerator, changing the water daily.

• Or store the herbs in plastic bags and place them in the vegetable crisper of the refrigerator.

• Buy herbs sold in plastic boxes or cellophane bags — they keep well if stored in the refrigerator.

• Preserve chopped fresh herbs by freezing them in a little water in ice-cube trays.

• For more detailed information, see Harvesting, preserving and storing, *page 152*. Delicate herbs such as basil do not dry well, but more robust herbs such as thyme and rosemary retain their flavor well and are a convenient alternative to fresh.

• When you are ready to use them, wash herbs in a bowl of cold water rather than running water, which can bruise them. Pat them dry with paper towels.

Dried herbs and spices

While you may prefer the taste of herbs picked fresh from the garden, there is always a place for dried or frozen ones as well as for dried spices. In Greek cooking, for example,

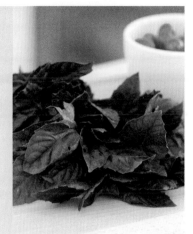

The must-haves

This selection of herbs and spices that you can grow yourself or buy is a useful culinary starting point. (If you enjoy making herbal teas, add chamomile, dandelion and lemon verbena.)

Basil, bay, chilies, chives, coriander, dill, garlic, ginger, lemongrass, lemon tree (it's an herb, too), lovage, marjoram or oregano, mint, parsley, rosemary, sage, tarragon, thyme and Vietnamese mint.

dried oregano (rigani) is used extensively in preference to fresh, while paprika, rather than fresh chilies, is an important ingredient in Hungarian food.

• Buy dried herbs and spices in small quantities to avoid waste, and store in airtight containers in a cool, dark place.

• Ignore the use-by date on commercial products, as the dried herb or spice may deteriorate long before the given date. The best way to check for freshness is by smell,

taste and appearance — for example, color fading is a good indicator of flavor loss.

• Whole spices, such as coriander and cumin seeds, retain their flavor and aroma longer than ground. Grind them in a spice grinder, or in a coffee-grinder kept specifically for the purpose, or use a mortar and pestle.

• Spices add color as well as flavor. Paprika adds a glorious red color, while saffron and turmeric transform a dish into a golden yellow.

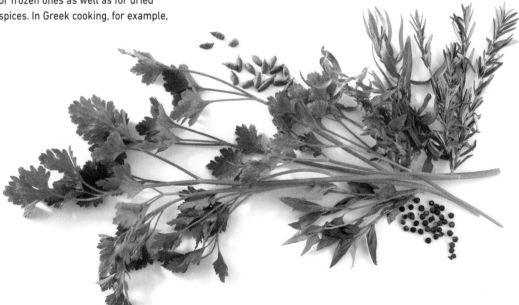

Harvesting, preserving & storing

Harvesting the flowers, leaves, seeds, roots and even bark of the herbs you've nurtured is one of gardening's true delights, and there's something just as special about gathering them in the wild. Follow our tips for collecting, preserving and storing herbs, as well as using them safely.

Safety

At best, mistaking the identity of a plant or using the wrong part could mean that your herbal remedy is ineffective, but at worst you could make yourself or someone else very ill by accidentally collecting a plant that's toxic.

Identification ▶ From a safety standpoint, there's nothing more important than ensuring that you only harvest an herb if you are confident you know what it is. This is reasonably straightforward in your own garden, but can get tricky if you're collecting plants you haven't planted yourself.

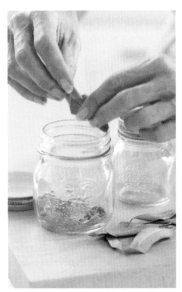
Dried leaves should be brittle and easily snap in your fingers. Store them in an airtight glass jar.

Once plants are dried, it becomes even more difficult to tell them apart, so harvest and dry only one herb at a time to prevent different batches of plants getting mixed up, and always tag or label them immediately, so they're easy to identify.

Use the correct part ▶ The chemical characteristics of different parts of each plant vary, and consequently have different effects on the body. For example, just as coriander leaves and seeds each bring different characteristics to a recipe, so too do the leaves and roots of the dandelion plant have different medicinal actions.

Before harvesting a plant for culinary or medicinal reasons, double-check which part of the plant you need to use. Once again, making a mistake could have dire consequences — for example, bark from the shrub called cramp bark (*Viburnum opulus*) is a very useful medicine, but the berries from the same plant are toxic and should not be eaten.

Harvesting and drying herbs

Freshly cut herbs add extra zing to your cooking and boost the refreshing flavor of herbal teas (see Infusions, *page 164*). But most of the time, you'll want to dry your herbal harvest so it's on hand to use when needed — regardless of the season.

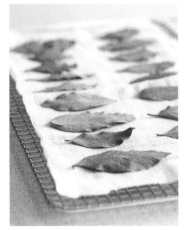
A cake rack is perfect for drying leaves.

Stored in labeled glass jars, in a cool dark spot, most dried herbs will keep for about a year. For more information on the best time and way to harvest specific herbs, consult the Herb Directory, *pages 8–131*.

Leaves ▶ The best time to collect leaves is on a dry, sunny morning before flowering has started. Choose a time after the dew has evaporated, but before the sun gets too hot and starts causing the essential oils in the plant to evaporate.

Use gardening scissors or pruning shears to snip sprigs or stems of young, healthy leaves, or gently pluck individual leaves from the plant by hand. Remove any dirt by gently brushing the leaves, but don't wash them in water. Discard any leaves that look diseased or damaged.

If you've collected sprigs of leaves, strip the lower leaves from each stem, tie the stems together and hang the bunches upside down. Spread individual leaves out to dry — a cake rack covered with kitchen paper is ideal.

Keep the leaves in a warm, airy place away from sunlight, and check them every day or so until they have completely dried.

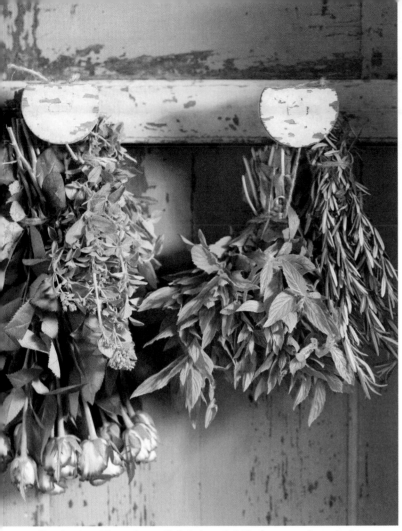
Hang bunches of flower stems, with their stems straight, where warm air can circulate around them.

Equipment checklist

Most of the equipment you'll need for harvesting herbs are everyday household items.

- **Sharp scissors, shears or garden knife** Help prevent damage to the plant by always using a sharp blade.

- **Gloves** Protect your hands from thorns, bristles and allergic reactions by wearing good-quality gardening gloves.

- **Basket** If possible, gather herbs in a tray or flat shallow basket, so you can spread out the samples, rather than pile them up. Avoid using bags or sacks that limit airflow or allow separate bunches of herbs to mingle.

- **Gardening fork** When digging up roots, use a gardening fork, not a spade or shovel, as it is less likely to damage the plant.

- **String** Tie bunches of herbs together with string.

- **Labels** The sooner you label your cut or dried herbs, the less likely you are to forget what they are.

- **Paper bags** Use paper bags for collecting seeds, and remember to label their contents as you go.

- **Rack or tray** Herbs dry best when there is good airflow around them, so a cake rack is perfect. You could also stretch mesh or netting over a frame.

- **Glass jars** Glass is airtight and moisture-proof, so it's perfect for storing dried herbs. If you notice condensation building up in the jar, the herbs may not be completely dry – remove them and allow them to dry further before storing.

Flowers ▶ Collect flowers shortly after the buds have opened and well before they start losing their petals. Flowers that grow in clusters — for example, elder flowers, angelica and meadowsweet — and those with long stalks, such as lavender and roses, can be picked on the stem, but it's preferable to collect individual flower heads of others, such as calendula blooms.

To dry flowers, follow the instructions for leaves (see opposite) and hang bunches of flowers or spread individual flower heads in a place where there is plenty of warm air circulating over a period of a few weeks. Flowers contain high levels of moisture, so to prevent mold from forming, make sure the petals aren't overlapping on the tray. Once the flowers are completely dried, they should feel stiff, not limp.

Store dried flower heads in a dark glass jar, or use in a potpourri. And once you remove flowers from dried stems, also store them in dark jars before they deteriorate.

Collecting wild herbs

Wandering fields, forests and footpaths as you collect wild herbs sounds rather romantic, but there are several important issues to be aware of before you start.

- **Identification** Identifying plants is a difficult skill, and even trained experts can make mistakes. Always carry a plant guide as a reference, and check both the photographs and the written description against each herb. If you are doubtful of a plant's identity, don't pick it. Prevent different plants from becoming jumbled or difficult to identify later by tying the samples into bundles and labeling them as you harvest. Make sure you collect the correct medicinal part of the plant, too.

- **Pollution** Many plants that seem to be growing in the clean, green countryside are actually exposed to large quantities of pollution, which can accumulate in their tissues and be passed on to those who consume them. Be aware that, in farming districts, agricultural chemicals are often sprayed on crops, and may drift to adjacent areas. Plants growing by the side of busy roads are constantly exposed to exhaust fumes. Even a patch of healthy-looking herbs that you discover in a country lane may have been sprayed with weedkiller just moments before you arrived. Wherever possible, gather information about any chemicals used in the area before you start collecting herbs, and always wash them thoroughly before using them.

- **Legalities** In some countries, it is illegal to collect plants without first seeking permission from the landowner. You'll also be in trouble if you harvest herbs in a national park, or if you gather plants that are endangered.

- **Ecology** Over-harvesting of wild crops of some medicinal herbs has resulted in them becoming endangered. The classic example is the North American herb goldenseal, which has a deserved reputation as a potent antimicrobial remedy. Unfortunately, golden seal is a difficult plant to cultivate, but is one of the most popular medicinal herbs in America. Over many years, this has led to an extremely lucrative market for wild-harvested (or 'wildcrafted') golden seal root, and consequently the plant is far less prevalent now than it was in days gone by; its trade is now strictly controlled. You can play your part in protecting our herbal heritage by finding out which, if any, plants are endangered in your own local area, and leaving them behind. Even when plants are plentiful, it's good practice to harvest only what you can use immediately, and to leave at least a third of each plant behind to regenerate.

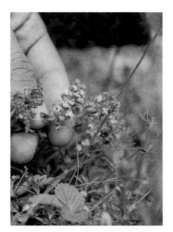

Always be sure to identify any herb you are going to pick.

Seeds ► When collecting seeds, the timing is vital. Harvest them in late summer in the short period between the ripening of the seed pod and the point when it bursts open to disperse the seeds into the air.

Keep a close eye on the plant, and when you judge that the seed pod is starting to ripen (its color will start changing from green to brown), cut the seed pods from the plant, taking plenty of the stem at the same time.

Gather the stems in a loose bunch, place the ends with the seed pods on them inside a brown paper bag, and use string to tie the opening of the bag around the stems. Hang the bag containing the herb in a warm, airy spot. As the seed pods ripen over the following week or two, the seeds will be released into the bag for you to collect. When the stems are dry, scrape any seeds still attached to the seed pods into the paper bag.

If you're going to use the seeds for planting, you can keep them in the same bag, as long as you tape it shut and clearly label the bag with the plant name and the date on which it was harvested. If you're using seeds for culinary or medicinal purposes, they will have a stronger flavor if you store them in glass, but again, make sure you label each one appropriately. Avoid storing seeds in plastic bags, because they allow moisture to build up and can cause mold to develop.

Roots and rhizomes ► Harvesting roots and rhizomes in autumn or winter maximizes the plant's ability to regenerate itself. Choose a time when the parts of the plant above the ground are starting to die back. That will also make it easier to identify them.

Using a gardening fork, dig out the whole plant and its roots. Carefully separate the portion of the root that you want to use, and replant the rest immediately.

Gently brush as much dirt as possible from the root. To clean more substantial roots and rhizomes, such as ginger and horseradish, scrub them with a vegetable brush; however, gently rinse finer and more delicate samples, such as valerian, under running water. Don't soak them, or they'll take up water and lose flavor, and perhaps develop rot.

Once the roots are clean, cut them into small pieces and dry them in the oven at a very low heat (120°F to 140°F or 50°C to 60°C). You may need to keep the oven door ajar to prevent the temperature from rising too much. Turn the root pieces regularly to ensure they dry out evenly; you'll know they're ready when they become brittle.

Allow the roots to cool before storing them in a dark glass jar.

Bark ▶ It's easy to kill or injure a tree when collecting its bark, so in many cases it's better to use commercially harvested varieties of these herbs. If you do decide to collect bark yourself, choose a damp day, and use clean, sharp tools to remove it from the tree in vertical strips at least a metre above the ground. Never take a horizontal band of bark from trees or collect bark from saplings, or they will die.

Clean the bark to remove any dirt, and then flatten it out as much as you can before leaving it in a warm, airy place to dry for a few weeks.

Freezing herbs

Although freezing herbs isn't suitable for those you are going to use medicinally, it is ideal for culinary herbs with very fine leaves or a very high moisture content, and for those that lose their taste when dried. Freezing herbs is a great way to retain their color and flavor. Good candidates include fennel and dill tips, tarragon, chives, parsley, chervil and basil.

For herbs you intend to use in small quantities or add to wet dishes, such as soups, casseroles and risotto, freezing herbs into ice cubes works perfectly. Rinse fresh herbs under cold running water before chopping them finely. Place a tablespoonful of the chopped herb into each segment of an ice-cube tray, add a little water, and then place the tray in the freezer. When the cubes are frozen, transfer them into a labeled plastic bag or container and they'll keep for months.

Freeze whole bunches of herbs to use in larger quantities or in recipes that won't benefit from the extra water of the melted ice. After rinsing the herbs, pat them dry with a paper towel and tie them loosely together. Place the whole bunch inside a sealed and labeled plastic bag and store it in the freezer. The frozen herbs will become quite brittle, so before you use them, just scrunch the bag with your hand to break the leaves into pieces.

Buying dried herbs

A wider variety of herbs than you could ever hope to dry or harvest yourself is available at your local health-food store. The more popular herbs are available in teabags, but while convenient, these sometimes contain a lower grade of herbal material, and tend to be more expensive by weight than loose herbs. Look for dried herbs that retain the color and shape of the plant and have a strong, pleasant scent. Reject those that are dusty, powdery or have little smell.

Freeze whole mint leaves or borage flowers in ice cubes and use them in fruit juices and cocktails.

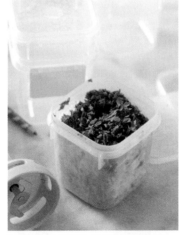

Another way to store chopped herbs is to freeze a large quantity in a small plastic container.

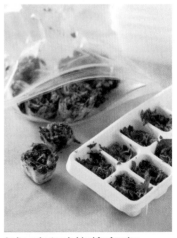

An ice-cube tray is ideal for freezing small quantities of herbs you tend to use sparingly.

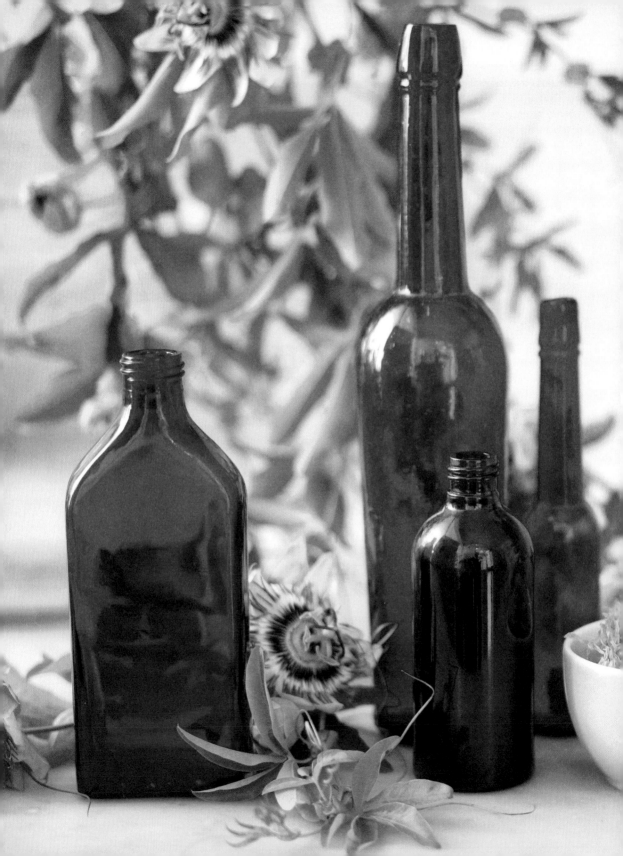

Herbal medicine

Treating common ailments and conditions safely and effectively with herbs is an area of growing interest as well as the focus of research around the world. Find out which herbs have healing properties and learn the best ways to use them.

Western herbal philosophy

The style of herbal medicine currently practiced in the Western world has its roots in the traditions of Europe and North America, but it has also adopted some key remedies from Africa and South America as well as from the practice of Chinese and Ayurvedic medicine.

Returning the body to balance

At its heart, Western herbal medicine retains some of the philosophies espoused by the Greek physician Hippocrates and his contemporaries more than 2,000 years ago. These teachings included the principle that a patient's diet, environment and mental state all contributed to his or her well-being.

Today's Western herbalists take a similar holistic approach to healthcare, prescribing dietary and other lifestyle changes as well as herbal remedies, based on the principle that the factors that contribute to ill health need to be removed in order for healing to occur.

This is an extension of their view that the body often repairs itself when provided with the optimal conditions in which to do so — another concept associated with the Hippocratic tradition, which taught the *vis medicatrix naturae*, or innate, self-healing capacity of the human body.

In many ways, this goal of returning the body to a state of balance is central to every decision the herbalist makes in treatment. Whereas the medical approach largely focuses on fighting disease and pathology, the Western herbalist mainly works toward optimizing the function of the organs and body systems so that the body can heal itself.

Of course, in all acute and serious conditions, medical intervention is entirely appropriate. The specific, targeted, disease-fighting approach is exactly what's required when dealing with dangerously high blood pressure, a life-threatening infection, a burst appendix or an anaphylactic allergic reaction — all of which require drastic and fast-acting treatment.

Gentle treatment for chronic health problems

On the other hand, herbs are often appropriate for chronic disease states, which develop over a longer period, and whose symptoms may be less well defined. These conditions are commonly linked with unhealthy dietary and lifestyle habits, and they often respond well to slower-acting, gentler herbal remedies — especially if healthier habits are adopted at the same time. By addressing these chronic states of ill-health, herbs may help prevent some conditions developing into more serious diseases that require acute intervention; in fact, disease prevention is often an important goal of treatment.

Digestive system

In order to restore the body to a state of balance, the Western herbalist considers the functioning of each of the body's major organs and body systems. Of central importance are the digestive system and the organs

Native American herbalism

It is said that when the Pilgrims arrived in North America, fewer than 90 diseases were known among Native American people, whose extraordinary fitness and vitality was noticed by European doctors in early Colonial days.

Native American healers were highly respected and played a valuable role in the physical and spiritual well-being of their society. They also had a rich herbal tradition on which to draw when treating illness or injury, and for midwifery and contraceptive purposes.

Today many of the remedies found in the Western herbalist's dispensary – including the very popular herbs echinacea (below), golden seal and black cohosh – were first introduced to settlers by the Native Americans.

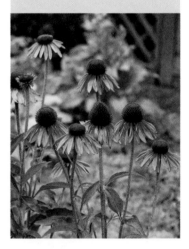

"Cure sometimes, treat often, comfort always."

Hippocrates, c. 460–c. 370 bce

of elimination: optimizing their ability to assimilate nutrients and process the bodily wastes is a major focus of many treatment protocols.

The herbalist may also prescribe remedies that:

- help the patient cope better with stress by either building up or calming down the nervous system;
- enhance resistance to infection or allergy by supporting the patient's immune system;
- normalize hormonal balance, relieving the symptoms of menopause or premenstrual syndrome and, where it is appropriate, priming the body for conception;
- relieve pain and inflammation; and
- support heart and blood vessel function.

Individualized care

Before determining an appropriate treatment, the herbalist considers each patient's individual circumstances and constitution. For example, in formulating a prescription for supporting weight loss, the herbalist may take into account factors such as the patient's bowel habits, energy levels, hormonal status and ability to cope with stress. This individualized approach to treatment — "treating the person, not the disease" — is the opposite of the "one size fits all" approach that can be characteristic of the medical or pharmaceutical model.

Combining science and tradition

To achieve these aims, the modern practice of Western herbal medicine, which is mainly based on the traditional practices of Europe and North America, has adopted an eclectic group of key remedies from Africa and South America as well as from traditional Chinese and Ayurvedic medicine.

Clinical trials

However, unlike Chinese and Ayurvedic herbalism modern Western herbalism does not incorporate a humoral or "elemental" approach to disease. For that reason, the herbal remedies the Western herbalist borrows from other traditions are rarely used in their original context.

The Western herbalist prescribing dan shen (*Salvia miltiorrhiza*), for example, is likely to be thinking of its clinically proven actions in angina and other heart problems, rather than its traditional Chinese attributes as a cooling herb.

In fact, Western herbalists are increasingly turning to scientific evidence such as this to validate their traditional knowledge. Notwithstanding that the scientific study of herbal medicines has to overcome a unique set of challenges, the double-blind, placebo-controlled, randomized clinical trial has become the gold standard of herbal medicine research — just as it is in medical science.

Given that relatively few herbs have been subjected to any scientific scrutiny, a prescription from your Western medical herbalist is likely to combine remedies that have been clinically proven with others whose use is based on traditional experience. In many cases, five or six different herbs — or more — are blended in one prescription.

Synergy

The prescription of combinations of remedies demonstrates the

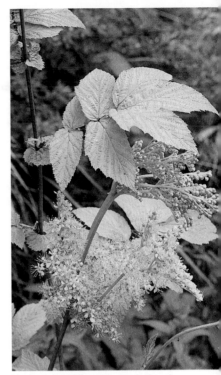

Meadowsweet (*Filipendula ulmaria 'Aurea'*)

herbalists' belief in synergy — the concept that different botanical medicines work together to produce an effect that is greater than any of the individual remedies acting alone.

Synergy also applies to the compounds within a plant, with Western herbalists believing that the whole remedy provides a safer, more effective medicine than its individual active constituents.

For example, aspirin, a salicylic acid compound originally derived from meadowsweet, sometimes causes side effects of gastric bleeding, whereas the herb in its entirety does not, and even seems to offer some protection from the gastric irritation caused by salicylates.

Eastern herbal philosophy

The ancient practices of traditional Chinese and Ayurvedic herbal medicine, both holistic approaches to healing, are based on the principle of humors or elements and focus on creating internal harmony or balance in the body.

An ancient tradition with spiritual roots

Chinese herbalism has a history that can be traced back thousands of years. The most famous of Chinese herb books, *The Yellow Emperor's Inner Classic (or Huang Di Nei Jing)*, may have been written in about 100 BCE, but its origins are even older: the emperor for whom it was named ruled from 2,698 to 2,596 BCE.

Since then, Chinese scholars have continued to document this complex and sophisticated method of healing, and traditional Chinese medicine continues to thrive today in mainland China, in other Chinese communities throughout Asia, and increasingly in the Western world.

The philosophy of traditional Chinese medicine (TCM) has its basis in the spiritual practice of Taoism (sometimes spelt Daoism), which teaches that human beings should strive to live in accordance with the rules of nature and emphasise the importance of balance and harmony. In keeping with the Tao teachings, the goal of all healing in TCM is to restore internal harmony.

This philosophy of returning the body to a state of balance in order to bring about healing is not unique to TCM — in fact, it is also central to the philosophies of Western herbalism and Ayurveda. But the methods used to achieve this aim in TCM are unique, and the concepts and practices involved can be quite difficult for Westerners to grasp, especially as they encompass not only herbal medicine, but also acupuncture, massage, diet therapy and healing exercises, such as *qi gong*.

The life force

The Chinese use the word *qi* (sometimes Westernized as chi or ki) to refer to the life force that inhabits not only the human body, but also all aspects of the environment and everything in it. *Qi* is a moving energy, sometimes defined as 'breath' or 'air,' which also has many characteristics of fluids.

In the human body, *qi* is believed to flow along channels called meridians. These are not physical anatomical structures like the blood vessels, but nevertheless TCM practitioners can identify their locations with pinpoint accuracy so they can insert acupuncture needles in any one of over 500 individual points, affecting the flow of *qi* through the body.

Yin and yang

Another important concept in TCM is that of yin and yang, two opposite but complementary qualities that can be attributed to all things. The familiar circular symbol made up of black and white tear-drop shapes, each containing a small piece of the opposing color, is called the *taijitu*. It represents the dichotomy of yin and yang by illustrating that any two opposites are dependent on each other, and cannot exist in isolation — each requires the other in order to make up the whole.

Yin is represented by the black segments of the *taijitu*. It is characterized as feminine, passive, dark, cooling and associated with night. Yang is depicted in white in the *taijitu*, and has active, masculine qualities associated with heat, lightness and daytime.

A state of harmony exists in the body when yin and yang are balanced, but a relative excess of one quality (and the consequent deficiency of the other) causes an imbalance that can lead to illness and disease. Herbs and foods are classified according to how yin or yang they are, and the

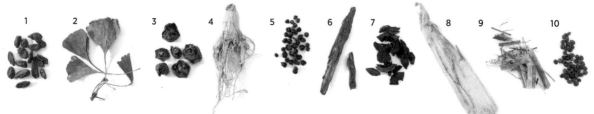

1. Boxthorn (*Lycium barbarum*) 2. Ginkgo (*Ginkgo biloba*) 3. Chinese haw (*Crataegus pinnatifida*) 4. Ginseng (*Panax ginseng*) 5. Schisandra (*Schisandra chinensis*) 6. Dan shen (*Salvia miltiorrhiza*) 7. Bitter orange (*Citrus aurantium*) 8. Dong quai (*Angelica polymorpha* var. *sinensis*) 9. Qing hao (*Artemisia annua*) 10. Chinese date (*Ziziphus jujuba*)

effects they have on the body, and these qualities are an important consideration in helping to restore harmony and health.

The five elements

Like several other ancient systems of medicine, TCM is based on a theory of elements or humors. Each of TCM's five elements or "phases" — in reference to their cyclical nature — has different qualities, governs different bodily functions and can be influenced by different medicines and foods, with the taste of each medicine giving insight into which element or elements it affects. In addition, each of the elements — fire, earth, metal, water and wood — interacts with and influences the others in many ways.

Visiting a TCM practitioner

A TCM practitioner uses tongue, facial and pulse diagnosis, as well as your description of your symptoms, to determine whether there is an imbalance in the five elements, in the yin and yang of the body, or the flow of qi. The terms used can be quite bewildering to a Westerner, who might be puzzled to hear their practitioner make a diagnosis of spleen qi deficiency when they came for a consultation about their persistent headaches!

Depending on your individual needs, your practitioner is likely to prescribe herbs for you, and sometimes also a course of acupuncture. Chinese herbal formulas often contain numerous herbs, which are boiled together for up to an hour to make a traditional decoction that concentrates the herbs' flavors and medicinal actions. The full course of your treatment may be dispensed to you in a series of paper packets, each containing your daily dose.

Ayurvedic medicine

Ayurveda, a traditional healing system from India, is an ancient holistic health practice with many similarities to traditional Chinese medicine (TCM). As with TCM, the aim of Ayurvedic medicine is to bring the body into balance. This is achieved through dietary change, the prescription of herbal medicines and also through meditation and yoga. "Ayurveda" is a Sanskrit word that literally means "the science of living," reflecting the principle that an individual's health is their own responsibility and that the physician can only guide their patients.

Again, like TCM, Ayurveda is based on a humoral philosophy, but there are three elements, called doshas, rather than five. You have all three of them in different proportions, and your constitution partly determines the ratio of each, but they are also affected by diet, climate and other lifestyle factors. Your doshas dictate your personality, the nature of the illnesses you experience and the types of food, herbal medicine and exercise that are best suited to you.

As with TCM, each of the doshas can be influenced by the tastes of the food and medicines you consume.

- Vata governs movement of the body and mind, and the functioning of the circulation, nerves, muscles and bones. It is associated with dryness, cold and wind. When vata is low, it can be stimulated by bitter, astringent and pungent tastes, while sour, sweet and salty tastes help bring it into balance.

- Pitta governs the power of trans-formation, such as the conversion of food into energy, and has moist, hot qualities. Associated with focus and concentration, it is stimulated by salty, sour, pungent tastes; sweet, bitter, astringent tastes reduce excess pitta.

- Kapha is binding, provides structure to the body and governs lubrication — for example, keeping the joints from getting stiff. Its qualities are earthy, watery and cold. Kapha is stimulated by sweet, salty and sour tastes, and suppressed by pungent, bitter and astringent flavors.

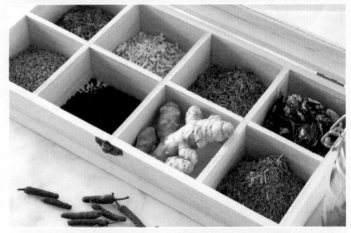

1. Fenugreek (*Trigonella foenum-graecum*) 2. Gymnema sylvestre 3. Nigella (*Nigella sativa*) 4. Winter cherry (*Withania somnifera*) 5. Turmeric (*Curcuma longa*) 6. Brahmi (*Bacopa monnieri*) 7. Gotu kola (*Centella asiatica*) 8. Tamarind (*Tamarindus indica*)

Using herbs safely

It's easy to fall into the trap of thinking that because herbs are natural they're also safe, but there are some important cautions you should be aware of. Always seek professional help if you suffer from a serious illness or severe symptoms, or if you are pregnant or breastfeeding, and if you're harvesting plants yourself, make sure you indentify the plant correctly. Finally, take care to choose a reputable professional herbalist.

Take the correct dose

The active constituents in herbs have the power to affect the physiological functioning of your body — some have a gentle impact while others are extremely potent medicines. As a rule of thumb, the stronger the action of the herb, the lower the dose required to cause a physical effect: Some herbs are so potent they are prescribed only in infinitesimal doses, because higher intakes are likely to cause serious adverse effects.

Our understanding of an appropriate dose for each herb is largely based on traditional and historical knowledge accumulated over hundreds of years and supplemented over recent times with a growing body of scientific study.

Always follow the dosage instructions, and do not exceed recommended doses or take a particular herb if there is a caution against its use in your circumstances. Seek professional advice before taking any herb over an extended period of time. In the majority of cases it is wise to seek professional advice before treating children or babies with herbs, because different doses may be required, depending on the child's age or condition. It is also important to keep herbal medicines safely out of the reach of children.

Identify the plant correctly

Identifying the correct herb to take as a medicine is not always easy, especially if you are harvesting plants yourself rather than buying commercially produced remedies. Plants that look alike sometimes have very different chemical makeups, and some plants from the same family have vastly different medicinal effects.

There are also many instances where the same common name is applied to several different species — for example, at least five different plants are referred to by the common name of balm of Gilead, making it very confusing, as well as potentially dangerous, for the amateur herbalist.

Herbalists overcome these problems by referring to plants by their botanical (Latin) names. This system of naming was developed by Linnaeus, the 18th-century Swedish botanist. The first word of a plant's botanical name refers to its genus — for example, all mint plants fall into the *Mentha* genus. The second word of the name refers to the plant's species, so the plant we commonly refer to as spearmint is named *Mentha spicata*.

Don't harvest or consume a plant if you have any doubt at all about its identity. Check which part of the plant to use before you harvest it, too — there is absolutely no point in collecting the leaves of a particular herb if the medicinal constituents are only present in the roots!

Avoid adverse effects

Even when they're taken at appropriate doses, both herbal and pharmaceutical medicines can sometimes cause adverse effects, which generally fall into one of three categories.

● **Side effects** are symptoms or physiological changes that can be predicted to occur in a percentage of all users of a particular medicine.

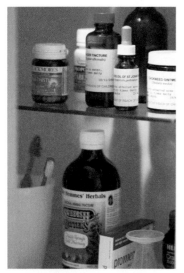

Like pharmaceutical medicines, herbal medicines should always be kept out of children's reach.

For example, herbalists can anticipate that a small number of patients who take valerian will report having vivid dreams, and similarly some that patients who take licorice will experience an increase in blood pressure. (Important side effects are listed on the relevant pages of this book.)

- **Drug interactions** may occur when a patient is taking two or more medicines simultaneously. For example, it is well documented that the herb St. John's wort interacts with numerous pharmaceuticals, reducing the efficacy of the drugs. Given the vast number of potential interactions between herbs and drugs, and between herbs and other herbs, not all of these types of adverse effects are predictable, while others are well documented. The Conditions section of this book, *pages 174–212*, details major potential drug interactions where appropriate, but should not be considered an exhaustive reference on this important issue. If you are taking pharmaceutical medications, talk to your pharmacist or doctor before adding herbs to your treatment regimen, even if you are using them to treat a different condition.

- **Allergies** occur when the immune system overreacts to a substance that is otherwise innocuous, and can range from minor inconveniences to severe, life-threatening problems. Some herbs are more likely to cause allergies than others; however, the real reason that allergies are unpredictable is that the underlying issue is in the patient's immune system, rather than the plant itself. If you are prone to allergies, take care with herbal medicines just as you would with other substances, and

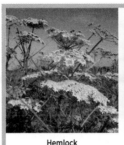
Hemlock
(*Conium maculatum*)

Mandrake
(*Mandragora officinarum*)

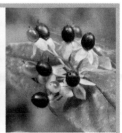
Belladonna
(*Atropa belladonna*)

Deadly Herbs

- **Hemlock** The Greek philosopher Socrates (c. 469–399 BCE) was found guilty of corrupting the youth of Athens and sentenced to death, so, according to Athenian law, he drank a cup of the poison hemlock. His student Plato recorded the effects of the poison, which started as a heavy sensation in Socrates's legs, gradually turning into a paralysis that crept up his body until his heart stopped beating.

- **Mandrake** The root of the hallucinogenic poisonous plant mandrake (*Mandragora officinarum*) is shaped like a crude impression of a person, and has been associated with magical qualities since biblical times. As

Harry Potter and friends learned in J. K. Rowling's *Harry Potter and the Chamber of Secrets*, legend has it that, when the root is unearthed, it emits such an ear-piercing shriek that anyone hearing it dies instantly.

- **Belladonna** In spite of its attractive, glossy black berries, belladonna is both poisonous and hallucinogenic. Also known as deadly nightshade, its common name (bella donna, or "beautiful woman" in Italian) derives from its former cosmetic use, dilating women's pupils to make them more attractive; however, prolonged use led to blindness. It was also believed to be used by witches in "flying ointments."

always patch-test topical remedies before using them.

If you develop any symptoms that could be due to an herb you are taking, stop using it immediately and, if necessary, seek medical treatment.

Choose a trained herbalist

Make sure you consult an herbalist who is appropriately trained. Do not be afraid to ask about their qualifications, whether they are a member of any professional associations, how long they've been practicing, or about the type of public liability insurance they carry. The

answers to these questions may depend to a certain extent on the legal status of herbal medicine in your country, but should give you an indication of the professionalism and experience of the practitioner.

It is also important to have a good rapport with your herbalist, just as you have with your doctor, so assess whether you feel comfortable and confident with them. For this reason, many people prefer to seek a referral to an herbalist. If no one you know and trust can recommend a local practitioner, ask your local health-food store proprietor or pharmacist.

Medicinal preparations

It's rewarding to make your own herbal medicines. Follow these step-by-step instructions to ensure you achieve the best results.

Infusions, decoctions, tinctures and syrups can all be prepared for internal use, while infused oils, compresses or poultices are more appropriate for topical applications. Some active constituents in herbs are readily soluble in water, while others require a more vigorous extraction process that involves alcohol.

Infusions

The word "infusion" is used to describe an herbal tea or tisane that is made by pouring boiling water over a quantity of fresh or dried herbal material. Every time you make a cup of tea with a tea bag, you are, in fact, making an infusion.

An infusion is an effective preparation method for delicate or fine plant parts, such as petals, leaves and other aerial parts. It is ideally suited to extracting water-soluble components from the plant and is often used for aromatic herbs that contain essential oils (such as peppermint, fennel and chamomile).

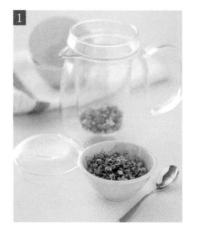

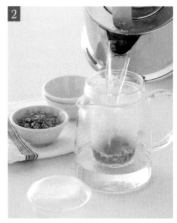

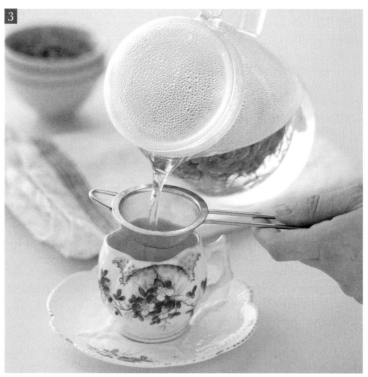

1 Place the recommended quantity of loose dried herb (dried chamomile is used here) or finely chopped fresh herb into a pre-warmed glass or china teapot or coffee plunger.

2 Pour about 1 cup (237 ml) freshly boiled water over the herb and stir. Place the lid on the teapot to trap the steam and prevent the essential oil evaporating. Allow the mixture to steep for 10 to 15 minutes.

3 Stir again before pouring through a strainer into your teacup.

Usage Drink one cup of tea three times a day over several weeks for chronic (longstanding) problems, or up to 6 cups a day in the shorter term for acute problems.

Storage Infusions do not store well, so it's always best to prepare a fresh pot of tea for each cup.

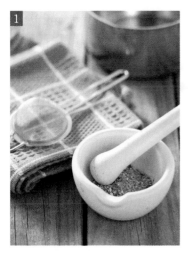

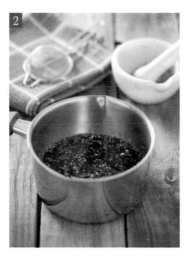

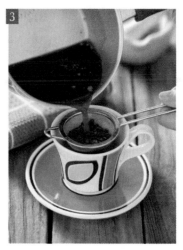

Decoctions

A decoction is an herbal tea made by boiling an herb in water. This method is most suitable for the woodier parts of a plant — such as the bark, roots, twigs and seeds — and is used to extract as many of the water-soluble active constituents as possible.

1 Grind the required quantity of dried herb (dried dandelion root is used here) into a coarse powder.

2 In a saucepan, cover the powder with about 2 cups (500 ml) cold (not hot) water; stir. Bring water slowly to the boil. Reduce heat to low and, with the lid still on, simmer for 10 to 15 minutes. (If your stovetop doesn't have a sufficiently low heat setting, use a double boiler.)

3 Stir again before pouring through a strainer into a teacup.

Usage Drink one cup three times a day over several weeks for chronic (longstanding) problems, or up to six cups a day in the shorter term for acute ones.

Storage Decoctions keep for a maximum of 3 days in the refrigerator. If you have the time, it's preferable to make a fresh decoction for each dose.

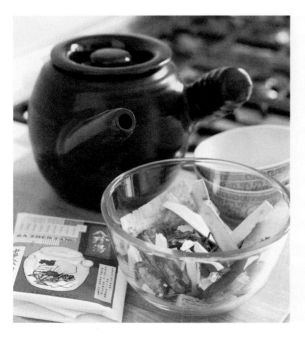

Chinese decoctions

Decoctions are revered by Chinese herbalists for their therapeutic effects and their versatility. They enable the herbalist to tailor remedies to the patient's needs, and allow the treatment to be amended as the patient's condition changes in response to the medicine.

The Chinese herbalist or pharmacist consults with the patient and determines the appropriate remedies to include in the prescription — the number of herbal ingredients (and their doses) is often larger than those used by Western herbalists.

Each daily dose of herbs is dispensed into a separate bag for the patient to prepare at home. The amount of water required, the boiling time and the quantity and frequency of medicine to be consumed may all vary.

Traditionally, ceramic clay pots with lids are used for Chinese decoctions, because chemical interactions can occur when herbs are exposed to metals such as iron, aluminium or copper.

Tinctures

Many of the active constituents in herbal medicines are readily soluble in alcohol, which is also an effective preservative. For this reason, professional herbalists use alcohol-based liquid herbal medicines to prescribe and dispense individualized herbal medicines for their patients.

For professional use, liquid extracts of herbs are made with a high concentration of pharmaceutical-grade alcohol (ethanol). Typically, 1 part of the herb is extracted in either 1 or 2 parts of alcohol.

Less concentrated preparations called tinctures are used for herbs that have a stronger taste (such as ginger or cayenne), and for those that are safest in very low doses (such as wormwood).

The recipes featured here use vodka in place of ethanol and a standard ratio of 1 part herb to 4 parts vodka. Note that while homemade remedies are often not as potent as the professional-strength remedies dispensed by an herbalist, they are still strong medicines and contain alcohol. Always store

tinctures in a safe place, out of reach of children, and always observe the dosage guidelines, taking care that they are not consumed in situations where alcohol intake is ill advised.

Herbal tinctures are suitable for nearly every plant and every plant part, with the exception of mucilage-containing herbs (such as marsh mallow root and slippery elm bark), which are better extracted in cold water.

Different methods are used to make tinctures from dried or woody herbs, or more delicate fresh herbs.

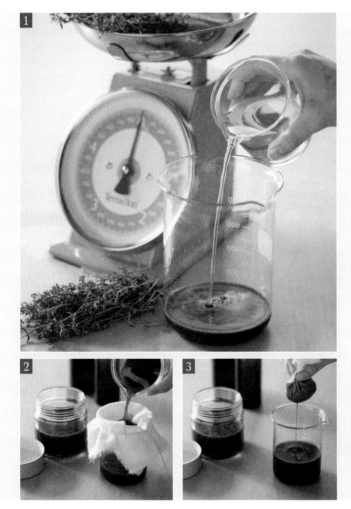

Fresh plant tincture

Use a kitchen scale to measure out 1.5 oz. (40 g) fresh herb (thyme is used here), then wash it carefully to remove any dirt. Chop the herb into small pieces, then blend to a pulp using a stick blender (add some water to aid the blending, if necessary). If you don't have a stick blender, chop the herb very finely.

1 Add ⅔ cup (160 ml) vodka to the pulped herb, and then blend again before pouring the mixture into a glass jar with a screw-top lid. Seal the bottle tightly and shake vigorously.

2 Store the bottle in a cool, dark place for 10 to 14 days, shaking it once or twice a day. Strain the mixture through a piece of fine muslin.

3 Squeeze as much moisture as possible from the remaining pulp. Pour into a dark glass bottle, seal and label with the name of the herb and the date on which you prepared the tincture. Makes about ¾ cup (200 ml).

Usage Using a dropper, dispense the required dose into ¼ cup (60 ml) water before drinking (this is usually taken three times daily).

Storage Refrigerate and store for 6 to 12 months. Make sure it is stored safely out of reach of children.

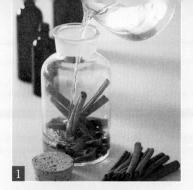
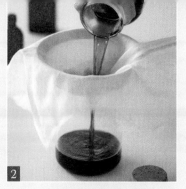
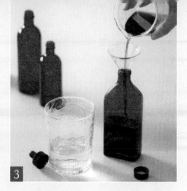

Dried herb tincture

1 Weigh 1.5 oz. (40 g) dried herb. Chop or grind into a coarse powder to create a larger surface area; this allows for greater penetration of the liquid. (Cinnamon quills, used here, have a large surface area so do not need chopping.) Place the herb in a large glass jar with a secure lid and pour ⅔ cup (160 ml) vodka over it, ensuring

that the herb is completely submerged. Stand the bottle in a warm place for 10 to 14 days, shaking it once or twice a day.

2 Strain the mixture through a piece of fine muslin. Squeeze as much moisture as possible from the remaining pulp.

3 Pour the tincture into a dark glass bottle. Seal and label with the name of the herb and the date you

prepared the tincture. Makes about ¾ cup (200 ml).

Usage Using a dropper, dispense the required dose into ¼ cup (60 ml) water before drinking (usually three times daily).

Storage Refrigerate and store for 6 to 12 months. Make sure it is stored safely out of reach of children.

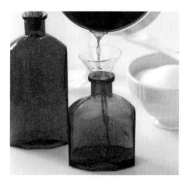

Syrups

Syrups are mostly used to ease coughs and sore throats, because the thick, sweet liquid has a very soothing effect. Commonly used herbs include marsh mallow, licorice, thyme and white horehound. Although syrups can also be made using an infusion or decoction, this recipe uses a tincture, so the result is a syrup with a stronger medicinal action.

Cough syrup from tincture

1 Stir together ½ cup (100 g) sugar (or honey) and ¼ cup (50 ml) water in a small saucepan over a low

heat until the sugar is dissolved and the mixture is thick but still runny. Remove from the heat and leave to cool. Add ¼ cup (50 ml) of the appropriate tincture; stir.

2 Pour the cough syrup into a dark glass jar and seal with a cork. Makes about ¾ cup (200 ml).

Usage Take the appropriate dose directly from the spoon without diluting it.

Storage Refrigerate the syrup for up to 3 months. The sugar may crystallize as a result of the

refrigeration, but the syrup will easily become liquid again if the bottle is allowed to stand in a bowl of hot water for a few minutes.

Caution

● Occasionally, when syrups are stored, fermentation occurs, so it's best to make a small quantity at a time and to use it quickly. Syrups are traditionally stored in bottles with a cork stopper so that the bottle will not explode if fermentation does take place.

Herbal creams

Herbal creams help to relieve itchy skin, soothe burns and irritations, relax tense muscles, encourage wound healing and treat infection.

To make medicated herbal creams at home, start with an unscented non-greasy cream base, such as sorbolene or vitamin E cream. Add some herbal tincture, using a ratio of 1 part tincture to 10 parts cream, or essential oil at 1 percent to 2 percent the weight of your base cream. Stir until your cream has an even consistency. (Some essential oils are unsuitable for topical use, so seek professional advice.)

Homemade herbal creams have a short life span, so make a small quantity as you need it and use it up quickly. To help extend the shelf life, add a few drops of lavender essential oil or the contents of some vitamin E capsules.

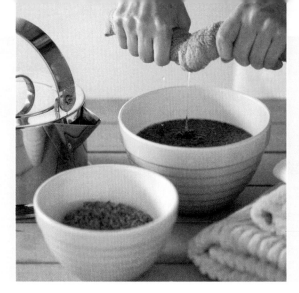

Compresses

A compress is a cloth that has been soaked in an infusion (or a diluted tincture) and applied to the skin. Compresses are used to relieve headaches and pain, disinfect wounds and soothe tired eyes. Make a fresh one each time.

Make a strong infusion of dried herb (lavender flowers are used here), using 2 to 3 teaspoons of dried herb per 1 cup (250 ml) water. Cover and steep for 10 to 15 minutes. Remove the cover and leave the infusion to cool to a temperature that is comfortable to the skin. Soak a face washer or flannel in the infusion and wring out the excess water.

Usage Apply to the affected part. As the compress dries out, it can be resoaked and reapplied.

Poultices

A poultice is a topical application of a fresh herb, which is most commonly used to encourage healing of injured muscles and bones (for example, strains, sprains and fractures), or to draw matter out of the skin (for example, to help remove a splinter or bring a boil to a head).

1 Chop sufficient fresh herb (comfrey leaves are used here) to cover the affected body part. Place in a container and blend using a stick blender, adding a little water to aid the blending, if necessary. The finished mixture should be of a mushy consistency.

2 Place the mixture on a piece of folded muslin. Use a spatula or the back of a spoon to spread the mixture thinly so that the surface area will cover the whole area of the affected body part.

3 Rub a little body oil onto the affected body part to prevent the poultice sticking to the skin. Apply the poultice, covering the muslin with plastic wrap to keep it in place. To make it more secure, if necessary, place a bandage around the poultice.

Usage Change the poultice about every couple of hours, or, if possible, leave it in place overnight.

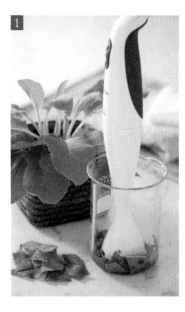

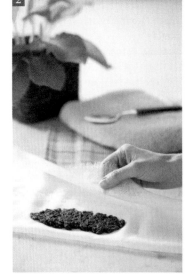

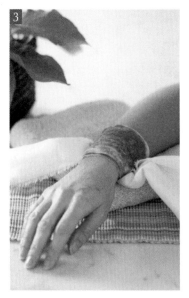

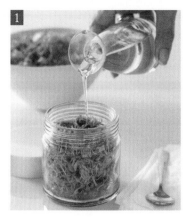

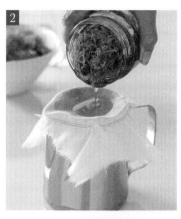

Infused oils

Oil-soluble components can be extracted by infusing an herb in oil over an extended period of hours or days. The pure infused oil is then used for topical applications or added to a cream or ointment. Medicated infused oils are similar to (although much stronger than) culinary infused oils. They are quite different to the essential oils used in aromatherapy, which are commonly extracted from plants by distillation.

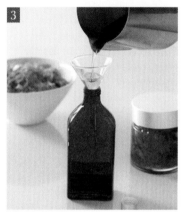

Cold infused oils

A cold infusion process (*shown above*) is used for fragile or delicate plant parts such as flowers, petals and leaves. Among the most popular cold infusions are calendula flowers (for eczema and other skin complaints), St. John's wort flowers (for the relief of nerve pain) and lavender flowers and rosemary leaves (both to help relieve muscle soreness).

1 Pack a wide-necked, clear glass jar with fresh or dried herb (fresh calendula flowers are used here), leaving about ½ in. (1 cm) space at the top of the jar. Pour vegetable oil (such as olive oil) over the herb until it is covered to a depth of about ¼ in. (5 mm). Stir gently.

2 Fold some fine muslin and place on top of the oil. Seal the lid tightly

and give the bottle a good shake. Store in a warm, sunny place for 3 to 10 days. Shake the bottle several times a day.

Filter the oil through fine muslin into a clean jug. Squeeze as much oil as possible through the remaining pulp. If any sediment remains in the oil, cover the jug and leave the oil to stand for a day or two until the sediment settles to the bottom.

3 Gently pour the oil into a dark glass bottle, taking care to leave the sediment layer behind. Seal; label with the name of the herb and the date on which you prepared the oil.

Usage Apply topically as is or add it to a cream or ointment.

Storage Store in a cool, dark place for up to 6 months, but discard at the first sign of rancidity or fermentation.

Hot infused oils

Hot infused oils are used for woodier, denser plant parts, and are used for plants with "heating" characteristics. Popular examples are hot infused oils of cayenne (chili pepper), black pepper and ginger, all of which are used to warm stiff, painful muscles and joints.

For dried herbs, use a ratio of 1 part herb to 3 parts oil. For fresh herb, the ratio is 1 part herb to 1.5 parts oil.

1 Coarsely chop or grind the herb (fresh bird's-eye chilies are used here). Add to a saucepan or glass bowl and stir in the required quantity of oil. Place the covered saucepan in a frying pan half filled with water (or use a double boiler). Simmer over very low heat for 2 to 3 hours. Do not allow oil to boil.

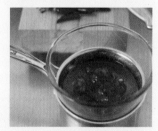

2 Allow to cool before straining through fine muslin into a clean jug. Squeeze as much oil as possible through the remaining pulp. Gently pour the oil into a dark glass bottle. Seal; label with the name of the herb and the date you prepared the oil.

Usage Apply topically or add to a cream or ointment. Do not use oils from hot-flavored plants on inflamed or sensitive skin. Do not get them in your eyes.

Storage Store in a cool, dark place for up to 6 months, but discard at the first sign of rancidity or fermentation.

Flower essences

A cross between herbal medicine and homeopathy, flower essences are subtle remedies that gently help resolve emotional problems.

Bach flower essences

Dr. Edward Bach was an eminent researcher in the fledgling science of immunology when he gave up medicine in 1930. A firm believer that mental and emotional issues were behind every illness, from then on he devoted his life to identifying gentle natural remedies to bring the heart and mind back to a state of balance.

Bach spent much of his time in the British countryside, where he "tuned in" to the healing properties of flowers, and where he developed a system of preparing his remedies — or flower essences — that is still in use today. He believed the subtle energetic qualities of the plant could be captured by floating freshly picked flowers in bowls of pure spring water, which were then allowed to sit in a sunny place for several hours before he used brandy to preserve and stabilize the essence.

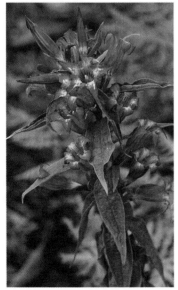

Gentian (*Gentiana ascelepiadea*)

This concentrated flower essence, called the "stock" remedy, can be further diluted with spring water and brandy for dispensing to patients, animals or plants. The stock is also sometimes added to creams and ointments.

Dr. Bach identified 38 flower essences that are still used throughout the world, and their indications are summarized below. Rescue Remedy, the most popular of his creations, is indicated during any emergency, large or small. This combination of the five flower essences — cherry plum, clematis, impatiens, rock rose and star of Bethlehem — helps to relieve fear, panic, stress and shock, and is mostly taken by mouth, but it can also be added to a bathtub, applied to the wrists or forehead, or administered in a cream.

Building on Bach's work, researchers have developed ranges of essences from flowering plants that are found in other parts of the world, including Australia, New Zealand, South Africa, Hawaii and even far-flung places such as Alaska, the Himalayan mountains and the Amazon jungle.

Introducing the remedies

Here's a list of the Bach Flower Remedies and their main indications.

Agrimony helps cheerful people who are secretly troubled to deal with their underlying problems.

Aspen supports those who are anxious or worried, but are unable to identify what frightens them.

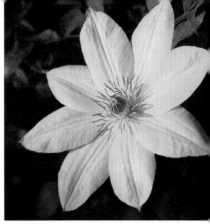

Clematis (*Clematis vitalba*) may also encourage great creativity and make you more alert.

Beech fosters a spirit of compassion in those who are intolerant of people who are different to them.

Centaury helps people who over-extend themselves helping others to learn to say no so they don't wear themselves out.

Cerato boosts self-confidence, teaching you to listen to your own counsel instead of others' opinions.

Cherry plum is for people who fear for their sanity, who feel they are heading for a nervous breakdown, or who are frightened they will harm themselves or others.

Chestnut bud teaches you to learn from your experiences, so you don't repeat the same mistakes again.

Chicory is for people who risk stifling their relationships by clinging too tightly to their loved ones.

Clematis brings those who are always dreaming about the future back down to earth to focus on the present.

Crab apple helps you to heal yourself of any feelings of unworthiness and uncleanliness.

Elm helps people who are overwhelmed by their responsibilities to feel able to cope again.

Gentian provides energy and enthusiasm after discouraging setbacks.

Gorse renews optimism in those who feel hopeless, and enables them to see the positive steps they can take.

Heather helps self-centered people who constantly seek attention from others to become less needy.

Holly helps release feelings of anger, aggression, jealousy and hatred, and encourages a positive, open outlook.

Honeysuckle is for people who are stuck in the past, reliving either their past mistakes or past happiness.

Hornbeam supports people who procrastinate because they are so overwhelmed by the tasks before them that they feel exhausted before they begin.

Impatiens is for critical, irritable or impulsive people who are easily frustrated by the slowness of others.

Larch builds self-confidence in those people who consider themselves inferior to others, and helps overcome an expectation of failure.

Mimulus helps heal fears and phobias, ranging from anxiety about public speaking to fear of illness or death.

Mustard brings clarity and light during times of despair and despondency.

Oak helps determined, driven people to realize when it is time to sit back and take a rest, or perhaps to realize that their goal is neither achievable nor worth striving for.

Olive brings renewed energy to those who are exhausted by struggle and ready to give up.

Pine is for those who feel guilty about their own perceived past failings, and always feel they could have done better.

Red chestnut releases excessive anxiety or fear for the well-being of others.

Rock rose brings calm during times of terror, panic or extreme fear.

Rock water is for those who deny themselves pleasure in favor of some higher goal and feel a failure when they cannot maintain their own impossibly high standards.

Scleranthus helps people who question themselves when making decisions to instead feel confident in their convictions.

Star of Bethlehem heals feelings of shock, regardless of whether the unpleasant event occurred recently or in the distant past.

Sweet chestnut strengthens those who feel they are in a hopeless situation and cannot go on.

Vervain brings flexibility and detachment to people who zealously try to convert others to their own beliefs, and who can become quite worked up by their own efforts.

Vine eases the need to dominate and control, and is for those who are prone to aggression and the abuse of power.

Walnut eases you through times of change and helps you confidently stand your ground when those around you have different opinions.

Water violet helps isolated or aloof people to reconnect with others.

White chestnut calms an overly busy mind, helping to settle circular or repetitive thoughts and allowing concentration and focus to return.

Wild oat helps those who can't decide their direction in life to identify their path.

Wild rose rekindles motivation in people who no longer strive for change because they have become resigned to their particular lot in life.

Willow helps people who feel overly sorry for themselves and resent the success and happiness of others to return to a more positive outlook.

Australian and South African flower essences

More than 65 essences are made from the flora of the Australian wilderness. Many Australian plants are unique in the world, and according to the manufacturers of the Australian Bush Flower Essences, these remedies draw on the wisdom of this ancient landscape to promote lasting emotional change.

The extensive range includes Sturt Desert pea for sadness and deep emotional pain, sunshine wattle to help people who are struggling with negativity to return to a positive outlook, and old man banksia to reenergize those who have become lethargic due to frustrations and setbacks.

Like the Bach Flower Remedies, the Australian Bush Flower Essences are created by "tuning in" to each plant's energetic qualities in its natural bushland setting. These energies are then captured and transferred to a liquid remedy that can be taken orally or added to creams.

Also available is a range of South African flower essences, which include agapanthus, blushing bride, keurtjie, nicotiana, sour fig and silverleaf.

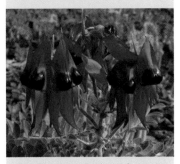

Sturt Desert pea (*Swainsona formosa*) has been proven to help alleviate deep emotional pain.

Medicinal herbs

Modern botanical medicine has become truly international, and herbalists now have access to the most effective herbs from all corners of the globe.

Albizia

Albizia lebbeck

Part used **Stem bark**

The traditional Ayurvedic applications for albizia include a range of inflammatory and allergic skin and respiratory conditions, and laboratory research indicates that it does indeed have anti-allergic properties. It appears to have particular benefits for mast cells, which play a major role in allergic reactions, so it may help some people become less sensitive to substances to which they are allergic.

Andrographis

Andrographis paniculata

Parts used **Leaves, aerial parts**

Andrographis features in the traditional medicine of China, Thailand, India and Korea. An extremely bitter herb, it is used as a digestive tonic in Ayurvedic medicine, while in traditional Chinese medicine, its cooling properties mean that it is indicated for dispelling heat and treating infections and toxins. Andrographis also has immune-stimulating properties, and is used to help prevent colds and flu and to treat their symptoms.

Astragalus

Astragalus membranaceus

Part used **Roots**

One of the most important *qi* tonics in traditional Chinese medicine, astragalus is taken to enhance vitality and increase energy. It has potent immune-boosting properties, so it may be prescribed to build resistance against infections as well as for more serious problems,

such as helping the body's defenses cope with the trauma of chemo- and radiotherapy. Herbalists also prescribe astragalus for a wide range of other conditions, including liver and kidney dysfunction, heart problems and for aiding recovery from blood loss (especially after childbirth).

Buchu

Agathosma betulina

Part used **Leaves**

The South African herb buchu is mainly regarded as a remedy for the urinary tract, although traditionally it was also used to treat digestion and joint problems. Its volatile essential oil has antiseptic properties and is considered responsible for the herb's benefits in treating infections of the kidneys, bladder, urethra and prostate. Buchu also has diuretic actions, so it is indicated for fluid retention.

Cat's claw

Uncaria tomentosa,
U. guaianensis

Part used **Vine bark**

Cat's claw grows in tropical South and Central America and takes its name from the shape of the long thorns that help it to climb over other plants in the jungle. It has been used for hundreds of years by Peruvians to treat inflammatory conditions, such as arthritis, asthma and skin problems, and is also a traditional remedy for infections, fatigue and cancer. Laboratory studies attribute it with a number of immune-stimulating and anti-inflammatory properties, which may be behind

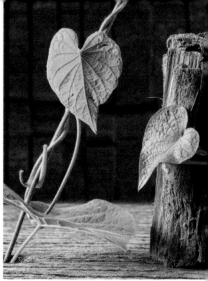

Cat's claw has hooklike thorns, which enable it to climb other plants rather voraciously.

many traditional applications; little research has been conducted in humans.

Dang shen

Codonopsis pilosula

Part used **Roots**

Chinese herbalists regard dang shen as a gentler version of the more famous stress and energy tonic, Korean ginseng. This distinction means that it can be prescribed for patients who are frail or debilitated, for whom ginseng is considered too stimulating. Dang shen is also traditionally used for treating digestive, respiratory and cardiac problems (especially when caused by stress) and as a nourishing blood tonic for nursing mothers and other anemic patients.

Devil's claw

Harpagophytum procumbens

Part used **Tubers**

Devil's claw grows in the grasslands of southern Africa and has been used there as a topical treatment for ulcers and wounds, and taken internally for fevers, allergies, digestive problems and as a pain reliever. Numerous scientific studies confirm its benefits, most notably as an effective analgesic and anti-inflammatory for arthritis pain and backache. Some studies have shown devil's claw to be as effective as pharmaceutical painkillers and anti-inflammatory drugs.

Golden seal

Hydrastis canadensis
Part used **Rhizomes**
Golden seal is named for its rhizome's characteristic yellow color, and it was used as both a dye and a medicine by Native Americans. It is still beloved by herbalists today, who regard it as a bitter digestive stimulant, an astringent tonic for the mucous membranes and a potent broad-spectrum antimicrobial remedy. Some of its most medically important alkaloids are also present in other plants (such as barberry and Indian barberry), and these are now largely used in its place, because golden seal has become endangered by over-harvesting.

Milk thistle

Silybum marianum
Part used **Seeds**
Milk thistle has such a remarkable ability to prevent and repair liver damage that certain constituents are sometimes used intravenously to treat death cap mushroom poisoning. It is also employed against more frequently encountered toxins, such as alcohol and environmental pollutants, and can help digestive and cholesterol problems, thanks to its effects as a liver and gallbladder tonic. The best-quality products are standardized for their silymarin content, which is considered to be responsible for most of the herb's medicinal benefits.

Pau d'arco

Tabebuia impetiginosa
Part used **Inner bark**
In the 1960s, pau d'arco developed an international reputation as a cancer cure, but it had been used as a traditional medicine in Brazil for hundreds of years before that. Some of the herb's constituents have been shown in a laboratory setting to inhibit the growth and activity of tumor cells. An immuno-stimulant action that may further help the body fight cancer (as well as fungal diseases and other infections) has also been documented. However, extensive research will be required before its potential is fully understood.

Senna

Senna alexandrina syn. Cassia angustifolia
Parts used **Leaves, pods**
Senna's purgative action is due to its content of anthraquinone glycosides, which stimulate intestinal peristalsis, triggering a bowel movement some 12 hours later. Probably the most popular laxative herb, senna has an effect that is strong and reliable, if a little drastic. Habitual use may lead to "lazy bowel syndrome," in which the colon becomes unable to function without the laxative.

Uva-ursi

Arctostaphylos uva-ursi
Part used **Leaves**
Uva-ursi's antimicrobial properties are specifically indicated for urinary tract infections, and seem to be more effective when the

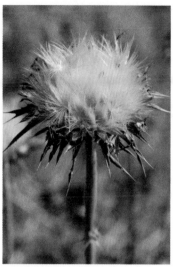

Each seed in the milk thistle bears a tuft of white hairs that help it to become airborne.

urine is alkaline. Since many urinary tract infections acidify the urine, the herb is sometimes prescribed with an alkalizing substance (such as bicarbonate of soda) to maximize its effects. The compounds that are responsible for the antibiotic action are not present in uva-ursi itself, but are formed from its content of phenolic glycosides after the herb is ingested.

Caution
● Do not take the herbs on these pages if you are pregnant or breastfeeding, except under the advice of a healthcare professional.

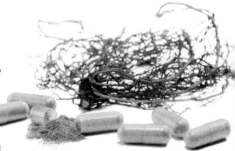

Cherokees pounded golden seal *(Hydrastis canadensis)* rhizomes with bear fat to make an insect repellent. Today the plant is dried and then ground to a powder for use in supplements.

Sore throats, colds & flu

The choice of an appropriate remedy to relieve a cold or a bout of flu is determined by the symptoms you're experiencing.

Sage

Salvia officinalis

Sore throat soother

Certain compounds in sage have been documented as having antimicrobial properties, which may help to explain the herb's traditional use as a gargle for sore throats and tonsillitis.

Dosage ▶ Make a strong infusion of dried sage; use as a gargle several times per day, as required.

Yarrow

Achillea millefolium

Fever remedy

Native Americans traditionally used yarrow to treat feverish conditions, and modern herbalists still follow their lead. It is often called for in the early stages of cold or flu, and is commonly combined with elder flower, which is also considered helpful in lowering high temperatures.

Dosage ▶ Infuse 1 teaspoon (4 g) dried yarrow (the flowers, seeds and leaves) in boiling water; drink 3 cups per day.

Elder

Sambucus nigra

Fever and flu relief

Elder flowers are used to treat upper respiratory infections with fevers or sinus congestion. The berries have long been used to make cordials and wines, but more recent research in Israel has established that a commercial preparation of elderberries, standardized for its content of anthocyanins — the purple compounds that give the berries their color — helps relieve the symptoms of flu and shorten the duration of the infection. The researchers in Israel hypothesize that the extract works by altering the surface of the virus, preventing it from taking hold in the body.

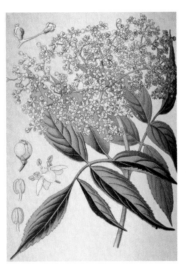

Elder flowers and berries have many applications in natural beauty preparations and in cooking.

Dosage ▶ Infuse 1 to 2 teaspoons (2 g to 5 g) dried elder flowers in boiling water; drink 3 cups per day. Alternatively, look for a commercial preparation made from elderberries and follow the manufacturer's instructions.

Andrographis

Andrographis paniculata

Clinically proven to reduce symptoms of respiratory infection

Used in many parts of Asia for the treatment of infectious and feverish conditions, andrographis has been investigated in several clinical trials. These studies document improvements in symptoms of cold, flu and pharyngo-tonsillitis, such as fatigue, sore throat, muscle aches, shivering, excessive nasal secretions, sinusitis and headache, and suggest that andrographis may also reduce the amount of sick leave patients need in order to recover. Like echinacea, astragalus and garlic, andrographis also appears to have some preventative action and, when taken over several months, may help reduce the incidence of colds.

Dosage ▶ For the best results, take andrographis as soon as possible after the onset of cold or flu symptoms. Look for commercial preparations standardized for their content of andrographolides, which are considered responsible for much of the herb's activity, and follow the manufacturers' instructions. Doses of up to 6 g dried herb per day are normally used to treat infection, while lower doses are taken for prevention.

Garlic

Allium sativum

Broad-spectrum infection fighter

In vitro research has shown that garlic and several of its constituents have broad-spectrum activity against a wide variety of disease-causing organisms, including strains of the virus that causes flu. Garlic also helps fight colds and flu by enhancing

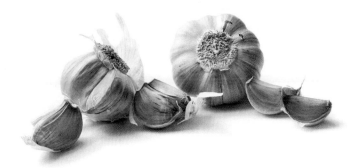

The main active constituent of garlic is allicin, which is released when you crush fresh cloves.

the activity of immune cells and, when taken prophylactically — that is, as a preventative medicine — may help protect you from catching a cold.

Dosage ▶ To treat infection, take up to 2 cloves fresh garlic per day. Chop them and leave them to sit for 5 to 10 minutes before cooking with them. This will allow the medicinally active component allicin to form. For prevention, aim for a dose of up to 3 cloves per week, or buy a commercial preparation that provides a standardized quantity of either alliin or allicin, and follow the manufacturer's instructions.

Thyme

Thymus vulgaris

Antimicrobial and antispasmodic

The essential oil of thyme is regarded as one of nature's most potent antimicrobial substances, so herbalists commonly prescribe the plant to help resolve respiratory tract infections, such as colds, flu, tonsillitis and laryngitis. It also has antispasmodic properties, so it can be used to help reduce coughing.

Dosage ▶ Infuse up to 1 teaspoon (4 g) dried thyme leaves or 2 teaspoons fresh leaves in boiling water; drink 3 cups per day.

White horehound

Marrubium vulgare

Loosens the mucus in unproductive coughs

White horehound has expectorant properties, helping to break up thickened phlegm and encouraging you to cough to remove it from the respiratory tract. It is particularly favored by herbalists when coughs are dry, hacking and unproductive.

Dosage ▶ Infuse up to 1 teaspoon (2 g) dried flowering tops of horehound in boiling water; drink 3 cups per day.

Marsh mallow

Althaea officinalis

Soothing expectorant for irritated airways

Both the roots and leaves of the marsh mallow plant can be used to treat coughs. However, herbalists prefer the root for its higher mucilage content, which is responsible for the herb's soothing actions on the respiratory mucous membranes. Marsh mallow is traditionally indicated to relieve irritated and inflamed throats and airways, and to help expel mucus when lungs are congested.

Dosage ▶ Infuse 2 g to 5 g dried marsh mallow root in cold (not hot) water, and steep for 8 hours to release mucilage; drink up to 3 cups per day.

Cautions

• Exceeding the recommended doses of yarrow, andrographis or white horehound may cause side effects and should be avoided.

• If you are taking blood-thinning or blood pressure medications, don't take garlic, andrographis or yarrow. Stop taking any of these herbs at least 2 weeks before undergoing surgery.

• Marsh mallow may interfere with the absorption of other medicines, so separate doses by 2 hours.

• Marsh mallow and andrographis may affect blood sugar levels, so they should not be taken by people with diabetes, except under professional supervision.

• Don't use yarrow if you are allergic to members of the Asteraceae family of plants (for example, chicory, daisies, echinacea and chrysanthemums).

• Do not consume the isolated essential oil of thyme. Use only the fresh or dried herb.

• Uncooked fresh elderberries may cause diarrhea and vomiting. Use only the dried or cooked berries.

• Andrographis may exacerbate pre-existing cases of heartburn and gastric ulcer. Garlic may cause minor gastric upset in some people, but these symptoms are less likely when the herb is cooked.

• Yarrow may very occasionally increase sensitivity to sunlight. If you develop this symptom, stop using it immediately and seek medical advice.

• Do not use large doses of elder flower over long periods of time.

• Black horehound (Ballota nigra) should not be used as a substitute for white horehound (Marrubium vulgare).

• With the exception of normal culinary quantities of sage, garlic and thyme, do not take the herbs on these two pages if you are pregnant or breastfeeding, except under professional advice.

Immune support

Help boost your body's defenses against disease-causing bacteria and viruses by taking immune-stimulating herbs.

Echinacea

Echinacea sp.

Strengthens resistance to infection

Laboratory studies into several different echinacea species and constituents isolated from the plant have identified a variety of immunological effects, and seem to validate the herb's usage to support immunity. The results of human clinical trials have not always demonstrated the anticipated effects, however, causing the popular use of echinacea as a preventative against colds and flu to become controversial.

But a meta-analysis published in 2007 may go some way in clarifying the situation. In this study, researchers pooled the results of 14 clinical studies and estimated that taking echinacea decreased the likelihood of developing a cold by 58 percent, and when a cold did occur, its duration was shortened by about 30 hours.

Dosage ▶ The most appropriate dose of echinacea depends on both the plant part and the species used, but it is important to start taking the herb as soon as possible after symptoms develop. Preparations made from the root of *Echinacea angustifolia* or *E. pallida* are generally taken at doses of about 1 g taken 3 times daily to treat colds or, in lower doses, as a preventative. For *E. purpurea*, either the whole plant (including roots) or the aerial parts may be used. The dose is up to 2 g taken 3 times daily as an infusion of dried herb, or .03 oz. (3 ml) juice made from the fresh plant and taken 3 times daily.

To make the juice, liquefy fresh aerial parts of *E. purpurea* with a little water in a home juicer or blender. The juice doesn't store well, so make only as much as you need to use immediately.

Astragalus

Astragalus membranaceus

Improves immunity in chronic conditions

In traditional Chinese medicine, the herb astragalus is attributed with warming properties and is regarded as a lung tonic. It is indicated for patients with longstanding illnesses and for those who are susceptible to recurrent infection, and appears to improve the functioning of the immune system so that the body can better defend itself against pathogens — especially viruses. Astragalus is a good herb to try if you're run down and tired and repeatedly catch colds or flu since, in addition to its immune-boosting properties, it is also traditionally used to raise overall vitality and energy.

Dosage ▶ Boil 3 g to 10 g dried astragalus root in ¾ cup (180 ml) water for 10 minutes before straining; drink the decoction in 2 doses during the day.

Alternatively, take tablets or capsules according to the manufacturer's instructions, up to a maximum dose of 7.5 g dried root per day.

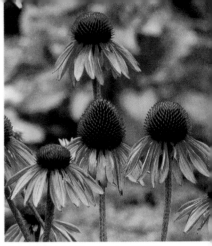

Three species of echinacea are cultivated for medicinal purposes — *Echinacea angustifolia, E. pallida* and *E. purpurea* (shown above).

Cautions

● Do not use echinacea if you are allergic to members of the Asteraceae family of plants (for example, daisies, chrysanthemums, chicory and chamomile); people with pollen allergies should also take care, as some preparations may contain pollen. Cases of contact dermatitis have also occasionally been reported.

● Talk to your doctor before taking echinacea if you have an autoimmune condition, such as lupus, or a progressive disease, such as multiple sclerosis or HIV/AIDS. Echinacea should not be used by patients taking immunosuppressive medications.

● Note that astragalus is recommended for chronic (longstanding) rather than acute infections; discontinue use if you develop an infection while taking it.

● The resistance-boosting effects of astragalus may help reduce the side effects of some immunosuppressive cancer treatments, such as radio- and chemotherapy, but should only be used in this way in consultation with your doctor.

● Do not use the herbs on this page if you are pregnant or breastfeeding, except under the advice of a healthcare professional.

Hay fever & sinusitis

Herbs can help provide relief from, and may even prevent, the debilitating pain of sinusitis and the symptoms of hay fever.

Horseradish
Armoracia rusticana
Relieves congested sinuses
If you've ever tasted horseradish (or its Japanese cousin wasabi), you'll know that it is a rapid decongestant, clearing the sinuses and easing breathing almost immediately after ingestion. This effect is due to the ability of compounds called glucosinolates to liquefy thickened mucus, making it easier to clear and relieving the pressure and head pain associated with sinus congestion. These are the same compounds that give horseradish its spicy taste. They also have antimicrobial properties, so horseradish helps fight sinus infections, too. In clinical trials in Europe, researchers found that a combination of horseradish and nasturtium (which also contains glucosinolates) was just as effective in treating sinus infection as antibiotics but produced fewer side effects.
Dosage ▶ Use horseradish paste or wasabi as a condiment. Alternatively, take commercially prepared tablets or capsules (with or without nasturtium) at a dose of up to 3 g per day.

Eyebright
Euphrasia officinalis
Traditional remedy for catarrh
Eyebright is traditionally used for respiratory conditions with watery discharges, so it's an ideal herb to take when you are suffering from hay fever symptoms, such as constant sneezing, a runny nose and watery or irritated eyes. It can also be used for colds and flu with similar symptoms.
Dosage ▶ Infuse up to 1 teaspoon (1 g to 4 g) dried aerial parts of eyebright in boiling water; drink 3 cups per day.

Albizia
Albizia lebbeck
Ayurvedic anti-allergy herb
Albizia lebbeck has a long history of use in Ayurvedic medicine, where it is prescribed for allergies and inflammatory conditions, including hay fever, asthma, hives and allergic conjunctivitis. Studies suggest that albizia works by stabilising the cells that release histamine and other allergic mediators, thereby relieving allergic tendencies and helping to manage allergy symptoms.
Dosage ▶ Look for commercial preparations providing the equivalent of 3 g to 6 g per day of the dried stem bark, and take it according to the manufacturer's instructions.

Perilla
Perilla frutescens
May prevent hay fever symptoms
Also known as shiso or beefsteak plant, perilla is a common ingredient in the traditional diet of Japan. Scientists there have also been integral in identifying its potential for preventing hay fever symptoms. Both the leaf and the seed of perilla contain compounds that help reduce allergy symptoms, such as sneezing, itchiness of the nose and scratchy, watery eyes. Preliminary research suggests that the herb (and particularly the constituent rosmarinic acid) may help seasonal allergy sufferers experience fewer hay fever symptoms during periods of high-pollen exposure.
Dosage ▶ Take up to 9 g of dried leaf per day in tablet or capsule form. For the treatment of seasonal allergies, it may help to start taking perilla about a month before the hay fever season.

Cautions
● Horseradish may irritate the digestive tract in some people and should be avoided by those with gastric ulcers; it may also cause irritation and burning if it comes into contact with the skin or eyes.
● If you suffer from thyroid disease or are taking blood-thinning medications, do not take horseradish at doses higher than normal culinary intake, except under professional supervision.
● Albizia and perilla should not be taken at the same time as pharmaceutical anti-allergy medications (such as antihistamines) except under professional supervision, as the effects of the drugs may be enhanced.
● Except for normal culinary quantities of horseradish, do not use the herbs on this page if you are pregnant or breastfeeding, except under the advice of a healthcare professional.

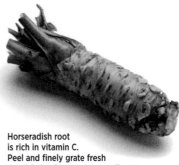

Horseradish root is rich in vitamin C. Peel and finely grate fresh wasabi root for use as a condiment.

Indigestion

The enjoyment of a meal quickly dissipates if the burning pain and discomfort of indigestion or dyspepsia follow.

Slippery elm

Ulmus rubra

Soothing and healing

The mucilage in slippery elm bark forms a gel that lines the gastrointestinal tract, acting as an anti-inflammatory and encouraging healing. Slippery elm is an ideal herb for indigestion sufferers, because the gel helps protect the stomach lining from the effects of excess acid.

Dosage ▶ Stir 1 teaspoon powdered slippery elm bark into water and drink 15 to 30 minutes before meals. (As slippery elm trees are becoming increasingly rare, it's preferable to buy bark in powdered form rather than collect it yourself.)

Meadowsweet

Filipendula ulmaria

Acid balance

Meadowsweet relieves indigestion, reflux and other problems of over-acidity. Taken over a period of several weeks, it helps to normalize stomach acid production while soothing inflamed gastric tissues and promoting healing.

Dosage ▶ Infuse 4 g to 6 g dried leaves and flowering tops of meadowsweet in boiling water; drink 3 cups per day.

Gentian

Gentiana lutea

Stimulates digestion

Bitter-flavored gentian improves digestion by stimulating the bitter taste receptors on the tongue, triggering the release of saliva, gastric acid and other digestive fluids. Gentian aids many of the symptoms that can occur due to poor digestion, including heartburn, flatulence, nausea and poor appetite. It is best taken before meals over several weeks, but a single dose after a heavy meal can also be beneficial.

Dosage ▶ Take 2 to 5 drops gentian root tincture in water, or infuse 1 g dried root and rhizome in boiling water. Take gentian 3 times per day, preferably 15 to 30 minutes before meals.

Anise

Pimpinella anisum

Relieves fullness and bloating

Anise helps to relieve the discomfort and pain of indigestion, and is particularly beneficial when wind or bloating are also present. Other aromatic herbs — such as caraway, fennel and dill — can be used in the same way.

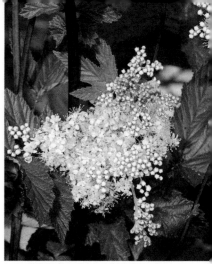

In the Middle Ages, meadowsweet flowers were a popular flavoring for wine and beer.

Dosage ▶ Grind up to 1 teaspoon (2 g) ripe anise seeds to release the essential oil before infusing them in boiling water. Drink up to 3 cups per day.

Cautions

● See your doctor if you experience indigestion or heartburn frequently, or if vomiting occurs.

● A heart attack sometimes mimics the symptoms of indigestion. Call for an ambulance immediately if your symptoms are accompanied by a pain that radiates down the arm or up the neck, or by dizziness, weakness or shortness of breath.

● Slippery elm may interfere with the absorption of other medicines, so separate doses by 2 hours.

● Do not take meadowsweet if you are taking blood-thinning or anticoagulant medications (including aspirin), or if you are allergic to salicylates.

● Do not confuse anise and star anise.

● Do not take gentian if you suffer from peptic or duodenal ulcer.

● With the exception of normal culinary quantities of anise, do not use the herbs on this page if you are pregnant or breastfeeding, except under the advice of a healthcare professional.

Herbal aperitifs

Many popular aperitifs are based on traditionally used bitter herbal medicines, such as wormwood, which not only stimulate stomach secretions but also act as tonics for the liver and gallbladder. Many other aperitifs, including ouzo from Greece and pastis from France, are dominated by the licorice-like aroma of anise or star anise. Taking a dose of one of the many bitter or aromatic herbs before your meal can have the same benefits; try peppermint, fennel, ginger or globe artichoke.

Nausea

Whether it's a 24-hour stomach bug, a case of food poisoning or a bout of seasickness, nausea makes you feel miserable.

Ginger
Zingiber officinale
Settles the stomach
If you're feeling queasy, reach for ginger first. Several clinical trials support its traditional reputation as an effective treatment and preventative for nausea from a variety of sources, including morning sickness, motion sickness and post-operative vomiting and nausea. For more information on ginger and morning sickness, see Pregnancy, *page 210*.
Dosage ▶ Add 20 to 30 drops ginger tincture to water, or infuse ½ teaspoon powdered ginger or 1 to 2 teaspoons grated fresh ginger root in boiling water; take 3 times per day. For children over the age of 4, add 10 to 15 drops of ginger tincture to lemonade or ginger beer.

To prevent seasickness and travel sickness, take 1 g dried ginger 30 minutes before the trip starts and every few hours during the journey. The same dose can be taken before surgery to reduce post-operative nausea (but discuss this with your surgeon first — see *Cautions* at right).

Peppermint
Mentha x piperita
Antispasmodic
Peppermint is specifically indicated when nausea is accompanied by churning sensations in the stomach or gripping pains in the bowel. Its antispasmodic actions in the gastrointestinal tract are due to its content of a menthol-rich essential oil.
Dosage ▶ Add 10 to 15 drops peppermint tincture to water, or

infuse 1 teaspoon fresh or dried aerial parts in boiling water; take 3 to 4 times per day. Children over 4 years can take a third to a half of the adult dose.

German chamomile
Matricaria recutita
Eases anxiety
The essential oil that gives chamomile its characteristic smell also imparts antispasmodic and anti-inflammatory properties, while its bitter principles help stimulate the secretion of gastric juices. This combination of actions, along with its renowned calming effects, make chamomile a very useful herb for the treatment of nausea, especially when it is due to, or accompanied by, anxiety and emotional upset.
Dosage ▶ Infuse 1 to 2 teaspoons dried chamomile flowers in boiling water; drink 3 to 4 cups per day. Children over the age of 4 years can take a third to a half of the adult dose.

Cautions
● In some cases, nausea and vomiting may be symptomatic of underlying disease. See your doctor if symptoms are severe, prolonged or occur frequently.
● Medical attention is also warranted if nausea is accompanied by severe abdominal pain, confusion, headache or a stiff neck, or is triggered by a head injury.
● Dehydration can occur as a consequence of vomiting. Watch out for symptoms such as dry lips and mouth, decreased urination and rapid pulse, especially in children. Rehydrate using an electrolyte replacement supplement

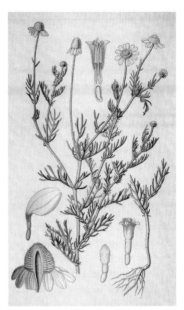

German chamomile grows wild throughout Europe, where it has long been used medicinally.

(available from pharmacies), and seek medical advice immediately.
● Ginger should not be taken for 2 weeks prior to undergoing surgery. However, in consultation with your physician, a single dose can be taken just prior to surgery to reduce post-operative nausea.
● Don't use peppermint if you suffer from gastroesophageal reflux disease (GORD) or hiatus hernia, because its antispasmodic effect may worsen your symptoms by relaxing the esophageal sphincter and allowing reflux to occur more readily. Ginger is also contraindicated in reflux and should not be used medicinally if you suffer from gastric ulcer or gallstones.
● Don't use chamomile if you are allergic to members of the Asteraceae family of plants (for example daisies, chicory, chrysanthemums and echinacea).
● With the exception of normal culinary quantities of peppermint and German chamomile, do not use any of the herbs on this page if you are pregnant or breastfeeding, except under the advice of a healthcare professional.

Wind, bloating & flatulence

A certain amount of wind every day is normal, but it can be uncomfortable and embarrassing if it occurs to excess.

Peppermint
Mentha x piperita
Irritable bowel relief

Known to relieve wind and gastro-intestinal spasm, peppermint is an ideal remedy for people with irritable bowel syndrome (IBS), a condition characterized by abdominal pain, bloating and excessive flatulence. Several clinical trials support the use of peppermint to relieve IBS symptoms, especially when taken as enteric-coated peppermint oil capsules that break down in the bowel, where their antispasmodic effects are most needed.

Dosage ▶ Add 10 to 15 drops peppermint tincture to water, or infuse 1 teaspoon fresh or dried aerial parts in boiling water; take 3 to 4 times per day. Alternatively, use commercial peppermint oil capsules and follow the manufacturer's instructions.

Star anise and colic

Chinese star anise (*Illicium verum*) has a long history of use in Spain, Latin America and the Caribbean as a treatment for colic, but following a number of severe adverse reactions in infants and young children, this practice should now be avoided. Some of these cases have been attributed to contamination by the related herb Japanese star anise (*Illicium anisatum*), which is toxic. However, Chinese star anise is also considered responsible for at least some of the reactions and even in low doses may cause severe reactions in young children.

Caraway
Carum carvi
Aromatic antispasmodic

Caraway is another herbal medicine that has been traditionally used to relieve wind, bloating and flatulence. Like peppermint, it helps to decrease spasm in the muscles of the digestive tract, and the essential oils of the two herbs are sometimes combined in commercial products.

Dosage ▶ Grind up to 1 teaspoon (2 g) caraway seeds to release the essential oil before infusing them in boiling water. Drink up to 3 cups per day. Alternatively, use commercial caraway oil capsules (often combined with peppermint) and follow the manufacturer's instructions.

Dill
Anethum graveolens
Soothes colic

Of the many herbs with calming actions on the digestive system, dill is the preferred remedy for the treatment of colic in babies and is equally beneficial for adults suffering from uncomfortable wind pain. As with other digestive remedies, it is the herb's essential oil that is responsible for its actions as a gastrointestinal antispasmodic, with the effect of releasing wind and reducing pain and discomfort.

Dosage ▶ Grind up to 2 teaspoons (4 g) dill seeds to release the essential oil before infusing them in boiling water. Drink up to 3 cups per day to relieve bloating and flatulence in yourself or colic in a breastfed baby. For babies over the age of

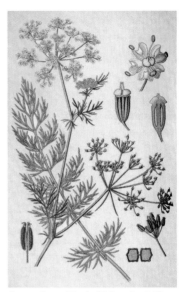

Caraway is combined with fennel and dill to make an infusion for treating intestinal problems.

3 months, allow the infusion to cool and give 1 to 3 teaspoons at a time up to 4 times a day.

Cautions

● Products containing the essential oils of peppermint and/or caraway are not recommended for infants, children, pregnant or breastfeeding women, or for people with gallbladder, kidney or gastroesophageal disease. Do not exceed the dose recommended by the manufacturer.

● If you are already taking prescribed medicines, talk to your doctor before taking peppermint oil capsules, because they may interact with some drugs.

● Caraway may cause an allergic reaction in some people. Stop using it if you experience any adverse effects, such as diarrhea or a runny nose.

● Do not use the herbs on this page in greater than culinary quantities if you are pregnant or breastfeeding, except under the advice of a healthcare professional.

Constipation & hemorrhoids

Ongoing problems with constipation can lead to hemorrhoids and an increased risk of diverticular disease and bowel cancer.

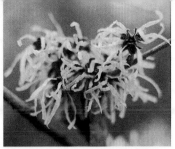

Witch hazel is native to North America, where it was used medicinally by Native American tribes.

Psyllium

Plantago ovata, P. psyllium
Soluble-fiber supplement

Mucilage-rich psyllium husks are a valuable source of soluble fiber, often lacking in the Western diet. In fact, psyllium is one of the few types of fiber supplement that have been proven to aid the management of chronic constipation problems.

Dosage ▶ Psyllium husks are available in tablets, capsules and soluble powders, and should be taken according to the manufacturer's instructions. A teaspoon of the powdered husks can also be sprinkled on fruit or breakfast cereal once a day. Every dose of psyllium should be taken with a large glass of water.

Witch hazel

Hamamelis virginiana
Hemorrhoid healer

In clinical trials, topical applications of witch hazel have been demonstrated to be as effective as other medications (including corticosteroids) for the relief of the pain, itching and bleeding of hemorrhoids. The herb is also traditionally taken internally for the treatment of hemorrhoids, but its astringent nature makes it unsuitable for people with a tendency to be constipated.

Dosage ▶ Rub witch hazel gel, ointment or tincture into the affected area once a day. Talk to a professionally trained herbalist, who can help determine whether internal use of witch hazel is appropriate for your circumstances.

Chinese rhubarb

Rheum palmatum
Strong laxative

Chinese rhubarb root is a strong laxative with a potent content of anthraquinone glycosides. In traditional Chinese medicine it is prescribed for constipation and is considered to promote bile secretion, improve appetite and act as a liver and gallbladder tonic.

Dosage ▶ Boil ¾ oz. (20 g) dried or 1½ oz. (40 g) fresh Chinese rhubarb rhizome in 3 cups (750 ml) water. Simmer until reduced to 2 cups (500 ml). Take ¼ to ½ cup (50 ml to 100 ml) of the decoction with your evening meal.

Yellow dock

Rumex crispus
Gentle cleanser

Yellow dock is a gentle digestive stimulant that is specifically indicated for sluggish liver or bowel function. While it does contain anthraquinone glycosides, its laxative action is less marked than that of Chinese rhubarb or other herbal laxatives such as senna and cascara.

Dosage ▶ Boil 1 g to 4 g dried yellow dock root in a cup of water for 10 minutes; drink the decoction up to 3 times daily.

Cautions

● Anthraquinone-containing herbs should not be taken in excessive doses, or for more than 10 days at a time.
● Do not use herbs to treat constipation in children, or if you are pregnant, breastfeeding, have undiagnosed abdominal pain or an intestinal or gallbladder blockage. Chinese rhubarb is also contraindicated in persons suffering from arthritis or kidney or urinary tract disease.
● Persons diagnosed with an intestinal illness should only use herbal medicines (including psyllium) on medical advice.
● Psyllium may interfere with the absorption of other medicines, so separate doses by 2 hours.
● Always drink lots of water when using psyllium, because cases of choking have occasionally been reported in people who have taken psyllium powders without adequate fluids.
● Rhubarb leaves are toxic and should not be consumed.
● Topical applications of witch hazel occasionally cause contact allergy. Stop using it immediately if you are concerned.
● With the exception of topical applications of witch hazel, do not use the herbs on this page if you are pregnant or breastfeeding, except under the advice of a healthcare professional.

A natural trigger

Laxative herbs tend to contain varying quantities of compounds called anthraquinone glycosides, which travel through the digestive system to the intestine. They stimulate peristalsis and trigger a bowel movement that usually occurs about 8 hours after consumed. They are traditionally taken in the evening, with the objective of developing a regular bowel habit in the mornings.

Liver & gallbladder support

Your liver and gallbladder are vital for your digestive and detoxification processes. Look after them, so they can look after you.

Milk thistle

Silybum marianum

Liver protection and repair

The seeds of milk thistle (also known as St Mary's thistle) contain a group of antioxidant compounds collectively referred to by the name silymarin.

Studies show silymarin helps protect liver cells from damage and aids the repair or replacement of injured cells. Under professional supervision, milk thistle and silymarin aid the management of a wide range of serious liver problems, including non-alcoholic and alcoholic liver disease and some forms of hepatitis.

Milk thistle can also be used to prevent or treat the effects of overindulgence in alcohol and fatty foods, to prevent liver damage from toxic exposure, and for headaches and skin problems associated with poor liver function.

Dosage ▶ Look for tablets or capsules that are standardized for their silymarin content (sometimes labeled as flavanolignans or silybin), and follow the manufacturer's instructions.

Schisandra

Schisandra chinensis

Liver support

Although there is less scientific evidence to support its use, schisandra may have similar liver-protecting properties to milk thistle. Laboratory studies demonstrate a number of antioxidant effects and suggest that it, too, has the ability to prevent cell damage by harmful substances and to reduce some of the symptoms associated with liver disease.

Dosage ▶ Take the equivalent of 500 mg to 1500 mg of the dried fruit 3 times per day, in either tablet or tincture form.

Dandelion root

Taraxacum officinale

Traditional hepatic tonic

As a bitter herb, dandelion root stimulates gastrointestinal function and is traditionally used for minor digestive ailments, especially sluggish liver and gallbladder function, indigestion and mild cases of constipation. An infusion of the roasted root is a popular caffeine-free alternative to coffee and a pleasant way to stimulate digestion before or after a heavy meal.

Dosage ▶ Infuse ½ to 2 teaspoons (2 g to 8 g) dried or roasted dandelion root in boiling water; drink 3 cups per day. If using the roasted root, add milk or soy milk to taste, but avoid sweeteners, because they may diminish the herb's effectiveness. Tablets, capsules and a tincture are also available.

Turmeric

Curcuma longa

Stimulates gallbladder function

Among its many other medicinal actions, turmeric helps to stimulate bile secretion and may offer some protection against the development of gallstones. Its effects on the liver and gallbladder may also be responsible for the herb's ability to help lower blood cholesterol levels.

Dosage ▶ Mix ½ teaspoon powdered turmeric with cold water and drink 2 to 3 times per day for up

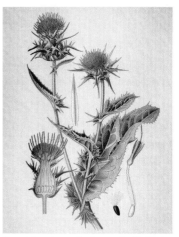

The white veins on the leaves of milk thistle were said to be milk from the Virgin's breast.

to 4 weeks at a time. Alternatively, take turmeric capsules, standardized for their content of curcumin.

Cautions

• If you suffer from liver or gallbladder disease (including gallstones), do not attempt to treat yourself using these or any other herbal medicines. Instead, seek the care of an appropriately trained healthcare professional.

• Minor gastrointestinal symptoms, such as nausea, diarrhea and flatulence, are sometimes experienced when these remedies are taken. If you experience any discomfort, discontinue use.

• Don't use milk thistle or dandelion root if you are allergic to members of the Asteraceae family of plants (for example, daisies, chrysanthemums and echinacea).

• If you have a gastric or duodenal ulcer, or are taking blood-thinning medications, do not take turmeric at doses higher than normal culinary intake.

• In traditional Chinese medicine, schisandra is contraindicated in the early stages of coughs and colds.

• With the exception of normal culinary quantities of turmeric, do not use the herbs on this page if you are pregnant or breastfeeding, except under the advice of a healthcare professional.

Detox

Feeling sluggish and run down? Maybe it's time to detox, especially if you've been overindulging or neglecting your diet.

Dandelion leaf

Taraxacum officinale

Herbal diuretic

Dandelion leaves have powerful diuretic activity: They promote the production and excretion of urine. They also have liver- and gallbladder-stimulating properties (although, traditionally, these actions are considered to be milder than the actions of the dandelion root).

Dosage ▶ Infuse 1 to 2 teaspoons (4 g to 10 g) dried dandelion leaves in boiling water; drink 3 cups per day.

Cleavers

Galium aparine

Lymphatic cleanser

Cleavers is traditionally regarded as a gentle yet effective tonic for the lymphatic system, which collects wastes and foreign material from the body and returns them to the bloodstream for disposal. It is specifically indicated when the lymph glands are chronically enlarged or congested, and when skin problems, such as acne or eczema, are present.

Dosage ▶ Infuse 1 teaspoon (4 g) dried aerial parts of cleavers in boiling water; drink 3 cups per day. Alternatively, juice the fresh herb and drink 5 ml to 15 ml 3 times daily.

Psyllium

Plantago ovata, P. psyllium

Facilitates excretion of toxins

Soluble fiber of the type found in psyllium husks is especially beneficial when you're detoxing because it forms a gel-like substance in the intestines, trapping toxic compounds so they can be excreted.

Dosage ▶ Psyllium husks are available in tablets, capsules and soluble powders, and should be taken according to the manufacturer's instructions. A teaspoon of powdered husks can also be sprinkled on fruit or breakfast cereal once a day. Take every dose of psyllium with a large glass of water.

Cautions

● Most people can safely undergo a gentle detox program by adopting a diet of fresh fruit and vegetables, drinking plenty of water, and avoiding caffeine, cigarettes, alcohol and processed foods for a few days. However, transient side effects do sometimes occur during a detox. These include gastrointestinal disturbances, headaches, joint and muscle pain, fatigue and skin rashes.

● The following people should not undergo detox regimens or take the herbs listed on this page except under the supervision of an appropriately qualified healthcare professional: children, teenagers, pregnant and breastfeeding women; people with chronic illness, diabetes, diagnosed intestine, kidney, liver or gallbladder disease; cancer patients; people taking prescribed medications; people with a history of eating disorders or alcohol or drug abuse; people who have had a higher than normal exposure to toxins (for example, through occupational exposure).

● Don't use dandelion leaf if you are allergic to members of the Asteraceae family of plants (for example, daisies, echinacea and chrysanthemums) or are taking potassium-sparing diuretics or ACE inhibitors.

● Psyllium may interfere with the absorption of other medicines, so separate doses by 2 hours.

● Always drink lots of water when using psyllium, because cases of choking have occasionally been reported in people taking psyllium powders without adequate fluids.

● Do not use any of these herbs if you are pregnant or breastfeeding, except under the advice of a healthcare professional.

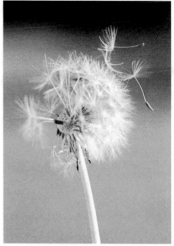

The roots of dandelion are dried and roasted to make a caffeine-free coffee substitute.

Eliminating toxins

Herbalists believe that it's difficult for the body to function at its best if the organs of elimination are overloaded. In the philosophies of many traditional healing systems, the resulting buildup of toxins can lead to symptoms as diverse as headaches, fatigue and skin problems. The liver and gallbladder play a major role in the formation and excretion of the feces, so remedies such as the ones detailed on this page tend to be central to any detox prescription, often with the support of herbs for the urinary and lymphatic systems.

Tension & stress

If you are feeling the pressure of too much to do in too little time, these herbs may help you to cope.

Korean ginseng
Panax ginseng
Improves performance under stress

The most highly valued of all Chinese herbs, Korean ginseng has a long-held reputation for helping the body and mind cope with stress. It has been the subject of numerous clinical trials, which have documented (among other effects) improvements in alertness, relaxation, mood and performance on various tests. Not all clinical trials have supported Korean ginseng's traditional reputation.

Dosage ▶ Take commercially prepared Korean ginseng tablets according to the manufacturer's instructions (up to a maximum of 1000 mg of dried root per day). Look for products standardized for their content of ginsenosides. Note that Korean ginseng is traditionally taken for 8 to 12 weeks at a time, followed by a break of several weeks; it is not appropriate for frail or anxious patients.

Oats
Avena sativa
Traditional restorative for the nervous system

The leaves, stems and other green parts (sometimes called "oat straw") of the oat plant are used to help restore a depleted or debilitated nervous system and aid with coping in times of stress or nervous exhaustion. Herbalists consider this herb a gentle and reliable nervous system tonic, capable of calming or energizing as required. Even the very frail or anxious patient can take this herb.

Dosage ▶ Infuse 1 to 1½ teaspoons (3 g) dried oats greens in boiling water; drink 3 cups per day. Children over 4 years can take up to half the adult dose.

Lemon balm
Melissa officinalis
Calming and relaxing

Lemon balm is traditionally used during times of tension, restlessness and anxiety, and is ideal when you are feeling uptight, agitated or overwrought. In clinical trials, people affected by stress have reported feeling increased levels of calmness and improved mood after just a single dose of lemon balm, but it can also be taken over a longer period when stress is ongoing.

Dosage ▶ Infuse 1 to 2 teaspoons of fresh aerial parts of lemon balm in boiling water; drink 1 cup 2 to 3 times per day. The herb has a mild sedative action, so if you are suffering from fatigue, take it only in the evening.

Cautions
● Do not take Korean ginseng if you have diabetes, cardiovascular disease (including high and low blood pressure), depression, anxiety, hyperactivity, mental illness (including bipolar disorder and similar conditions), insomnia, blood clots or bleeding disorders.
● Korean ginseng is known or suspected to interact with many pharmaceutical

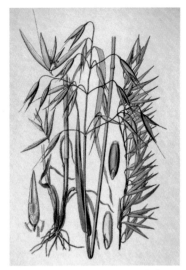

An infusion of oats seed is used topically to soothe itchy skin.

medications — including antidepressants, antipsychotic medications, anticoagulants, insulin and hormonal therapy — so consult with your physician or pharmacist before taking it. Do not take it at the same time as stimulants such as caffeine.
● Korean ginseng is traditionally contra-indicated during acute infections.
● Side effects are occasionally reported with the use of Korean ginseng. These may include headache, disturbed sleep and skin problems. If this occurs, stop taking the herb.
● Do not use oats if you have celiac disease or gluten intolerance.
● Lemon balm may interact with some pharmaceutical medications, including certain sedatives, and a group of medicines referred to as cholinergic (or parasympa-thomimetic) drugs, which are prescribed for Alzheimer's disease and a range of other conditions — if you are taking prescribed medicines, talk to your doctor before using lemon balm.
● Do not take any of these herbs if you are pregnant or breastfeeding, except under the advice of a healthcare professional.

Depression & anxiety

Used appropriately, herbs can help lift your mood or calm your nerves when you find things difficult to deal with.

St. John's wort

Hypericum perforatum

Herbal antidepressant

Clinical research has proven the anti-depressant effects of St. John's wort, with some studies demonstrating a level of efficacy in mild to moderate depression that is similar to that of important pharmaceutical anti-depressants, but with a better safety profile. Interestingly, the way the herb works in the body is also similar to the mechanisms of action of some of these pharmaceutical medicines.

Dosage ▶ Look for supplements that are standardized for their contents of hypericin and hyperforin (considered to be the main active constituents) and with a daily dose of 900 mg per day of the concentrated (6:1) extract, equivalent to 5.4 g of dried herb.

Lavender

Lavandula angustifolia

Aromatherapy to relieve anxiety

The scent of lavender has long been attributed to promoting relaxation, and there is a growing body of evidence to support this traditional practice. Studies indicate that inhaling lavender essential oil helps ease anxiety and improves feelings of calmness and well-being in a range of stressful situations, including dental waiting rooms and intensive-care units. Research also shows that lavender inhalation has the effect of reducing the body's production of the stress hormone cortisol.

Dosage ▶ To enjoy the anti-anxiety effects of lavender, use a ratio of 4 drops lavender essential oil for every 10 ml carrier oil and massage into the shoulders and temples. Or, inhale the steam from 4 drops essential oil diluted in 20 ml hot water (for example, in an oil burner). You can also drink an infusion made from ½ teaspoon (1 g to 1.5 g) of the dried flowers twice a day, and again at bedtime.

Cautions

● St. John's wort is known or suspected to interact with many pharmaceutical medications (including antidepressants, cardiovascular medicines and contra-ceptives), so consult your physician or pharmacist before taking it.

● Depression is a serious condition and is not suitable for self-treatment. Do not stop taking prescribed antidepressants except under the advice and supervision of your doctor. A 2-week wash-out period is advised if you are switching from pharmaceutical antidepressants to St. John's wort.

● Research into the use of St. John's wort in severe depression has not yet demonstrated safety or efficacy and so should be avoided unless medically prescribed. It should not be used by people with bipolar disorder.

● The effects of St. John's wort take 2 to 4 weeks to develop. If there is no noticeable improvement after 6 weeks, this herb may not be suitable for you; consult your doctor.

● St. John's wort occasionally causes minor side effects (for example, gastrointestinal upset, headache). The most common of these is photosensitivity, a condition in which the skin becomes more prone to sunburn. Avoid sunbathing or prolonged sun exposure while taking St. John's wort and consult your doctor if you develop this symptom.

● Stop taking St. John's wort at least 2 weeks prior to undergoing surgery.

● Unless advised to do so by your doctor, do not take St. John's wort if you are pregnant or breastfeeding, and do not give it to children.

● Do not ingest lavender essential oil and do not use it during pregnancy or breastfeeding, except under the advice of a healthcare professional.

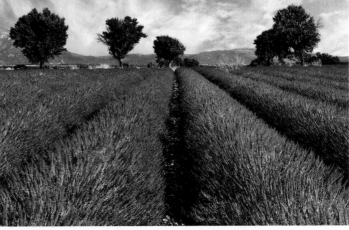

Soothing and aromatic, lavender flowers are cultivated commercially.

Tiredness & fatigue

If your energy levels are flagging, a stimulating herbal pick-me-up may be all that you need.

Siberian ginseng

Eleutherococcus senticosus

Extra energy during stressful times

Herbalists recommend Siberian ginseng as a stimulating herb for people who are tired and run down, especially those affected by stress. It is traditionally used to help rebuild energy levels during the recovery period following an illness, and may be beneficial for some sufferers of chronic fatigue syndrome when professionally prescribed.

Dosage ▶ Take commercially prepared Siberian ginseng tablets according to the manufacturer's instructions (up to a maximum of 3 g per day) for a period of up to 6 weeks, followed by a 2-week break.

Withania

Withania somnifera

Blood-building herb

In Ayurvedic medicine, withania (also known as ashwagandha or Indian

ginseng) is used to enhance energy and stamina and to help the body cope with stress, so it's considered especially beneficial for patients who are physically or emotionally exhausted. Withania contains iron, so it can also be helpful for fatigue caused by anemia or low iron levels. A small number of studies indicate that it helps to promote blood-cell formation and raise the level of hemoglobin in the blood.

Dosage ▶ Take commercial withania tablets according to the manufacturer's instructions. Look for a product providing the equivalent of 3 g to 6 g of the dried root per day.

Astragalus

Astragalus membranaceus

Energy tonic with immune support

Astragalus is one of the most important energy tonics in traditional Chinese medicine. It is used to help increase the vitality of patients who are debilitated, and is specifically indicated for cases of fatigue accompanied by poor appetite. Astragalus is particularly useful if you are constantly feeling run down as well as tired, since it also supports the immune system, helping the body to fight off infections, such as colds and flu.

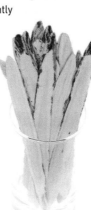

Native to Mongolia and parts of China, astragalus is also called milk vetch.

Dosage ▶ Boil 3 g to 10 g dried astragalus root in ¼ cup (60 ml) of water for 10 minutes before straining; drink the decoction in 2 doses during the day. Alternatively, take tablets or capsules according to the manufacturer's instructions, up to a maximum dose equivalent to 7.5 g dried root per day.

Cautions

● Do not exceed the recommended dose of Siberian ginseng.

● Siberian ginseng is unsuitable for people with hyperactivity disorders, bipolar disorder or similar conditions. If you have cardiovascular disease (including high and low blood pressure), or if you are taking anticoagulant medication, only use it under professional supervision.

● Siberian ginseng and astragalus are contraindicated during acute infections.

● Stop using Siberian ginseng at least 2 weeks before undergoing surgery.

● If you are diabetic, do not use Siberian ginseng, except under medical supervision.

● If you are taking tranquilizers, sedatives, antidepressants, thyroid medication, chemotherapy or immunosuppressant medication, do not take withania, except under professional supervision.

● Resistance-boosting astragalus may help reduce the side effects of some immunosuppressive cancer treatments, but should only be used in this way in consultation with your doctor. Siberian ginseng may also interact with chemotherapy.

● Do not take withania if you are sensitive to plants belonging to the Solanaceae family (for example, potato, tomato, eggplant).

● Do not use these herbs if you are pregnant or breastfeeding, except under the advice of a healthcare professional.

Why am I so tired?

Fatigue is your body's way of telling you that it's time to rest. Although most causes of fatigue are related to lifestyle factors, such as the amount of sleep, exercise and healthy food you are getting each day, tiredness can also present as a symptom of an underlying health problem, such as anemia, underactive thyroid conditions or mononucleosis. As well as the herbs detailed on this page, the remedies for Tension & stress (see page 184) and Insomnia (see page 188) may also be useful.

Memory & concentration

If you keep forgetting where you put the car keys or your glasses, it could be time to mix up a memory tonic.

Ginkgo

Ginkgo biloba

May delay the progression of dementia

Ginkgo is the world's most popular memory tonic, and is believed to work via a number of mechanisms, including improving blood flow to the brain, acting as an antioxidant and helping to prevent injury to blood vessels. It may help delay the progression of Alzheimer's disease and other forms of dementia, so has the ability to improve the quality of life for sufferers of these debilitating conditions. Ginkgo can also be taken for more minor memory problems or as a supportive tonic during study periods. However, there is little scientific evidence available to help us understand whether the herb is also beneficial in healthy people.

Dosage ▶ Look for supplements standardized for their content of the important active constituents ginkgo flavone glycosides, ginkgolides and bilobalides, with a daily dose of 120 mg of a concentrated (50:1) extract, providing the equivalent of 6 g of the dried herb. Ginkgo takes a month or two to reach its maximum effect, so use it for 6 to 12 weeks before assessing whether or not it is helping you.

Brahmi

Bacopa monnieri

Aid for learning

Brahmi appears to enhance the way the brain processes new information, which makes it a perfect herbal tonic for students. It also helps relieve anxiety, so it can be of real benefit at exam time — but it does take up to 3 months to start working, so don't leave it too late!

Dosage ▶ Infuse 1 g to 2 g dried brahmi in boiling water; drink 3 cups each day. Alternatively, take commercial preparations, up to a maximum of 6 g per day, according to the manufacturer's instructions.

Rosemary

Rosmarinus officinalis

Traditional memory tonic

Rosemary has had a reputation as a memory tonic since the time of the ancient Greeks, and it can help increase alertness, reduce anxiety and encourage a calm mind.

Dosage ▶ Add a few drops of rosemary essential oil to an oil burner in the room or area where you are studying or working.

Cautions

● If your memory problems worsen or become serious, it is essential to discuss your concerns with a doctor.

● If you have been diagnosed with Alzheimer's disease or any other form of dementia, do not take ginkgo or brahmi without first talking to your doctor.

● Ginkgo is known or suspected to interact with many pharmaceutical medications (including antipsychotic medications, anticonvulsants, anticoagulants and anticholinergic medications), so consult your doctor or pharmacist before taking it. Stop taking ginkgo at least 2 weeks before undergoing surgery.

● Always use commercially prepared ginkgo products from a reputable company. Do not consume unprocessed ginkgo leaves, as they may cause an adverse

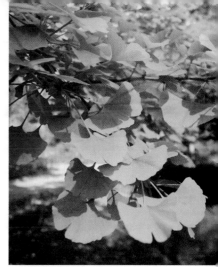

Ginkgo trees, which date back to the Jurassic period, can live for more than a thousand years.

reaction. Do not eat large quantities of the seeds or allow children to do so.

● Ginkgo sometimes causes mild adverse reactions, which may include dizziness, gastrointestinal upset, headache and allergic skin reactions. More severe reactions have occasionally been recorded, including bleeding problems and seizures. If symptoms occur, stop taking the herb and seek medical advice.

● Brahmi occasionally causes gastrointestinal irritation (for example, reflux). It should not be taken with anticholinergic medications.

● Do not take ginkgo if you suffer from a bleeding disorder.

● Do not take brahmi if you suffer from celiac disease, malabsorption syndromes, gallbladder blockage or gastric reflux problems.

● Both brahmi *(Bacopa monnieri)* and gotu kola *(Centella asiatica)* are sometimes referred to by the name "brahmi" in Ayurvedic herbal texts, so make sure you don't confuse the two.

● Do not take ginkgo or brahmi, or apply rosemary essential oil to the skin, if you are pregnant or breastfeeding, except under the advice of a healthcare professional.

Insomnia

Missing out on a good night's sleep can be enough to ruin your whole day. The right herb may prevent that from happening.

Valerian

Valeriana officinalis

Clinically proven herbal sedative

A number of clinical studies support valerian's traditional reputation as a sedative herb. It helps insomnia sufferers to fall asleep more quickly, wake less often during the night and generally experience a better night's sleep. In contrast to some pharmaceutical sedatives, it is very rarely associated with side effects, and doesn't tend to cause sleepiness and difficulty waking in the morning.

Dosage ▶ Infuse 3 g dried valerian rhizome in boiling water and drink 1 cup an hour before bedtime. Alternatively, take commercial preparations according to the manufacturer's instructions. Valerian works best when it is taken every night over a period of several weeks, rather than when taken occasionally.

Hops

Humulus lupulus

Traditional sleep inducer

Although more famous as an ingredient in beer, hops has a long history of being used to help treat insomnia and sleep disorders. This herb is also traditionally regarded as helpful in treating anxiety and restlessness, although there is conflicting evidence about its effects on depression. In many cases, hops is taken in combination with other sedative herbs, such as valerian and passionflower.

Dosage ▶ Infuse up to 1 g dried hops in boiling water and drink 1 cup an hour before bedtime. Dried hops can also be used to make pillows to

aid restful sleep in the same way that lavender is sometimes used.

Passionflower

Passiflora incarnata

Sleep problems with anxiety

Passionflower is traditionally taken to aid insomnia — especially when sleep troubles are accompanied by nervousness or anxiety — so it is ideally suited to those whose insomnia has an emotional basis. Although there hasn't been much scientific research into passionflower's actions, there is some preliminary data to support its traditional applications.

Herbalists commonly prescribe passionflower in combination with other relaxing herbs, such as valerian.

Dosage ▶ To treat insomnia, infuse 2 g dried passionflower leaves in boiling water and drink 1 cup an hour before bedtime. For anxiety, take the

same dose twice more during the day. Like valerian, passionflower may take several weeks to achieve optimal effect.

Cautions

● Do not exceed the recommended dose of the herbs listed here.

● If you are taking pharmaceutical tranquilizers, sedatives or antidepressants, do not take the herbs listed here, except under professional supervision. If you are taking anticoagulant medication, do not use passionflower except under professional supervision.

● If valerian worsens insomnia and/or causes exceptionally vivid dreams, discontinue it and try an alternative herb.

● If you suffer from depression, do not use hops, except on professional advice.

● Allergic symptoms sometimes occur from contact with hops, and may include dermatitis and respiratory symptoms.

● Do not use hops if you have a history of hormone-sensitive tumors or are taking anti-estrogenic medication.

● Do not use these herbs if you are pregnant or breastfeeding, except under the advice of a healthcare professional.

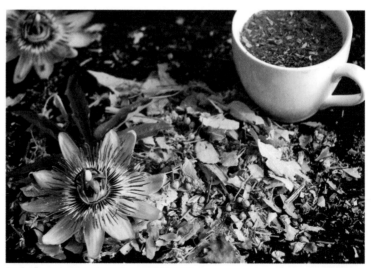

Passionflower leaves make a tea to treat insomnia.

Headache & migraine

Whether you suffer from headache or migraine frequently or occasionally, an herbal alternative may bring welcome relief.

Feverfew

Tanacetum parthenium

Reduces migraine frequency and symptoms

Feverfew is the most famous of all herbs for treating headache, and is one that migraine sufferers find particularly effective. If taken over several months, it lowers the frequency of migraines and reduces symptoms, such as headache, nausea and vomiting, as well as decreases the duration of the attacks.

Dosage ▶ You can take feverfew either by eating 2½ fresh leaves every day (with or after food) or by using commercial preparations according to the manufacturer's instructions. It may take from 1 to 4 months before the effects become evident — perhaps even longer if you are taking the fresh leaves.

White willow bark

Salix alba

Herbal aspirin

White willow bark contains compounds called salicylates, which are similar to the active ingredient in aspirin. It has traditionally been used to relieve headaches of all types, especially those accompanied by fever. In one small-scale preliminary study, white willow bark was also combined with feverfew for the prevention of migraine, producing highly significant improvements in the frequency, intensity and duration of the attacks.

Dosage ▶ Boil 1 g to 3 g dried white willow bark in a cup of water for 5 to 10 minutes; drink the decoction up to 3 times daily.

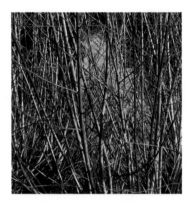

White willow bark is harvested from young branches in late winter and spring.

Alternatively, take commercially prepared products according to the manufacturer's instructions.

Peppermint oil

Mentha x piperita

Rapid relief for tension headaches

Applying peppermint essential oil to the forehead and temples has been scientifically proven to be as effective as paracetamol (acetaminophen) for the relief of tension headaches. This effect occurs very quickly — a significant reduction in the headache's intensity may be noted as quickly as 15 minutes after the oil has been applied.

Dosage ▶ Apply a solution containing 1 part peppermint oil diluted in 9 parts alcohol (or water if alcohol is not available) to the forehead and temples every 15 to 30 minutes after the onset of symptoms. Take care not to allow the solution to come into contact with the eyes. Using both peppermint oil and paracetamol simultaneously may enhance the effects of both treatments.

Cautions

- Severe or frequent headaches may require medical investigation — always consult your doctor.
- Feverfew sometimes causes allergic side effects, most commonly mouth symptoms, such as mouth ulcers and soreness of the tongue. These symptoms are more likely to occur in people chewing fresh leaves (as opposed to taking tablets or capsules).
- Do not take feverfew if a rash develops after coming into contact with the plant or if you are allergic to other members of the Asteraceae family of plants (for example, chicory, daisies, chrysanthemums, sunflower and echinacea).
- Do not take white willow bark if you are allergic to salicylates (including aspirin).
- Do not take feverfew or white willow bark with antiplatelet or anticoagulant medication, or if you suffer from a blood disorder.
- Peppermint oil should always be diluted before application. It should not be used on or near the face of children and babies (even in its diluted form).
- Do not take feverfew or white willow bark, or apply peppermint oil to the skin, if you are pregnant or breastfeeding, except under the advice of a healthcare professional.

Is it a migraine?

The word "migraine" is often used to describe a particularly severe headache, in medical terms a migraine is a specific type of debilitating headache that may be accompanied by other symptoms, such as nausea and vomiting, blurred vision or other visual disturbances, and tingling or numbness of the limbs. Sufferers may also be particularly sensitive to noise or light during an attack, and may retreat into a dark, quiet room until the episode has passed.

Acne

Breaking the cycle of skin eruptions can be a living hell. Try these herbal solutions for treating problem skin.

Tea-tree oil

Melaleuca alternifolia

Nature's powerful pimple healer

With a combination of broad-spectrum antimicrobial properties and anti-inflammatory activity, tea-tree oil is an ideal topical treatment for acne. In a recent study, people with mild to moderate acne experienced reductions of more than 40 percent in both the number of acne lesions and the severity of their acne when they used a tea-tree oil gel over a 6-week period. A previous study had already shown that tea-tree gel had a similar level of efficacy to benzoyl peroxide (also used topically for the treatment of acne), but with a much lower incidence of side effects.

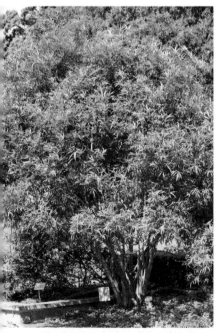

The chaste tree is also called monks' pepper because it was once used to suppress libido.

Dosage ▶ In these scientific studies, a gel containing 5 percent tea-tree essential oil was used — a more concentrated preparation may have yielded even more impressive results, but may also have increased the risk of side effects (see *Cautions*). To replicate the study conditions at home, apply tea-tree gel to the affected area twice a day, washing it off with water after 20 minutes.

Cleavers

Galium aparine

Skin and lymphatic detoxifier

In the Western herbal tradition, skin problems, such as acne, are considered an indication that toxins in the bloodstream are being excreted via the skin. Cleavers is one of a wide range of blood-cleansing herbs that are used to detoxify the blood and lymph and support the body's organs of elimination, thus improving skin health.

Dosage ▶ Infuse 4 g (1 teaspoon) of dried aerial parts of cleavers in boiling water; drink 3 cups per day. Alternatively, juice the fresh herb (excluding the root) using a stick blender, and drink 5 ml to 15 ml 3 times daily.

Chaste tree

Vitex agnus-castus

Herbal hormone balancer

Hormonal imbalance can be an important factor in the development of acne — not just in teenagers, but also for many adults. To restore hormonal balance and help resolve problem skin, herbalists often prescribe chaste tree. This herb,

Vitex agnus-castus, is more widely known for its role in the treatment of premenstrual syndrome (PMS) and female reproductive issues, but can also be taken by both males and females for treating acne. It is especially useful for premenstrual acne flare-ups.

Dosage ▶ Take tablets, capsules or tincture according to the manufacturer's instructions. Look for products that are standardized for their content of the compounds casticin and/or agnuside. Results may take up to 12 weeks or longer to become noticeable.

Cautions

- Tea-tree oil sometimes causes reactions, such as contact dermatitis, itching, burning or scaling of the skin, especially if used in high concentrations or on inflamed or eczematous skin. Use diluted preparations to reduce the likelihood of these reactions occurring, and patch-test on an unaffected area of skin 24 hours before applying to any infected or inflamed area.
- Do not ingest tea-tree oil.
- Chaste tree occasionally causes mild, reversible side effects, such as headache, nausea and gastrointestinal upset. Stop taking it if you experience these symptoms.
- Do not take chaste tree at the same time as the oral contraceptive pill, hormone-replacement therapy (HRT) or drugs containing progesterone, except under professional advice. People with a history of hormone-sensitive tumors should not take chaste tree, because safety in people with these conditions has not been established.
- Do not take chaste tree or cleavers, or apply undiluted tea-tree oil to the skin, if you are pregnant or breastfeeding, except under the advice of a healthcare professional.

Eczema & psoriasis

Herbalists use a combination of internal and topical treatments to relieve itchy, inflammatory skin conditions.

Chickweed
Stellaria media
Soothing relief from the garden
You probably have some chickweed growing in your garden — it's one of the most common weeds in the world. Chickweed is traditionally used to relieve itchy and inflamed skin conditions, including eczema, dermatitis and psoriasis. It's gentle enough to use on the most delicate and inflamed skin, and is even suitable for use on babies (see *Cautions* at right before using).
Dosage ▶ Juice the fresh aerial parts of the chickweed plant, then mix into a cream or ointment base using a ratio of 1 part chickweed to 5 parts base cream. Apply to the affected area as required. Alternatively, use a commercially prepared cream in the same way.

Flaxseed oil
Linum usitatissimum
Herbal source of omega-3 fatty acids
Without fats and oils in your diet, your skin can become dry, flaky, scaly and itchy, so the quality and type of fats you eat is very important. The omega-6 group of fatty acids (found in safflower, sunflower, corn and grapeseed oils) can exacerbate inflammation. On the other hand, omega-3 fatty acids, such as those found in flaxseed (as well as other seeds, nuts and seafood), enhance the body's production of anti-inflammatory compounds, and can be beneficial in the treatment of psoriasis, eczema and other inflammatory skin conditions.

Dosage ▶ Take flaxseed oil in either capsules or liquid form, according to the manufacturer's instructions. Alternatively, grind fresh whole seeds and serve them with breakfast cereal, smoothies or yogurt. Note that the oil is more unstable than other culinary oils, so keep it refrigerated to ensure its freshness.

Turmeric
Curcuma longa
Ayurvedic anti-inflammatory
In Ayurvedic medicine, turmeric has been used for centuries as a topical treatment for psoriasis and other inflammatory skin disorders. Modern Western herbalists sometimes also prescribe it internally for the well-documented antioxidant, anti-inflammatory and immune-stimulating properties of both turmeric and a yellow pigment it contains, called curcumin. As the herb is also a liver and gallbladder tonic, this use reflects the traditional view that cleansing the body of toxins can help to resolve chronic skin problems.
Dosage ▶ Mix ½ teaspoon powdered turmeric with cold water and drink it 2 to 3 times per day for up to 4 weeks at a time. For topical use, mix ½ cup (50 g) turmeric powder with 1 teaspoon baking soda and some hot water and apply as a poultice. For more detailed instructions, see *page 168*.

Cautions
● Chickweed and turmeric occasionally cause allergic skin reactions. Patch test on an unaffected area of skin 24 hours

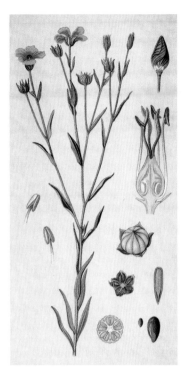

The stalks of the flax are used to make linen, while its seed oil is used in herbal medicine.

before applying to inflamed skin or before using either herb on infants or children.
● Although they are made from the same plant, flaxseed oil is a different preparation from the refined oil sold as "linseed oil" and used for industrial purposes (for example, in paints), which should not be consumed.
● If you are taking anticoagulant or blood-thinning medications, talk to your doctor before taking high dosages of flaxseed oil or other omega-3 fatty acids.
● Turmeric is a safe herb, although high doses can cause minor gastrointestinal symptoms. Do not use it at higher than culinary doses if you have liver and gallbladder disease (including gallstones), gastric or duodenal ulcer, or take blood-thinning medication, except under professional advice.
● Do not use flaxseed oil or turmeric in greater than culinary quantities if you are pregnant or breastfeeding, except under the advice of a healthcare professional.

Athlete's foot & fungal infections

**Once a fungal infection takes hold, it can be hard to get rid of.
Try these herbal options, but be prepared to wait for results.**

Tea-tree oil

Melaleuca alternifolia

Proven tinea treatment

Tea-tree oil is effective against a vast number of disease-causing fungi. Clinical trials also support its use, especially in foot conditions, such as tinea pedis (athlete's foot) and onchomycosis, a fungal infection of the toenail that is very difficult to treat and can lead to destruction of the nail.

In order to be effective, the tea-tree oil needs to be used at just the right concentration — in one study, a solution containing 50 percent tea-tree oil killed the fungal infection in 64 percent of tinea sufferers after 4 weeks. However, in another study that used tea-tree at a concentration of only 10 percent, the tinea symptoms improved but the infection remained present.

With fungal nail infections, applying 100 percent tea-tree oil for a minimum of 3 months has been shown to achieve similar results to pharmaceutical topical agents, with about half of all people experiencing improvements in symptoms and the appearance of the affected nails.

Dosage ▶ To treat athlete's foot (tinea), make a solution containing 25 to 50 percent tea-tree oil in water, and apply to the affected area twice daily for several weeks. Alternatively, add 15 drops of pure tea-tree oil and some salt to an electronic foot bath (the heat and salt may enhance the antifungal activity of the essential oil), and use for 20 minutes twice a day. For onchomycosis, apply 100 percent tea-tree oil to the affected area twice daily for at least

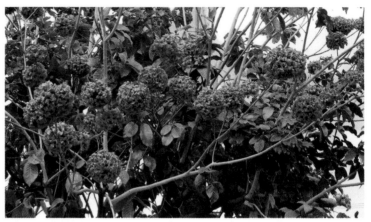

Native to mountainous regions of South America, pau d'arco prefers a tropical to subtropical climate.

3 months. Specially formulated tea-tree oil products can also be useful for some other types of fungal infections — talk to your medical herbalist.

Pau d'arco

Tabebuia impetiginosa

Antifungal remedy from the Amazon

The wood of the South American tree pau d'arco is famously resistant to fungi. In the traditional medicine of Brazil, a poultice or decoction made from the tree's inner bark is applied to the skin to treat fungal infections as well as conditions such as eczema, psoriasis and skin cancer. Laboratory studies support a number of pau d'arco's traditional uses, including fungicidal activity.

Dosage ▶ Add 10 g inner bark of pau d'arco to 2½ cups (600 ml) water and simmer gently for 15 minutes. Cool it to a comfortable temperature and then use the decoction as a compress or poultice on the affected

area twice daily. For more detailed instructions, see *page 168*.

Cautions

● Tea-tree oil may cause reactions, such as contact dermatitis, itching, burning or scaling of the skin in as many as 1 in 25 people with tinea, especially if used at high concentration or on inflamed or eczematous skin. Use diluted preparations to reduce the likelihood of these reactions occurring, and patch test on an unaffected area of skin 24 hours before applying to any infection or inflammation.

● Pau d'arco can be taken internally to support the immune system during systemic fungal infection. However, such conditions are not suited to self-treatment, especially because certain components of pau d'arco may be toxic if taken in excessive amounts. Consult a professionally trained herbalist for more information before using.

● Do not use any of the herbs listed on this page if you are pregnant or breastfeeding, except under the advice of a healthcare professional.

Cold sores, gums & mouth health

Whether you're suffering from the pain of cold sores, toothache or bleeding gums, herbs can help keep your mouth healthy.

Lemon balm
Melissa officinalis
Cold-sore treatment

Clinical studies show that lemon balm is an effective topical remedy for cold sores, helping to decrease healing time, prevent lesions from spreading and relieve symptoms. Symptomatic relief is particularly impressive on the second day of the outbreak, which is usually the time when symptoms are at their most acute. These effects aren't surprising, since laboratory tests show that the herb, and particularly its fragrant essential oil, has the ability to quickly kill the herpes simplex viruses 1 and 2.

Dosage ▶ The lemon balm cream used in the clinical studies mentioned was extremely concentrated (containing the equivalent of 700 mg of lemon balm extract per gram). Look for commercial preparations of the same strength, or ask a medical herbalist to make some for you. Alternatively, try making a strong infusion of lemon balm and use the liquid in a compress. For more detailed instructions, see *page 168*.

Clove oil
Syzygium aromaticum
Rapid toothache relief

Clove oil is a remarkably effective painkiller and anaesthetic. When applied to toothache or inflamed gums, it reduces pain within minutes — although only for a relatively short time. It works by decreasing the affected tissue's perception of pain, and also has anti-inflammatory and antibacterial properties.

Dosage ▶ Dab a small quantity of clove essential oil directly onto the site of the pain. If the essential oil is not available, gently rub powdered cloves or clove buds on the affected area, but take note that they may not be as effective as the essential oil, which is rich in eugenol, the most important active constituent.

Myrrh
Commiphora myrrha
Traditional antiseptic for gums

The gum (or resin) of the myrrh tree is used for the treatment of mouth and gum problems in many of the world's traditional healing systems. It's a useful, fast-acting treatment for mouth ulcers, gingivitis, periodontitis and bleeding gums because it is an effective antiseptic, helps reduce swelling and inflammation, has a local anaesthetic action and encourages wound healing.

Dosage ▶ Myrrh is normally used as a tincture, which is available from an herbalist. It can be painted onto

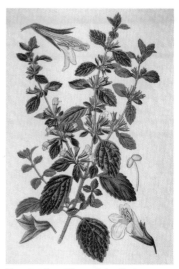
If you brush past lemon balm, the leaves release a delicious lemon-and-mint scent.

mouth ulcers and infections without being diluted, or added to water (30 to 60 drops at a time) for use as a mouthwash or gargle for more generalized gum problems.

Cautions
- Only apply clove oil as a topical treatment to teeth and gums. Do not take it internally.
- Clove oil sometimes causes contact dermatitis or worsens irritation of the gums and mucous membranes. If this occurs, stop using it and rinse your mouth thoroughly with water.
- Use clove oil only as an emergency or short-term remedy until you are able to access professional dental care. Avoid using it repeatedly or for long periods of time, as it may damage gum tissue.
- Do not confuse myrrh (*Commiphora myrrha*) with *Myrrhis odorata* (sweet cicely).
- Do not use any of the herbs listed on this page if you are pregnant or breastfeeding, except under the advice of a healthcare professional.

A biblical herb

Myrrh has long been a valuable trading commodity, and was often worth more than its weight in gold. Uses throughout the ages include: mummification; the preservation of wine; a treatment for snake bite, intestinal worms and scurvy; and as an aphrodisiac. It is known to kill various pests that carry human parasites, including mosquitoes and ticks; pellets of myrrh were burned in ancient Egyptian homes to help rid them of fleas.

First aid

Stock your herb garden and medicine cabinet with the right remedies and you'll be ready to handle all life's little mishaps.

Aloe vera

Aloe vera, A. ferox

Speedy burn repair

Keep an aloe vera plant (*Aloe* sp., including *Aloe vera* and *A. ferox*) on your kitchen windowsill so that it's handy if you accidentally burn yourself while cooking. Not only does the cooling aloe vera gel soothe the pain of burns, it also reduces inflammation. And if the skin is broken, aloe vera helps protect the burn site from infection as well as encourages the skin's collagen to repair itself. The result is that burns (and other kinds of wounds) heal more rapidly when aloe vera is used; in fact, researchers estimate that using aloe vera gel speeds up burn healing time by more than 8 days.

Dosage ▶ Apply the mucilaginous gel from the center of the aloe vera leaf to the affected area 3 times per day, or use a commercially prepared gel that contains a high percentage of aloe vera. Avoid using small, young leaves, as the active

constituents are most prevalent at about 3 years old. When shopping for commercial products, choose those certified by the International Aloe Science Council (IASC), which ensures that the product is of high quality.

Arnica

Arnica montana

Bumps and bruises

Arnica has a long history of use as a topical treatment for bruises and for helping them to heal quickly. Users often report that their bruises change color more quickly and consider this an indication that the healing process is enhanced. It is also traditionally indicated for the treatment of swollen or sprained tissue. Homoeopathic preparations of arnica can be taken internally for the same conditions.

Dosage ▶ Apply arnica cream, ointment or infused oil to the affected area 3 times per day. Choose a product that contains 10 to 20 percent arnica tincture or oil.

Calendula

Calendula officinalis

Skin healer

A traditional remedy for burns, wounds, grazes and rashes, calendula has been documented as encouraging skin healing in a range of circumstances, and may also be useful in helping stop bleeding.

Dosage ▶ For broken skin, first cleanse the wound with an antiseptic solution to ensure that it's clean, then apply calendula tincture to the affected area 3 times per day.

For closed wounds, grazes, rashes and burns, apply calendula cream, ointment or infused oil to the affected area 3 times per day.

Chickweed

Stellaria media

Soothes itches and relieves rashes

Cooling chickweed is a traditional remedy for all manner of itchy skin conditions, so it's useful to have on hand to relieve rashes and bites. It may also be useful in soothing the irritation and itch of urticaria or hives.

Dosage ▶ Juice the fresh aerial parts of the chickweed plant, and mix into a cream or ointment base using a ratio of 1 part chickweed to 5 parts base cream. Apply to the affected area as required. Alternatively, use a commercially prepared cream in the same way.

Lavender oil

Lavandula angustifolia

Takes the sting out of insect bites

Lavender essential oil can quickly relieve inflammation and swelling when applied to insect bites and stings. It also has antimicrobial activity to help prevent wounds from becoming infected. Its use in burns is reputed to have started when the French scientist Gattefosse (one of the pioneers of aromatherapy) stuck his hand in a nearby bowl of lavender oil after burning himself in his laboratory, and was intrigued by how quickly his skin healed.

Dosage ▶ Dab undiluted lavender oil onto insect bites or stings as quickly as possible after they occur. For wounds and burns, first cleanse the wound with an antiseptic solution to ensure that it's clean, then apply undiluted lavender oil to the affected area 3 times a day.

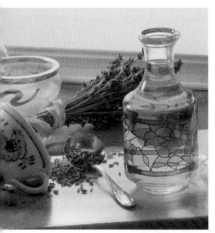

Lavender oil (*Lavandula angustifolia*)

Slippery elm

Ulmus rubra

Drawing agent for splinters and boils

In the same way that slippery elm is used internally to reduce inflammation in the gastrointestinal tract, its soothing properties can also be applied to irritated and inflamed skin. Mixed with water, it forms a gel-like layer that protects the wound and allows it to heal. Slippery elm poultices can also be used to draw splinters and other foreign bodies from the skin, and to encourage boils and abscesses to come to a head.

Dosage ▶ Mix slippery elm bark powder with hot water until it has a pastelike consistency, and use it as a poultice on wounds, to draw foreign bodies out of the skin or to hasten the resolution of boils and abscesses. For more detailed instructions, see *page 168.*

Tea-tree oil

Melaleuca alternifolia

Nature's potent antiseptic

Tea-tree oil is one of nature's most important antiseptics, and its activity against an extensive variety of bacteria, viruses and fungi is well documented. Since it also has anti-inflammatory properties, it's very useful for cuts, grazes and deeper wounds, and can help prevent them from becoming infected.

Dosage ▶ Tea-tree oil can be used undiluted to help cleanse wounds at risk of infection or on tougher skin surfaces (for example, the soles of the feet), but will often make an open wound sting and smart, so in most cases a solution containing 15 percent tea-tree oil is more appropriate. Creams and lotions containing tea-tree oil are also available.

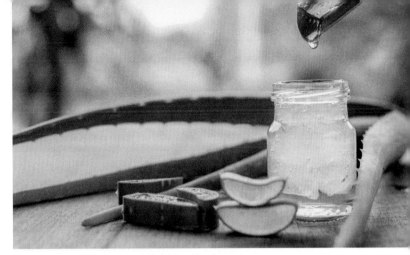

Aloe vera is a very useful herbal medicine for skin treatment.

Cautions

● Do not consume essential oils of tea-tree or lavender.

● Do not consume aloe vera gel unless in a commercial form that is specifically intended for internal use.

● Do not take arnica internally, except in its very dilute homoeopathic form. Do not apply it to broken skin or near the eyes or mouth. Do not use topical applications of arnica for more than 10 days at a time.

● Topical applications of any herb can some-times cause reactions, such as dermatitis, or itching and burning sensations, so perform a patch test at least 24 hours before use. Discontinue use if a reaction develops. Take particular care with arnica and calendula if you are allergic to the Asteraceae family (for example, daisies, chrysanthemum and echinacea) and with arnica if you are allergic to the Lauraceae family (for example, sassafras, avocado, camphor laurel). Take note that topical use of essential oils may also irritate the skin, especially if it is already inflamed.

● With the exception of topical applications of calendula and aloe vera, do not use the herbs listed on these pages if you are pregnant or breastfeeding, except under the advice of a healthcare professional.

New Zealand tea tree

The essential oil of the New Zealand tea tree or manuka (*Leptospermum scoparium*) is strongly antimicrobial and can be diluted and used to disinfect wounds. A particularly important remedy is honey from bees that graze on manuka. Manuka honey contains a compound called Unique Manuka Factor (UMF), which super-charges its ability to heal infections. Extensive research at the University of Waikato in New Zealand has demonstrated that high-UMF honey disinfects wounds and also encourages them to heal, making it an ideal dressing for leg ulcers and other slow-healing skin infections. High-UMF honey is labeled as "active manuka" honey. Other manuka honeys without the "active" label (or a UMF rating of at least 10) are not likely to be as potent.

Sports injuries, sprains & strains

Taken a nasty knock? These herbs can help you get up and about and back on the playing field.

Arnica
Arnica montana
Reduces bruising and repairs swollen or injured tissue
Topical applications of arnica have traditionally been used to reduce bruising and stimulate the healing of muscles and other soft tissues after trauma. As long as the skin is not broken, arnica can be rubbed into sprains, strains, swollen joints, fractures and dislocations. It is also used internally in extremely dilute homoeopathic preparations, and although this use is controversial in the medical world, several clinical trials have been published that suggest arnica may have a beneficial effect. For example, marathon runners have been documented to experience less muscle soreness when they take homoeopathic arnica pills in the days before and after a race.
Dosage ▶ Apply arnica cream, ointment or infused oil to the affected area 3 times per day. For internal use, take commercially prepared homoeopathic arnica pills or liquid in the strength 30x (sometimes labeled 30D) according to the manufacturer's instructions.

Comfrey
Symphytum officinale
Traditionally used to heal strains, sprains and fractures
Comfrey was once widely used internally as well as externally to encourage broken bones to heal, and was so highly regarded for this use that it was also known by the names "knitbone" and 'boneset." However, following the revelation that

some of its compounds (known as pyrrolizidine alkaloids) are potentially toxic, these days its use is restricted to topical applications. As well as being used for fractures, comfrey helps soothe and take the swelling out of strains and sprains.

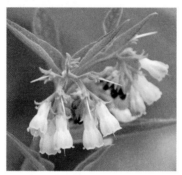

The hairy foliage of the comfrey plant may cause skin irritation in some people.

Dosage ▶ Juice the fresh aerial parts of the comfrey plant, and mix into a cream or ointment base using a ratio of 1 part comfrey to 5 parts base cream. Apply to the affected area as required. Alternatively, blend a few fresh leaves from a comfrey plant into a pulp and make a poultice from them. For detailed instructions, see *page 168*. If you don't have access to a comfrey plant, commercial cream and ointments are also available.

Witch hazel
Hamamelis virginiana
Stems bleeding and reduces swelling
With its high concentration of tannins, witch hazel is highly regarded as an astringent remedy with the ability to stop bleeding and reduce inflammation — especially the

localized swelling caused by sprains and other injuries. It is also used to encourage the healing of bruises.
Dosage ▶ Apply commercially prepared witch hazel cream or ointment to strains, sprains, grazes or bruises 2 to 3 times per day. Alternatively, prepare a decoction using 1 to 2 teaspoons of the dried leaves or bark, and use the liquid to make a compress for the affected part. For detailed instructions, see *page 168*.

White willow bark
Salix alba
Aspirin-like pain relief
Studies show that white willow bark preparations, standardized for their content of salicin, provide effective relief of lower back pain, with up to 40 percent of volunteers becoming pain-free after taking the herb for 4 weeks. These results are not surprising, since salicin (which has aspirin-like properties), has well-documented anti-inflammatory and analgesic effects.
Dosage ▶ Take commercially prepared white willow bark tablets or capsules (standardized to contain 240 mg of salicin per day), according to the manufacturer's instructions.

Devil's claw
Harpagophytum procumbens
Highly effective anti-inflammatory
This African herb has a long history of use to reduce pain and inflammation in muscles and joints, and is traditionally prescribed for joint, back and tendon pain caused by injury and overuse. These traditional applications are supported by

scientific studies in which devil's claw reduced muscle stiffness when taken for 4 weeks, and reduced back pain and increased mobility in 4 to 8 weeks.

Dosage ▶ The most important active constituent of devil's claw is a compound called harpagoside, and according to researchers, preparations standardized for their content of harpagoside are more effective than non-standardized preparations. Look for commercial tablets or capsules providing at least 50 mg harpagoside per day, and take according to the manufacturer's instructions.

Cramp bark
Viburnum opulus
Muscle relaxant and anti-spasmodic

If you're prone to tension or spasms in your muscles, cramp bark may be just the herb you're looking for. Native Americans used it to relieve cramps and other types of muscle pain, and herbalists still prescribe it today. With an ability to reduce both long- and short-term muscle tension, it is considered particularly effective for overuse injuries and backache.

Dosage ▶ Take commercially prepared cramp bark tablets or tincture, up to a maximum dose of 1 g, 3 times per day.

St. John's wort
Hypericum perforatum
Topical treatment for nerve pain

Topical applications of St. John's wort historically have been used to treat nerve pain of various kinds, but especially the pain of sciatica. This traditional use is supported by laboratory tests that demonstrate both anti-inflammatory and painkilling properties.

Dosage ▶ Rub the infused oil of St. John's wort flowers into the affected part, 2 to 3 times per day. For instructions on how to make infused oils, see *page 169*.

Cautions

- Arnica and comfrey should not be taken internally (except in their very dilute homoeopathic forms), and should not be applied to broken skin or near the eyes. Avoid using comfrey for more than 10 days at a time.
- Topical applications of any herb can sometimes cause reactions, such as dermatitis or itching and burning sensations, and ideally a patch test should be performed at least 24 hours prior to use; discontinue if a reaction develops. Take particular care with arnica if you are allergic to the Asteraceae (for example, daisies, chrysanthemum, echinacea) or Lauraceae families of plants (for example, sassafras, avocado, camphor laurel).
- Cramp bark berries are poisonous and should not be ingested.
- Do not take white willow bark if you are allergic to salicylates (including aspirin). If you are taking antiplatelet or anti-coagulant medication, or if you suffer from a blood disorder, only take it under professional supervision.
- Devil's claw may occasionally cause digestive problems, such as diarrhea, and should not be used by people with pre-existing gastrointestinal complaints, such as ulcers, gallstones or diarrhea, except under professional advice.
- Do not take devil's claw if you are taking warfarin or antiarrhythmic drugs, except under professional advice. Stop taking devil's claw at least 2 weeks before undergoing surgery.
- Devil's claw does not appear to be effective for back pain that radiates down the legs, a symptom that may indicate nerve involvement. It should be investigated by a healthcare professional.

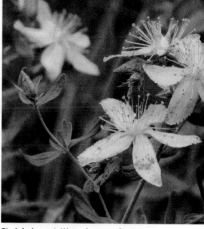

St. John's wort (*Hypericum perforatum*)

- With the exception of topical applications of St. John's wort and witch hazel, do not use any of these herbs if you are pregnant or breastfeeding, except under the advice of a healthcare professional.

Take action

The actions you take immediately after a soft tissue injury have a direct influence on how quickly the problem heals.

- **Reduce** blood flow and slow both swelling and bleeding by resting the injured part as quickly as you can.
- **Apply** an ice pack to the injured area to reduce inflammation, pain and tissue damage, but always make sure you protect your skin from ice burn by placing a wet towel or cloth beneath the ice and your skin.
- **Apply** a firm, wide bandage, known as a compression bandage, over the injured area to help reduce bleeding and swelling.
- **Raise** the injured part so it is higher than the heart, further reducing blood flow to the area.
- **Consult** a physiotherapist or doctor as soon as possible, because many soft tissue injuries require professional treatment.

Arthritis & gout

Don't let the stiffness, debilitating pain and inflammation of arthritis cramp your style. Try some herbal remedies.

Boswellia

Boswellia serrata

Relief from rheumatoid and osteoarthritis

The resin from the boswellia tree has been used in Ayurvedic medicine for the treatment of inflammatory and rheumatic conditions for centuries. With a combination of anti-inflammatory, analgesic and immune system-modifying effects, it is particularly relevant for rheumatoid arthritis, an autoimmune form of arthritis that is both debilitating and difficult to treat.

In a review collating the results from 12 rheumatoid arthritis studies, researchers concluded that boswellia was just as effective as some medicinal treatments (for example, gold therapy), and could be particularly useful for sufferers whose arthritis responds poorly to more conventional medication, for those who have had the disease for a long time, and for children with juvenile chronic arthritis. Boswellia also offers improvements in osteoarthritis, and is documented to help decrease pain and swelling,

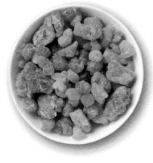

Resin made from boswellia extract has been used for centuries in Asian and African folk medicine

improve range of motion and increase walking distance in people with osteoarthritis of the knee.

Dosage ▶ Look for commercial preparations standardized for their content of the active constituents boswellic acids, and take according to manufacturer's instructions or as professionally prescribed. The research into osteoarthritis used the equivalent of 1000 mg of boswellia resin (sometimes referred to as oleo-gum or gum resin) per day, standardized to contain 40 percent (400 mg) boswellic acids. Research indicates that it may take up to 2 months for significant effects to be felt, but that they persist for some time after the herb is stopped. Rheumatoid arthritis is a complex condition that is not well suited to self-treatment — ask your healthcare professional to assess whether boswellia is an appropriate treatment for you, and only take it according to the prescribed dosage.

Devil's claw

Harpagophytum procumbens

Clinically proven for arthritis pain

Devil's claw has anti-inflammatory and analgesic properties, and is a proven treatment for osteoarthritis, with several studies demonstrating its benefits — particularly for osteoarthritis of the knee and/or hip. In some of these studies, devil's claw was compared to pharmaceutical analgesics, with researchers concluding that the herb was just as effective as the drug, but with a lower incidence of side effects. Laboratory tests suggest that devil's

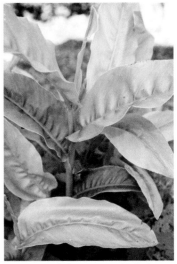

The rhizomes of the leafy ginger plant are harvested at least a year after planting.

claw may provide more than just symptomatic relief — it also appears to inhibit some of the processes that both damage cartilage and trigger the joint changes characteristic of osteoarthritis. Clinical trials indicate that pain and other symptoms of osteoarthritis start to abate after about 2 months of taking the herb.

Dosage ▶ The most important active constituent of devil's claw is a compound called harpagoside, and according to researchers, preparations standardized for their content of harpagoside are more effective than non-standardized preparations. Look for commercially prepared tablets or capsules providing at least 50 mg harpagoside per day, and take according to the manufacturer's instructions.

Ginger

Zingiber officinale

The spicy anti-inflammatory

The humble spice ginger is also a potent medicine with impressive anti-inflammatory capabilities. Laboratory tests show that ginger inhibits a number of the compounds that promote inflammation in the body — including several of the enzymes that are targeted by pharmaceutical anti-arthritis medications. As a result, it provides relief from arthritis pain, and some studies have even found it to be as effective as the non-steroidal anti-inflammatory drug ibuprofen.

Dosage ▶ Add 20 to 30 drops of ginger tincture to water, or infuse ½ teaspoon powdered ginger or 1 to 2 teaspoons of grated fresh ginger root in boiling water; take 3 times per day. Concentrated ginger tablets may also be useful.

White willow bark

Salix alba

Herbal pain reliever

The bark of the white willow tree is believed to have been used as an herbal painkiller since at least the time of Hippocrates. Laboratory tests have demonstrated the anti-inflammatory and analgesic properties of its aspirin-like substances. Most (but not all) clinical trials also support its role in relieving the pain of osteoarthritis, but there has not been enough research to confirm its effectiveness in the treatment of rheumatoid arthritis.

Dosage ▶ Take commercial white willow tablets or capsules standardized to contain 240 mg of salicin per day according to the manufacturer's instructions.

White willow bark
(*Salix alba*)

Celery seed

Apium graveolens

Handy gout remedy

Celery seed is a traditional remedy for all kinds of arthritis, but it is considered particularly effective for the treatment of gout. This extremely painful form of arthritis classically affects a single joint, such as the big toe, which rapidly becomes hot, swollen and inflamed.

Dosage ▶ Boil 0.5 g to 2 g dried celery seed in a cup of water for 10 minutes; drink the decoction up to 3 times daily. Alternatively, take a commercially prepared tincture, tablet or capsule according to the manufacturer's instructions.

Cautions

● Boswellia occasionally causes mild adverse effects, such as diarrhea or hives. If this happens, discontinue its use. Little is known about potential interactions between boswellia and other medications, so if you are taking prescription drugs, talk to your doctor or pharmacist before using it.

● Devil's claw may occasionally cause digestive problems such as diarrhea, so should not be used by people with pre-existing gastrointestinal complaints, such as ulcers, gallstones or diarrhea, except under professional advice.

● Do not take devil's claw if you are taking warfarin or anti-arrhythmic drugs, except under professional advice. Stop taking devil's claw at least 2 weeks before undergoing surgery.

● Do not take white willow bark if you are allergic to salicylates, including aspirin. If you are taking antiplatelet or anticoagulant medication, or suffer

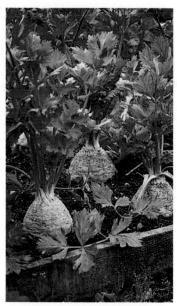

Celery seed (*Apium graveolens*) promotes the elimination of uric acid and waste products and so is helpful in cases of gout.

from a blood disorder, take it only under professional supervision.

● Ginger should not be taken in medicinal doses by people suffering from gastric ulcer or gallstones, or those taking warfarin or antiplatelet medication, except under professional advice. Stop taking it at least 2 weeks prior to undergoing surgery.

● Celery seed may interact with medications, including warfarin and thyroxine. It may also increase the risk of side effects associated with some forms of ultraviolet light therapy. Consult your doctor before use.

● Do not use celery seed if you have a kidney disorder, or if you have low blood pressure.

● Celery occasionally causes allergic reactions. Do not take the seed if you are allergic to the plant or vegetable, and exercise caution if you are allergic to dandelion or wild carrot.

● With the exception of ginger, do not take these herbs if you are pregnant or breastfeeding, except under the advice of a healthcare professional.

Circulation problems & varicose veins

Inadequate circulation – particularly in the legs – can become a persistent and debilitating problem as you age.

Horse chestnut

Aesculus hippocastanum

Relieves symptoms of chronic venous insufficiency

The term "chronic venous insufficiency" is used medically to describe leg veins that are having trouble pumping blood back up to the heart. In time, and with the effects of gravity, the legs become heavy and swollen, and can feel itchy, tense and painful. Varicose veins may also develop. At least 17 clinical trials have examined the effects of horse chestnut seed extract (HCSE), standardized for its content of escin, on the symptoms of chronic venous insufficiency. Collectively, this research demonstrates that HCSE can help to relieve the pain, swelling and itchiness associated with chronic venous insufficiency. It appears to do this by helping to maintain the integrity of the blood vessel walls.

Dosage ▶ Take commercial tablets or capsules of HCSE that are standardized for their content of escin (sometimes spelt aescin). Look for a product that provides 100 mg to 200 mg of escin per day, and always take it with food.

Grapeseed

Vitis vinifera

Antioxidant support for blood vessels

Grapeseed extract is rich in a potent group of antioxidants collectively referred to as oligomeric proanthocyanidins (OPCs). OPCs help to maintain the integrity of the blood vessels and stabilise the capillary walls, so they may be beneficial for a wide range of circulatory problems. In people with chronic venous insufficiency, grapeseed extract has been shown to relieve symptoms such as itchiness and leg pain in as little as 10 days, and it's likely to have even more benefits for the circulatory system when taken over a longer period of time.

Dosage ▶ Look for commercial grapeseed tablets, or capsules that are standardized to provide 150 mg to 300 mg OPCs per day, and take them according to the manufacturer's instructions.

Ginkgo

Ginkgo biloba

Tonic for peripheral circulation

Although most famous for its action as a memory tonic, ginkgo is also an important circulatory tonic. For example, it helps relieve symptoms of both Raynaud's syndrome and intermittent claudication — two conditions associated with peripheral circulation issues. Raynaud's syndrome is characterized by coldness of the extremities and intermittent claudication by severe cramping pain in the legs that is triggered or exacerbated by walking.

Dosage ▶ Look for supplements standardized for their content of the active constituents ginkgo flavone glycosides, ginkgolides and bilobalides, with a daily dose of 120 mg of a concentrated (50:1) extract, providing the equivalent of 6 g of the dried herb. Higher doses may be required for intermittent claudication — for more information, talk to your healthcare professional.

Cautions

● Horse chestnut, ginkgo and grapeseed are known or suspected to interact with some prescription medications, so consult your doctor or pharmacist before taking them. Stop taking ginkgo and grapeseed at least 2 weeks before surgery.

● HCSE occasionally causes side effects including gastrointestinal symptoms, nausea, headaches and itchy or irritated skin. If this occurs, stop taking the herb and seek medical advice.

● Do not take homemade horse chestnut or ginkgo preparations, as they may contain toxic compounds and/or cause adverse reactions.

● Do not use horse chestnut if you are allergic to latex, as cross-reactivity may occur.

● Do not take HCSE if you have diabetes, liver or kidney problems, or celiac or other intestinal diseases, or if you are taking anti-platelet or anticoagulant medication, except under professional supervision.

● Grapeseed may reduce iron absorption, so separate doses by 2 hours.

● Ginkgo may cause mild adverse reactions, including dizziness, gastrointestinal upset, headache and allergic skin reactions. More severe reactions, including bleeding problems and seizures, have occasionally been recorded. If symptoms occur, stop taking the herb and seek medical advice.

● Do not take ginkgo if you have any kind of bleeding disorder.

● Do not use any of the herbs listed on this page if you are pregnant or breastfeeding, except under the advice of a healthcare professional.

Leg ulcers

A leg ulcer that won't heal can have a negative impact on your quality of life. Use herbs to aid the healing process.

Horse chestnut
Aesculus hippocastanum
Helps heal ulcers from the inside

According to a small clinical trial, a standardized extract of horse chestnut seed (HCSE) has been demonstrated to enhance the standard medical treatment of leg ulcers. Australian researchers found that compared to those taking a placebo, the wound dressings on the legs of people taking HCSE could be changed less frequently, resulting in a significantly lower cost of treatment. These effects are probably an extension of the actions of horse chestnut on peripheral circulation (see opposite), as about half of all leg ulcers occur as a result of chronic venous insufficiency.

Dosage ▶ Take commercial tablets or capsules of HCSE that are standardized for their content of escin. Look for a product that provides 100 mg to 200 mg of escin per day, and always take it with food.

Gotu kola
Centella asiatica
Nature's tissue healer

Gotu kola contains compounds that encourage wounds, ulcers and scars to heal, and can be used both internally and externally for this purpose. Taken internally, it can also aid symptoms of chronic venous insufficiency so, like horse chestnut, it may encourage the healing of ulcers.

Dosage ▶ Take commercially prepared tablets or capsules of gotu kola extract according to the manufacturer's instructions. For topical use, add gotu kola tincture

to a cream or ointment base (for detailed instructions, see *page 167*), and apply to the affected area 2 to 3 times per day.

Calendula
Calendula officinalis
Accelerates ulcer healing

Calendula ointment was recently the subject of a small-scale clinical trial that suggests it may play a valuable role in helping to heal leg ulcers. In this study, ulcers were treated with either calendula ointment or saline solution dressings for 3 weeks. At the end of the trial, the ulcers treated with calendula ointment had shrunk in size by more than 40 percent, while those treated with saline had only decreased by about 15 percent.

Dosage ▶ Apply calendula ointment to the affected area 2 to 3 times per day, or soak dressings with calendula tincture and then apply to the affected area. You can also use fresh calendula flowers to make a poultice (see *page 168*). If the skin is broken, disinfect the wound by washing it with an antiseptic before using calendula.

Cautions

● Ulcers are not well suited to self-treatment, as they may be symptomatic of underlying vascular problems. Always seek medical advice before commencing any self-prescribed treatment, including topical applications.

● HCSE occasionally causes side effects, including gastrointestinal symptoms, nausea, headaches and itchy or irritated skin. It should not be taken by people with a latex allergy.

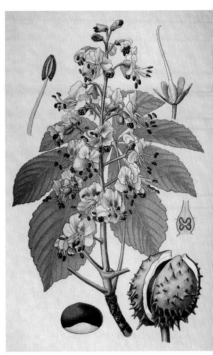

Horse chestnut is also known as buckeye, because the seeds resemble the eyes of deer.

● Do not consume homemade horse chestnut preparations, as they may contain toxic compounds.

● Do not take HCSE if you have diabetes, liver or kidney problems, or celiac or other intestinal diseases, or if you are taking anti-platelet or anticoagulant medication, except under the supervision of a healthcare professional.

● The skin around leg ulcers is particularly prone to dermatitis and rashes. Ideally, a patch test should be performed at least 24 hours before any topical application. If a reaction develops, discontinue use and seek medical advice. Take particular care with calendula if you are allergic to the Asteraceae family of plants (for example, daisies, chrysanthemum and echinacea).

● With the exception of topical applications of calendula, do not use any of the herbs listed on this page if you are pregnant or breastfeeding, except under the advice of a healthcare professional.

High blood pressure & high cholesterol

Blood pressure and cholesterol levels are important indicators of heart health, as well as your risk of cardiovascular disease.

Hawthorn

Crataegus laevigata, C. monogyna, C. pinnatifida

Classic heart tonic

Herbalists regard hawthorn as the most important of all cardiovascular remedies, with a protective action on the heart and its function. It is prescribed for a range of cardiovascular problems, including high blood pressure, high cholesterol, angina, irregular heartbeat and heart failure. Numerous clinical trials support the use of hawthorn as an adjunctive treatment for heart failure, and in this context it is documented to help reduce blood pressure as well as improve other symptoms, such as tiredness and shortness of breath. Some of hawthorn's active constituents have potent antioxidant activity, and these compounds may be responsible for the herb's cholesterol-lowering effects, helping to prevent the oxidation of LDL-cholesterol (so-called "bad" cholesterol), and decreasing both the production and absorption of cholesterol.

Dosage ▶ Ask your healthcare professional to assess whether hawthorn is an appropriate treatment for you, and take it according to the dosage prescribed. To ensure you receive a guaranteed dose of the herb's key active constituents, your practitioner may stipulate a standardized hawthorn preparation. Take it for at least 2 months before assessing whether it's working effectively. Western herbalists have long used *Crataegus laevigata* and *C. monogyna* to treat cardiovascular problems. In traditional Chinese medicine, *C. pinnatifida* has an extensive history of use as a digestive tonic, but its application has extended to heart complaints, in line with the promising results attributed to the European species.

Garlic

Allium sativum

Protects the heart and blood vessels

There's good evidence to suggest that the more garlic you include in your diet, the less likely you are to suffer from cardiovascular disease. And when taken as an herbal medicine, it's been shown to lower blood pressure, reduce total cholesterol levels and the development of plaque in the arteries, and inhibit the formation of blood clots. Some of these actions in the body are only mild, temporary or applicable to certain groups of people, but because it works via several pathways, the collective effect is a degree of protection for overall cardiovascular health.

Dosage ▶ The scientific research into garlic's potential as a treatment for high blood pressure and cholesterol is controversial — not least because different commercial garlic preparations have different chemical characteristics, and some may not retain the medicinally effective compounds, which can degrade quickly after the garlic bulb is cut or crushed. If you decide to take garlic tablets or capsules, opt for those that are enteric-coated and labeled with a guaranteed yield of the compound allicin, or standardized for their content of alliin. Other high-quality supplements may be standardized for their content of S-allyl-L-cysteine (SAC). Follow the dosage recommendations of the manufacturer. If you prefer to consume garlic as a food, aim to eat at least 3 cloves per week, or even more if you are at particular risk of cardiovascular disease. Chop or mince the cloves, then leave them to stand at room temperature for 5 to 10 minutes, so that enzymatic reaction allows the biologically active compounds to develop.

Turmeric

Curcuma longa

Cholesterol-clearing spice

Turmeric is another culinary spice that supports heart and blood vessel health. It contains a yellow-colored pigment called curcumin — the compound that is credited with most of the herb's medicinal activity. For example, curcumin has been shown to lower levels of total cholesterol, increase levels of HDL-cholesterol ("good" cholesterol), and protect both HDL- and LDL-cholesterol from the damaging effects of free radical activity. In laboratory and animal studies, it has also been shown to help lower blood pressure and reduce the ability of cholesterol to form plaque on artery walls.

Dosage ▶ Add up to 3 g of grated or powdered turmeric root to your cooking each day. Alternatively, look for a commercial preparation that has been standardized to contain 95 percent curcumin, and take it according to the manufacturer's instructions, up to a maximum of 300 mg per day.

Psyllium

Plantago ovata, P. psyllium

Lowers cholesterol levels

Psyllium is an important source of water-soluble fiber, which forms an absorbent gel in the bowel, trapping cholesterol and facilitating its excretion from the body. Combining psyllium with a low-fat diet for as little as 8 weeks has been shown to reduce LDL-cholesterol without adversely affecting HDL-cholesterol levels. Under professional supervision, psyllium may be particularly beneficial for patients with Type 2 diabetes, because it can also help control their blood glucose and insulin responses after meals.

Dosage ▶ Psyllium husks are available in tablet, capsule and soluble powder form, and should be taken according to the manufacturer's instructions (note that the dose of psyllium used in cholesterol research is generally about 10 g per day). Every dose of psyllium should be taken with a large glass of water.

Lime flowers

Tilia cordata, T. platyphyllos, T. x europaea

Calming blood pressure remedy

Lime flowers are a traditional European medicine for high blood pressure, especially when it is accompanied by heart palpitations or hardening of the arteries. They are also a gently calming remedy for anxiety and restlessness, so are particularly useful when high blood pressure is caused or worsened by worry.

Dosage ▶ Infuse 1 teaspoon of dried lime flowers in boiling water and drink up to 3 cups per day.

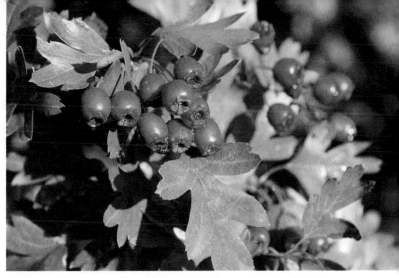

With its white flowers followed by red berries, the hawthorn makes a pretty hedge.

Cautions

- Heart disease and other cardiovascular conditions are potentially serious issues, and should not be self-treated. Always follow the advice of your doctor, and if you experience any symptoms that may indicate a heart attack, such as chest pain (which may radiate to the jaw, back or arms), shortness of breath, or a general feeling of discomfort in the upper body, call for an ambulance without delay.

- Hawthorn, garlic and turmeric are known or suspected to interact with many prescription medications (including heart, blood pressure, cholesterol and blood-thinning drugs), and may alter the dosage requirements of your existing medication, so consult your doctor or pharmacist before taking these particular herbal remedies.

- Occasionally, adverse effects of hawthorn have been reported in clinical trials, but they tend to be mild and transient. The symptoms may include digestive problems, headache, dizziness, sleepiness and palpitations. If you experience any of these symptoms, consult your healthcare professional.

- Garlic can cause side effects, including gastrointestinal discomfort, nausea, indigestion, offensive breath and body odor. Some of these effects can be minimized by eating cooked rather than raw garlic.

- Turmeric sometimes causes side effects of gastrointestinal upset when taken in large doses. Except under professional advice, it should not be used at higher than culinary doses by people with liver and gallbladder disease (including gallstones), gastric or duodenal ulcer, or people taking blood-thinners.

- Persons with diagnosed intestinal illness should only use psyllium on medical advice.

- Psyllium may interfere with the absorption of other medicines, so separate doses by at least 2 hours.

- Always drink plenty of water when using psyllium, as occasionally cases of choking have been reported when psyllium powders have been taken without adequate fluids.

- Lime flowers may reduce the absorption of iron, so separate doses by at least 2 hours.

- Contact allergies to lime flowers have occasionally been reported.

- If you are pregnant or breastfeeding, do not take hawthorn, lime flowers or psyllium, except under professional supervision. Do not take garlic or turmeric in greater than culinary quantities.

Premenstrual syndrome

There is gentle herbal help available for treating hormonal imbalances, period pain, mood swings and cravings.

Chaste tree
Vitex agnus-castus
Clinically proven to reduce PMS symptoms

In clinical trials, chaste tree extracts have shown a remarkable ability to relieve many of the symptoms of premenstrual syndrome (PMS), including depression, anger and irritability, mood swings, food cravings, bowel problems, and headaches. It achieves these effects by helping to normalize the complex hormonal fluctuations that govern the female menstrual cycle, and can help set up a regular pattern of menstruation. In clinical practice, herbalists also prescribe chaste tree (often in combination with other herbs) for women who are experiencing difficulties conceiving.

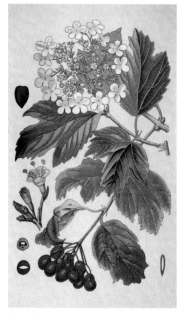

Chaste berries are used as a pepper substitute and in Middle Eastern spice mixes.

Dosage ▶ To relieve the symptoms of premenstrual syndrome, take tablets, capsules or tincture throughout the month, according to the manufacturer's instructions. Look for products that are standardized for their content of the compounds casticin and/or agnuside. Results may take 12 weeks or longer to become noticeable. If you're experiencing difficulty conceiving, consult a medical herbalist who has been professionally trained and who can help to determine whether chaste tree is appropriate for you.

White peony
Paeonia lactiflora
Hormone balancer

In the traditional medicine of China and Japan, white peony root is combined with other herbs to treat period pain, heavy bleeding, uterine fibroids and other issues that, in Chinese medical philosophy, are associated with pelvic congestion. It is commonly prescribed with licorice for conditions such as polycystic ovarian syndrome (PCOS) and endometriosis and, like chaste tree, is thought to exert its effects via a balancing influence on hormone levels.

Dosage ▶ Talk to a professionally trained herbalist, who can help to determine whether white peony is appropriate for your individual needs.

Dong quai
Angelica polymorpha var. *sinensis*
Chinese tonic for female problems

Dong quai is another herb prescribed in traditional Chinese medicine

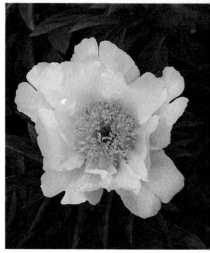

White peony is revered in traditional Chinese medicine.

for female reproductive disorders. Among other indications, and generally in combination with other herbs, it is prescribed for a range of gynaecological conditions, including painful, irregular, scanty or absent periods. To date there has been little clinical research to confirm whether the high regard in which it is held in China is justified.

Dosage ▶ Boil 1 g to 3 g dried dong quai root in a cup of water for 10 minutes; drink the decoction 3 times daily. Alternatively, take commercial tablets or capsules, according to the manufacturer's instructions.

St. John's wort
Hypericum perforatum
Proven antidepressant

PMS causes many women to experience depression, increased anxiety and also difficulty in relating to family and friends. Since its efficacy for the treatment of depression from other causes is well established, it's likely that St. John's wort is also an effective treatment for these PMS symptoms. In a small pilot study published in 2000, women taking St. John's wort reported that the severity of their mental and emotional PMS symptoms had improved by more than 50 percent after just two menstrual cycles. Further investigation is required to determine whether longer-term use has additional health benefits.

Dosage ▶ Look for supplements that are standardized for their content of hypericin and hyperforin, which are considered the main active constituents, and with a daily dose of 900 mg per day of the concentrated (6:1) extract, which is equivalent to 5.4 g of the dried herb. Take the supplements throughout the month.

Cramp bark
Viburnum opulus
Pain relief for cramps and spasms
Women who experience period pain will find cramp bark invaluable because, as its name suggests, it has a long history of use for the relief of cramps. It is traditionally used for any type of spasmodic or cramping pain, including uterine, ovarian, abdominal, back and leg pains that occur during the premenstrual phase of the monthly cycle.

Dosage ▶ Take commercially prepared cramp bark tablets or tincture, up to a maximum dose of 1 g, 3 times daily, as required for symptomatic relief.

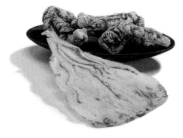

Dong quai (*Angelica polymorpha* var. *sinensis*) naturally gnarled root is flattened out for medicinal use.

Clary sage
Salvia sclarea
For period pain and emotional upsets
The essential oil of clary sage is one of the most popular aromatherapy treatments for PMS, especially as it is also considered to have antidepressant, anti-fatigue and stress-relieving properties. Laboratory research supports the oil's use by demonstrating an antispasmodic action on uterine tissue, but the efficacy of this treatment has only recently been tested in human studies. In 2006, researchers conducted a clinical trial in which college students who suffered from period pain and menstrual cramps used either aromatherapy massage oil containing clary sage, lavender and rose essential oils; massage without aromatherapy; or no treatment at all. The symptoms of the women who received the aromatherapy massage were significantly less severe during the first 2 days of their period than the women in either of the other treatment groups.

Dosage ▶ To relieve period pain, make a massage oil using 1 drop of clary sage, 1 drop of rose and 2 drops of lavender essential oil per 5 ml of almond oil, and rub into the abdomen or lower back as required. For premenstrual mood swings or emotional problems, clary sage can also be added to an oil vaporizer.

Cautions
● The herbs featured on this page have known or suspected hormonal activity and should not be taken at the same time as the oral contraceptive pill, hormone replacement therapy or other medications that affect hormonal balance, except under professional supervision. People

who have a history of hormone-sensitive tumors should only take these herbs under professional advice.

● Chaste tree occasionally causes mild, reversible side effects, such as headache, nausea and gastrointestinal upset. If you experience any of these symptoms, stop taking it.

● Do not take white peony or dong quai if you are taking warfarin or other blood-thinning or anticoagulant medicines.

● Dong quai is traditionally contraindicated in women with bleeding disorders, heavy periods or a history of recurrent miscarriage. It should not be used during bouts of diarrhea or acute viral infection.

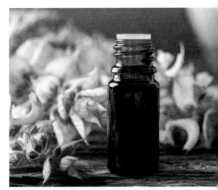

Clary sage blossoms with essential oil.

● Cramp bark berries are poisonous and should not be ingested.

● Clary sage essential oil is very potent and should always be diluted and used sparingly. It may cause headaches or sedation in some people, and may also cause contact dermatitis or skin irritation. Do not apply it to inflamed skin or open wounds, and do not use it topically if you are prone to dermatitis.

● For the safe and appropriate use of St. John's wort, see Depression & anxiety, *page 185*.

● Do not use any of the herbs listed on this page if you are pregnant or breastfeeding, except under the advice of a healthcare professional.

Fluid retention & cystitis

Try using these herbs to keep your fluids in good order and to prevent inflammations and infections such as cystitis.

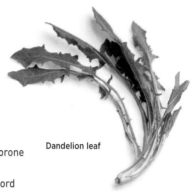
Dandelion leaf

Cranberry

Vaccinium macrocarpon

Prevents cystitis

Cranberry is famous for its ability to help prevent cystitis, a bladder infection that causes burning pain on urination. It works by preventing the bacteria *E. coli* (which causes the vast majority of cystitis cases) from taking hold on the bladder wall and setting up an infection. This herb is particularly useful for women who experience recurrent urinary tract infections (UTIs), as clinical trials indicate that, over a 12-month period,

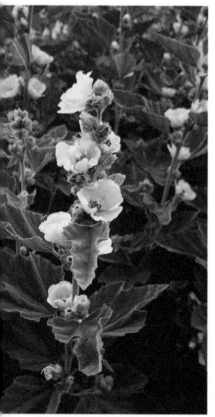

Marsh mallow (*Althaea officinalis*)

the frequency of UTIs in women taking cranberry is significantly reduced. Other people who are prone to recurrent UTIs — such as the elderly and people with spinal cord injuries — may also benefit from taking cranberry as a prophylactic against cystitis, but there is not as much scientific data available to confirm its efficacy in these groups of people.

Dosage ▶ Cranberry can be taken in juice, tablet or capsule form. Many people prefer to take the tablets or capsules, as up to 1¼ cups (300 ml) per day of pure juice may be required in order to reach therapeutic levels. Few commercial juice products contain 100 percent cranberry juice, so if you do decide to take the juice for medicinal purposes, you'll need to calculate how many glasses of juice you require, depending on the percentage of cranberry that's present in the product. Alternatively, cranberry tablets and capsules are made from concentrated juice, and are generally taken at doses of approximately 30 g (30,000 mg) per day, in divided doses.

Marsh mallow

Althaea officinalis

Soothes inflamed mucous membranes

With its rich content of mucilage, marsh mallow provides soothing relief to irritated mucous membranes of the urinary tract. Herbalists often prescribe it to ease the pain and discomfort of infections or inflammation of the bladder and kidneys.

Dosage ▶ Infuse 2 g to 5 g of dried marsh mallow root in cold (not hot) water, and steep for 8 hours to release the mucilage; drink up to 3 cups per day.

Dandelion leaf

Taraxacum officinale

Nature's diuretic with plenty of potassium

Dandelion leaf is traditionally regarded as one of the most important herbal remedies for the elimination of excess fluid, regardless of its cause. Although there is little data available to confirm its efficacy in humans, a small number of animal studies suggest that it may be as effective as some commonly prescribed pharmaceutical drugs. Dandelion leaf is a natural source of potassium; therefore, it doesn't tend to cause the adverse effects associated with potassium depletion that are sometimes observed with the use of pharmaceutical diuretics.

Dosage ▶ Infuse 1 to 2 teaspoons of dried dandelion leaf in boiling water; drink 3 cups per day.

Grapeseed

Vitis vinifera

Relieves premenstrual fluid retention

Hormonal fluctuations during the menstrual cycle can cause

troublesome fluid retention in some women. Although predominantly considered a remedy for the blood vessels, grapeseed extract has also been documented to effectively reduce premenstrual fluid retention and associated symptoms, including weight gain and abdominal pain and swelling.

Dosage ▶ Look for grapeseed tablets or capsules that are standardized to provide 150 mg to 300 mg oligomeric proanthocyanidins (OPCs) per day, and take them during the second half of the menstrual cycle. You may need to take them for several months before experiencing the full benefits.

Cautions

● UTIs are potentially serious — consult your doctor at the first sign of symptoms or if your symptoms worsen during treatment. Always investigate UTIs in children immediately.

● Fluid retention is sometimes a symptom of heart problems or other serious health conditions, in which case

medical treatment is required. Always talk to your doctor before commencing self-treatment.

● High doses of cranberry juice may cause diarrhea and other gastrointestinal symptoms — if this occurs, discontinue use immediately.

● If you are taking warfarin or have a history of kidney stones, do not take medicinal quantities of cranberry except under professional supervision.

● If you have diabetes, avoid drinking high quantities of sugar-sweetened cranberry juice and do not take marsh mallow except under professional supervision, as it may affect blood sugar levels.

● Marsh mallow may interfere with the absorption of other medication, and grapeseed may reduce iron absorption, so separate doses by at least 2 hours.

● Don't use dandelion leaf if you are allergic to members of the Asteraceae family of plants (for example, daisies, echinacea).

● Grapeseed and dandelion leaf (and, particularly, the potassium found in dandelion) may interact with some medications, so check with your doctor or pharmacist before taking them.

● Do not use dandelion if you suffer from liver or gallbladder disease (including gall stones).

● Stop taking grapeseed at least 2 weeks before undergoing surgery.

● With the exception of normal culinary quantities of cranberry, do not take the herbs on this page if you are pregnant or breastfeeding, except under the advice of a healthcare professional.

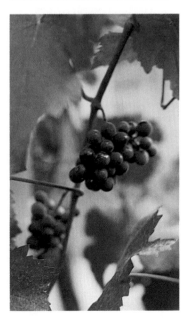

Grape 'Black Hamburgh' (*Vitis vinifera*). There are hundreds of cultivars of the grape vine, grown for fruit (fresh and dried) as well as wine.

Self-help for cystitis

Cranberry is an effective preventative medicine for cystitis, but once an infection takes hold, you may need to take stronger medicine. Your doctor may prescribe antibiotics, or your professionally trained medical herbalist may treat you with urinary antiseptics, such as the herb uva-ursi. Meanwhile, these steps can help.

● **Act quickly** While cystitis is generally a relatively mild and self-limiting condition, if it is left untreated, the infection can spread to the kidneys – with much more serious consequences.

● **Increase your fluid intake** Although the intense pain during urination may discourage you from drinking more, it's vital that you do. At the first sign of symptoms, increase your fluids to about 1 liter per hour, if possible. This helps flush bacteria from the bladder, and can help prevent infections from becoming more serious. Choose water or soothing herbal teas (such as marsh mallow), and avoid alcohol, caffeine and fizzy soft drinks, which may aggravate the problem.

● **Empty your bladder** every time you go to the toilet. Wait a few moments after urinating, and then try again to expel the last few milliliters of urine from the bladder. Afterward, women should take care to wipe from front to back to ensure that bacteria from the anus aren't accidentally transferred to the urinary tract.

● **Alkalize your urine** Reducing urinary acidity may help to relieve burning symptoms, and can also make it more difficult for bacteria to survive. Avoid acidic foods, such as citrus and tomatoes, and consider taking a commercial urinary alkalizer (available from pharmacies). A home remedy of a teaspoon of baking soda in water is also an effective urinary alkalizer.

Menopause

There are natural herbal remedies that will help support your body through the demands of menopause, or the change.

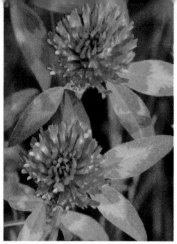

Red clover (*Trifolium pratense*)

Black cohosh

Actaea racemosa

Proven treatment for hot flashes

An extract of the North American herb black cohosh has been used to relieve menopause symptoms for more than 50 years. As the subject of numerous clinical trials, black cohosh extract has demonstrated significant improvements in symptoms such as hot flashes, night sweats, insomnia, depression and anxiety. Of these, it is probably most effective against hot flashes, which many women consider the most troublesome aspect of menopause. Some research indicates that hot flashes may be reduced by more than 50 percent after just 4 weeks of therapy with standardized black cohosh extract. When taken under medical supervision, this extract may also be beneficial for some women who, for medical reasons, are unable to use menopause treatments that are estrogen-based, or who prefer to use natural alternatives.

Dosage ▶ Take black cohosh tablets standardized for their content of triterpene glycosides according to the manufacturer's instructions, or as prescribed by your doctor. You may need to take black cohosh for up to 3 months before your symptoms start to improve.

St. John's wort

Hypericum perforatum

Relieves anxiety and depression

While black cohosh is very effective for the treatment of hot flashes, night sweats and insomnia, its effects against the anxiety and depression that sometimes come with menopause are less marked. Consequently, herbalists often prescribe it with St. John's wort for women whose menopausal symptoms include emotional upset. When the two herbs were taken together during a 2006 study, significant improvements were noted in both the psychological and physical symptoms. In other research, St. John's wort alone demonstrated a significant ability to reduce menopausal symptoms in women whose primary concerns were mood-related.

Dosage ▶ Buy supplements that are standardized for their content of hypericin and hyperforin, which are considered to be the main active constituents, and with a daily dose of 900 mg per day of the concentrated (6:1) extract, equivalent to 5.4 g of the dried herb. Take supplements throughout the month.

Red clover

Trifolium pratense

Herbal phytestrogens

Red clover is an interesting example of an herb whose modern application is largely different to its historical uses. While the flower heads have long been regarded as a detoxifying remedy for skin problems, the relatively recent discovery that the leaves contain phytestrogens similar to those found in soybeans means that red clover is now predominantly thought of as a treatment for menopause. Clinical trials investigating the effects of phyto-estrogens from red clover have yielded ambiguous results, so more research is needed to clarify their effects, but there are some indications that they may help to prevent the decline in cardiovascular and bone health that many women experience after menopause.

Dosage ▶ Take commercially prepared red clover isoflavones in doses of 40 mg to 86 mg per day, or as prescribed by your doctor.

The old French name for sage was *toute bonne*, meaning "all is well."

Sage

Salvia officinalis

Traditionally used to reduce hot flashes

Sage is not only a popular culinary herb, but also a widely used traditional remedy for the relief of hot flashes. The plant is rich in tannins, giving it astringent properties and supporting its use to reduce excessive bodily secretions. In addition to hot flashes, these drying properties may benefit other menopausal symptoms such as night sweats and heavy periods. Laboratory studies have demonstrated that some compounds in sage possess estrogenic effects, which may further help to explain its traditional use in menopause.

Dosage ▶ Infuse 1 g to 4 g of dried sage in boiling water; drink 3 cups per day.

Lemon balm

Melissa officinalis

Helps anxiety, insomnia and concentration

As a traditional remedy for restlessness and anxiety, lemon

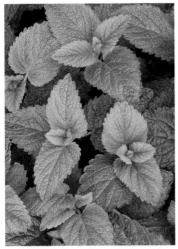

Popular in dried form for teas, lemon balm was called the "elixir of life" by Paracelsus.

balm is ideal for women who find themselves worrying more or becoming more sensitive to stress during and after menopause. Its relaxing properties can also help with sleep disturbances. Lemon balm helps promote feelings of calmness and can be beneficial as a mood lifter when you're feeling emotionally flat. It has also been used to promote mental function, and preliminary research indicates that it may help memory and concentration.

Dosage ▶ Infuse 1 to 2 teaspoons of fresh aerial parts of lemon balm in boiling water; drink 1 cup 2 to 3 times per day, with the last cup 30 to 60 minutes before bed.

Cautions

● Do not take any of the herbs listed on these pages if you have a history of hormone-sensitive tumors, endometriosis or uterine fibroids, except under the supervision of a healthcare professional.

● Do not take black cohosh if you are taking any prescription medication, except under medical supervision.

● Do not take black cohosh except under medical supervision if you have a history of liver disease, as some authorities believe that black cohosh may occasionally cause severe liver damage. These instances are extremely rare, but potentially very serious. If you experience minor side effects, such as mild, reversible stomach upset and skin problems, stop using the herb and seek medical advice.

● Do not confuse black cohosh with blue cohosh (*Caulophyllum thalictroides*), which you should only take under medical supervision.

● Do not take red clover isoflavones if you are taking warfarin or anticoagulant medication, except under medical supervision.

Menopause and soy products

Soy foods are a major dietary source of phytestrogens, plant compounds that have mild estrogen-like effects in the body. Soy phytestrogens can help to reduce menopausal symptoms and appear to have protective effects against some of its associated health problems.

Soybeans, soy flour, miso, tofu and tempeh can all help to top up the small quantities of phytestrogens you obtain from other dietary sources.

Alternatively, supplements that contain concentrated phyto-estrogens (also referred to as isoflavones) are now widely available, and most (but not all) research indicates that they are an effective strategy for reducing hot flashes and night sweats.

Consuming soy phytestrogens at levels higher than normal culinary intake may cause problems for women with some health conditions or who are taking certain types of medications, so talk to your doctor before taking a soy supplement.

● Due to its astringent nature, sage tea has sometimes been reported to cause dryness and irritation of the mouth. If this occurs, try reducing the dose of sage relative to the amount of water used, and make sure you drink plenty of water throughout the day.

● Sage may reduce the absorption of minerals such as calcium and iron, so separate doses by at least 2 hours.

● Lemon balm may interact with some pharmaceutical medications, so consult your doctor or pharmacist before taking it.

● For the safe and appropriate use of St. John's wort, see Depression & anxiety, *page 185*.

● Do not use the herbs on this page if you are pregnant or breastfeeding, except under the advice of a healthcare professional.

Pregnancy

Only the safest of herbal medicines are recommended for women to use during pregnancy and breastfeeding.

Ginger
Zingiber officinale
Reduces morning sickness
Many women are understandably reluctant to take drugs to help deal with the nausea and vomiting of morning sickness, so it's reassuring to know that ginger, which has been used medicinally for thousands of years, is both safe and effective to use. Ginger has been compared to other drugs and placebos in a number of clinical trials, with overwhelmingly positive results. It does occasionally cause minor, self-limiting side effects in some women, but the results of these scientific studies indicate that ginger doesn't have any negative effects on the baby's health.
Dosage ▶ Clinical trials for morning sickness have generally used doses of 1 g to 2 g of ginger in tablet or capsule form, in divided doses throughout the day. Ginger tea made from freshly chopped or powdered ginger may also be effective, but different preparations of ginger have different chemical characteristics, so if your homemade ginger remedy doesn't work, try a commercial preparation.

Witch hazel
Hamamelis virginiana
Relieves hemorrhoids and varicose veins
Bowel habits can become less regular during pregnancy — yet another effect of the hormonal changes your body is going through. Aside from being uncomfortable, constipation sometimes leads to hemorrhoids,

or piles, which are actually varicose veins in the blood vessels supplying the anus and rectum. Swollen, itchy and painful varicose veins can also appear in the legs or around the genitals. Topical applications of witch hazel may help relieve the pain and itchiness of both varicose veins and hemorrhoids, and can also stop hemorrhoids from bleeding.
Dosage ▶ Rub witch hazel gel, ointment or tincture into the affected area once a day. It may take up to 3 weeks before you notice any improvements.

Calendula
Calendula officinalis
Great all-around healer
Calendula has many uses during pregnancy. If your gums become prone to bleeding, try a strong infusion of the flowers as an antiseptic mouthwash. Calendula cream, ointment or infused oil are traditionally rubbed into aching or itchy hemorrhoids and varicose veins, and bring relief to cracked nipples. Occasionally, herbalists and midwives even use the tincture to encourage the healing of vaginal tears or caesarean section scars after delivery.
Dosage ▶ For hemorrhoids, varicose veins and cracked nipples, apply calendula cream, ointment or infused oil to the affected area 3 times a day; the infused oil is preferred for use on the nipples if you are breastfeeding, as it is safe for your baby to consume in small quantities. For bleeding gums, prepare a strong infusion of dried

calendula, and use it as a mouthwash after brushing your teeth. Don't use calendula tincture on surgical wounds or vaginal tears without talking to your doctor or midwife first, as it's vital to ensure that the wound is clean and free of infection before you start. Tissue treated with calendula heals remarkably quickly, so, it is important to check that no infection remains beneath the treated wound.

Rosehip oil
Rosa canina
May help prevent stretch marks
Rosehip oil is growing in popularity as a remedy for the prevention of stretch marks — including those of pregnancy. The herb has a rich content of anti-inflammatory compounds, including vitamins A and C and essential fatty acids, all of which are important for skin health. So, although its efficacy hasn't yet been scientifically confirmed, there may be some substance to its reputation.
Dosage ▶ Massage commercially prepared rosehip oil into the abdomen twice daily.

Raspberry leaf
Rubus idaeus
Prepares the uterus for childbirth
The traditional use of raspberry leaf to help the body prepare for labor is supported by laboratory studies indicating that the herb has a range of effects on the pregnant uterus. Although very little clinical research has been conducted, in one small study, researchers concluded that raspberry leaf may help to shorten labor time and decrease the likelihood of babies being born either prematurely or after their due date. This study also suggested that taking raspberry leaf may help to

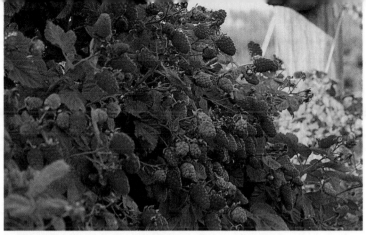

Raspberry leaves are rich in vitamins and minerals. They provide B vitamins, vitamin C and a number of minerals, including potassium, magnesium, zinc, phosphorus and iron.

reduce the risk of forceps or vacuum delivery, or caesarean section. In a second study, 192 women with low-risk pregnancies took either raspberry leaf or a placebo from the 32nd week of pregnancy. In this trial, the second stage of labor was about 10 minutes shorter in those women who took raspberry leaf, and fewer forceps deliveries were required. At 1.2 g of raspberry leaf twice daily, the dose used in this study is only 10 percent of that recommended by herbal authorities, so it's possible that more remarkable results could be obtained with higher doses.

Dosage ▶ Infuse 4 g to 8 g dried raspberry leaf in boiling water; drink 3 cups per day from the 32nd week of pregnancy. Alternatively, take raspberry leaf tablets or capsules according to the manufacturer's instructions, at a dose equivalent to 4 g to 8 g of dried herb, 3 times daily.

Cautions

● Self-treatment with herbal medicine is only appropriate for women whose pregnancies have been assessed as low-risk. Use of any herbal medicine during pregnancy and breastfeeding, including those mentioned here, is best carried out under professional supervision. Seek immediate professional care for

any but the most minor problems during pregnancy, or if you are concerned about the health or well-being of your baby. Always inform your doctor or midwife of any herbal medicines you are taking.

● Ginger occasionally causes minor, self-limiting symptoms, such as heartburn and gastrointestinal discomfort. If this occurs, stop taking the herb, or try taking it in a different form.

● Ginger has documented blood-thinning effects, and should not be taken concurrently with anticoagulant or anti-platelet medication, except under professional supervision. Women who are at risk of hemorrhage should not take ginger in greater than culinary quantities.

● Ginger should not be taken for 2 weeks prior to undergoing surgery. However, in consultation with your physician, a single dose can be taken just prior to surgery to reduce post-operative nausea.

● Topical applications of any herb can some-times cause reactions, such as dermatitis or itching and burning sensations, and ideally a patch test should be performed at least 24 hours before use. Discontinue use if a reaction develops. Take particular care with calendula if you are allergic to the Asteraceae family of plants (for example, daisies and echinacea).

● Like ginger, raspberry leaf has traditionally been used as a treatment for morning sickness. However, it is

Breech babies and Chinese medicine

Toward the end of pregnancy, most babies position themselves so that they'll exit the birth canal head first. The term "breech" is used to describe those babies that are not in this position, and who are therefore at increased risk of complications during labor. If your baby is breech, your doctor will probably suggest that he or she manually adjust the baby into a more appropriate position – a procedure that's both very safe and highly effective.

Alternatively, you could consider traditional Chinese medicine, which has a good success record for turning breech babies. Your acupuncturist will use an acupuncture needle on a specific point on your little toe and simultaneously burn the herb mugwort (*Artemisia vulgaris*) near the skin in the same place. While this process, called moxibustion, may seem peculiar if you haven't experienced acupuncture before, research in both Asia and Europe suggests that it is quite effective at encouraging breech babies to turn. In one trial conducted in Japan, 92.5 percent of babies whose mothers had acupuncture and moxibustion subsequently rotated into the headfirst position, compared to only 73.7 percent of those whose mothers did not. Other researchers have monitored unborn babies' reactions to this procedure and reported that it does not appear to cause any fetal distress.

best avoided during the first trimester of pregnancy, as there is no research to confirm its safety at this time.

● Raspberry leaf may reduce the absorption of minerals, such as calcium and iron, so separate doses by at least 2 hours.

● Do not use raspberry leaf if you are suffering from constipation, peptic ulcer, or any inflammatory disease of the digestive system.

Sexual & prostate health

The traditional use of herbs to support male reproductive health is being increasingly backed up by medical science.

Saw palmetto
Serenoa repens
Clinically proven for prostate problems

With prostate problems affecting about hall of all men ages 50 and over, saw palmetto is one of the world's most popular herbs for male health. It's been the subject of numerous clinical studies, the majority of which show it to be an effective treatment for mild cases of benign prostatic hyperplasia (BPH), and specifically for symptoms such as reduced or hesitant urinary flow and the need to urinate overnight. It has been compared with several of the key pharmaceutical treatments for the same condition and shown to have a similar level of efficacy, but with fewer side effects. Research also suggests that, unlike some pharmaceutical medications, saw palmetto does not interfere with the measurement of a marker called prostate-specific antigen (PSA), the levels of which are used by doctors to predict the presence of prostate cancer.

Dosage ▶ Most research has used a special extract from saw palmetto berries that is standardized for its content of free fatty acids and other oily compounds, referred to as a liposterolic extract. Take 160 mg of the concentrated liposterolic extract in capsule form, twice daily with meals. It may take 1 to 2 months before your symptoms improve.

Nettle root
Urtica dioica
Support for mild prostate conditions

Like saw palmetto, nettle root has been clinically trialed for the relief of mild BPH, and the two herbs are often taken in combination. Nettle is documented to improve a range of BPH symptoms, including nighttime urination, frequent urination and incomplete emptying of the bladder. In a study of over 2,000 patients taking a formula containing nettle root and saw palmetto, improvements were noted in both symptoms and pathological changes — an indication that the herbal combination helps treat the disease, rather than simply suppresses the symptoms.

Dosage ▶ Look for tablets or capsules that provide the equivalent of up to 6 g of dried nettle root per day, and take them according to the manufacturer's instructions.

Korean ginseng
Panax ginseng
Potent male tonic

In traditional Chinese medicine, Korean ginseng is regarded as the most important herbal medicine

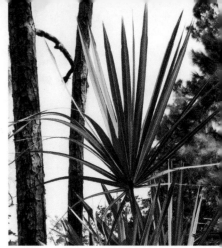

The berries of the saw palmetto were used by both Native Americans and European settlers.

for men, and ginseng roots with a shape resembling a man's body are highly prized. Its traditional indications include replenishing vital energy (referred to in Chinese as *qi*), helping the body and mind to cope with stress, and as a tonic to promote general health and longevity. Ginseng is also widely used to enhance men's sexual performance, and has been shown in a few clinical trials to have a beneficial effect on erectile dysfunction. Results of these trials, as well as animal studies, suggest that the effects on sexual performance cannot be attributed to a purely hormonal effect, but may be caused at least in part by the herb's impact on the central nervous system and on the blood supply to the penis.

Dosage ▶ Take Korean ginseng tablets up to a maximum of 1,000 mg of the dried root per day, according to the manufacturer's instructions. (Higher doses may sometimes be appropriate under professional supervision.) Look for products that are standardized for their content of ginsenosides. Traditionally, Korean ginseng is taken for 8 to 12 weeks, followed by a break of several weeks. This herb is not appropriate for frail or anxious people.

The herb Panax ginseng (shown as capsules and leaves) may help restore sexual function in men.

Ginkgo

Ginkgo biloba

Stimulates circulation

With its documented ability to improve circulation, ginkgo can be a useful remedy for cases of male sexual dysfunction that are known or suspected to be due to reduced blood flow to the penis.

Problems with both libido and sexual performance are fairly common side effects of some groups of pharmaceutical medicines, and there is a small amount of evidence that treatment with ginkgo can help to resolve these issues in some patients when taken under the supervision of a professional.

Dosage ▶ Look for supplements standardized for their content of the important active constituents ginkgo flavone glycosides, ginkgolides and bilobalides, with a daily dose of 120 mg of a concentrated (50:1) extract, providing the equivalent of 6 g of the dried herb.

Ginkgo takes a month or two to reach its maximum effect, so use it for 6 to 12 weeks before assessing whether or not it has helped you. If you suspect you are experiencing any adverse effects of your prescribed medication, talk to your doctor before taking ginkgo, and refer also to the Cautions section that follows.

Cautions

- The symptoms of BPH and prostate cancer can be very similar, so it's important to see your doctor for a diagnosis before commencing self-treatment. Only mild cases of BPH are suitable for self-treatment. All men over 50 years of age should consider regular screening for prostate cancer, which can easily go undetected without testing.
- Do not take saw palmetto or nettle root if you are taking pharmaceutical medication for BPH or prostate cancer, except on professional advice.
- Saw palmetto occasionally causes mild adverse effects, such as digestive upsets and headaches. Nettle root infrequently causes mild adverse effects; if this occurs, stop taking the herb.
- Nettle plants cause urticaria, or hives, if they touch the skin, so if you harvest nettle root, take appropriate precautions. Do not take nettle root if you have had an allergic reaction to the nettle plant.
- Do not take Korean ginseng if you have diabetes, cardiovascular disease (including high and low blood pressure), depression, anxiety, hyperactivity, mental illness (including bipolar disorder and similar conditions), insomnia, blood clots or bleeding disorders, except under the advice of a healthcare professional.
- Korean ginseng and ginkgo are known or suspected to interact with many pharmaceutical medications (including antidepressants, antipsychotics, digoxin, anticoagulants, anticonvulsants, insulin and hormonal therapy), so consult your physician or pharmacist before taking them.
- Do not take Korean ginseng at the same time as stimulants such as caffeine.
- Korean ginseng is traditionally contraindicated in people suffering from acute infections.
- If you have been diagnosed with Alzheimer's disease or any other form of dementia, do not take ginkgo without first talking to your doctor.
- Stop taking ginkgo at least 2 weeks before undergoing surgery, and do not take it if you have a bleeding disorder.
- Always use commercially prepared ginkgo products from a reputable company. Do not consume unprocessed ginkgo leaves as they may cause adverse reactions. Do not eat large quantities of the seeds or allow children to do so.
- Ginkgo sometimes causes mild adverse reactions, which may include dizziness, gastrointestinal upset, headache and allergic skin reactions. More severe reactions have occasionally been recorded, and have included bleeding problems and seizures. If symptoms occur, stop taking the herb and seek medical advice.
- Do not use any of the herbs on this page if you are pregnant or breastfeeding, except under the advice of a healthcare professional.

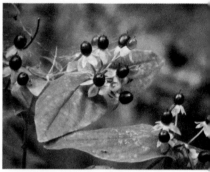

Ginkgo biloba leaves turn a bright yellow in the fall right before they all fall off.

Tomatoes for a healthy prostate

Tomatoes – along with other red- and pink-colored fruit and vegetables, such as guava, watermelon and pink grapefruit – contain a pigment called lycopene, which has important benefits for men's health. Population studies suggest that men whose diets are highest in tomatoes have up to 40 percent less chance of developing prostate cancer than those men whose tomato consumption is low. As a potent antioxidant, lycopene also supports the heart and blood vessels and may help to reduce the risk of cardiovascular disease. For optimal absorption, lycopene needs to be consumed at the same time as a little oil, so tomato-based products such as pasta sauces and tomato paste are valuable inclusions in your diet.

Index

Bold page numbers refer to photo captions; *italic* page numbers refer to recipes; underlined page numbers refer to main remedy sections.

A

abrasions, 8
abscesses, 48, 195
achillea (yarrow), 131, **131**, 174, 175
Achillea filipendulina, 131
Achillea millefolium, 131, **131**, 174
Achillea omentosa, 131
Achillea ptarmica, 131
Achilles (ancient Greek), 131
acid reflux, 78, 178
acne, 20, 63, 110, 122, 183, <u>190</u>
aconite, 128
Aconitum sp., 128
Actaea racemosa, 208, 209
Adam and Eve, 68
Aesculus hippocastanum, 136, **136**, 200, 201, **201**
African marigold, 24
African (lemon) savory, 109
Agastache cana, 11
Agastache foeniculum, 11, **11**
Agastache rugosa, 11, **11**
Agastache rupestris, 11
Agastache urticifolia, 11
Agathosma betulina, 172
age spots, 72
agrimony (flower essence), 170
ajmud, 25
ALA (alpha-linolenic acid), 48, 105
albizia, 172, 177
Albizia lebbeck, 172, 177
Alcea ficifolia, 75
Alcea rosea, 75, **75**
alecost (costmary), 118
alfalfa (lucerne), 93
Algerian oregano, 76
allergies to herbs, 163
allergy remedies, 172, <u>177</u>.
 See also hay fever
allheal. See yarrow
Allium ampeloprasum, 50, 52
Allium canadense, 50
Allium cepa, 50
Allium cernuum, 50
Allium chinensis, 50
Allium fistulosum, 52
Allium odorum, 50
Allium porrum, 50
Allium sativum, 50, 52, 174–175, 202, 203
Allium schoenoprasum, 50, 53, **53**
Allium scorodoprasum, 50
Allium sp., 50–53, **51**, **52**

Allium tricoccum, 52
Allium triquetrum, 50, **50**
Allium tuberosum, 50
Allium ursinum, 50
Aloe barbadensis, 8
Aloe ferox, 8, 194, 195
aloe vera (*Aloe vera*), 8, **8**, 194, 195, **195**
Aloe vulgaris, 8
Aloysia citriodora, 71, **71**
alpha-linolenic acid (ALA), 48, 105
Alpinia caerulea, 49
Alpinia galanga, 49, **49**
Alpinia officinarum, 49
Alpinia oxyphylla, 49
Althaea officinalis, 75, **75**, 175, 206, 207
Alzheimer's disease, 55, 107, 187, 213
American ginseng, 56
American highbush cranberry, 128
American sloe. See viburnum
anal fissures, 88
ancho chili, 33
andrographis, 172, 174, 175
Andrographis paniculata, 172, 174
anemia, 56, 172
Anethum graveolens (dill), 39, **39**, 155, 180, **180**
angelica, 9, **9**, 146, 153
Angelica archangelica, 9, **9**
Angelica atropurpurea, 9
Angelica gigas, 9
Angelica pachycarpa, 9
Angelica polymorpha, **160**, 204, **204**, 205
angel's water, 114
angel wing jasmine, 64, **64**
angina, 86, 107, 202
anise, 10, **10**, 143, 178
'Anise Basil,' 14
anise hyssop, 11, **11**
anise mint, 11
anise myrtle, 114
Anthemis tinctoria, 28
anthocyanins, 174
Anthriscus cerefolium (chervil), 29, **29**, 155
antibacterials. See disinfectant herbs
antimicrobials. See disinfectant herbs
ant repellents, 80, 118, 125
Antwerp hollyhock, 75
anxiety remedies, <u>185</u>
 German chamomile, 179
 gotu kola, 57
 hops, 59
 hyssop, 62
 lavender, 68
 lemon balm, 69, 209
 lime, 73
 passionflower, 84

poppy, 89
 St. John's wort, 104, 208
 valerian, 126
aperitifs, herbal, 178
aphid repellents, 10, 30, 41
aphrodisiacs, 74, 95
Apium graveolens, 27, **27**, 199, **199**
Apium nodiflorum, 129
Apium prostratum, 27
Apollo (sun god), 17
apothecary rose, 96
appetite stimulants
 angelica, 9
 coriander, 36
 cumin, 132
 gentian, 178
 parsley, 83
 perilla, 87
 rocket, 95
 tarragon, 119
 white horehound, 130
 yarrow, 131
apple geranium, 110
apple (pineapple) mint, 79, **79**, **146**
apple sage, 106
Arabian jasmine, 64
archangel. See angelica
Arctium lappa, 23, **23**
Arctium minus, 23
Arctostaphylos uva-ursi, 173
Armistice Day, 89
Armoracia rusticana, 60, **60**, 177
arnica, 12, **12**, 194, 195, 196, 197
Arnica chamissonis, 12
Arnica montana, 12, **12**, 194, 195, 196, 197
artemisia (*Artemisia* sp.), 13, **13**
Artemisia abrotanum, 13
Artemisia absinthium, 13
Artemisia afra, 13
Artemisia annua, 13, **160**
Artemisia arborescens, 13, **13**
Artemisia dracunculoides, 119
Artemisia dracunculus, 119, **119**
Artemisia ludoviciana, 13
Artemisia pontica, 13
Artemisia vulgaris, 13, 211
arthritis herb. See gotu kola
arthritis remedies, <u>198–199</u>
 cat's claw, 172
 celery seed, 27
 devil's claw, 173
 evening primrose oil, 44
 ginger, 54
 juniper, 134
 nettle, 81
 parsley, 83
 rosemary, 101
 roseships, 97
 sorrell, 112
 turmeric, 125
 white willow, 136
arugula (rocket), 94–95, **94**, **95**
asafetida, 132, **132**

ashwagandha (withania), 56, **161**, 186
Asian ginseng. See Korean (Chinese) ginseng
Asiatic pennywort. See gotu kola
Aspalathus linearis, 120
aspen (flower essence), 170
aspic oil, 66
aspirin origins, 78
asthma, 15, 55, 134, 172
astragalus, 172, 176, 186, **186**
Astragalus membranaceus, 172, 176, 186, **186**
atherosclerosis, 52, 73, 125
athlete's foot, <u>192</u>
Atropa belladonna, 163, **163**
Australian Bush Flower Essences, 171
Avena sativa, 184, **184**
Ayurvedic medicine, 161
Azores jasmine, 64
Azores (orange peel) thyme, 123
Aztec sweet herb, 71

B

Bach, Edward, 170
Bach flower essences, 170–171
bachu, 172
Backhousia anisata, 114
Backhousia citriodora, 114
Backhousia myrtifolia, 114
back pain, 136, 173, 196, 197
Bacon, Sir Francis, 108
bacopa (*Bacopa monnieri*), 22, **22**, **161**, 187
bai shao. See peony
Ballota nigra, 130, 175
banana chili, **31**
Barbados aloe. See aloe vera
Barbarea verna, 129
bark, harvesting and storing, 155
basil, 14–16, **14**, **15**, *16*, **16**, 143, 150, 155
basil oil, *16*, **16**
bathroom cleaning spray, 124
bay, 17–18, **17**, *18*, **18**, **19**, **150**
bay laurel. See bay
bay rum tree, 17
bear's garlic (ramsons), 50
beauty treatments
 age spot removal, 72
 eye care, 45
 hair care, 103, 110
 skin care, 8, 44, 98, 110
bedwetting, 61
bee balm (bergamot), 20
bee balm (lemon balm). See lemon balm
beech (flower essence), 170
beefsteak plant. See perilla
beggar's buttons, 23
belladonna (deadly nightshade), 163, **163**

beneficial insects, 9, 10
benign prostatic hyperplasia (BPH), 134, 212, 213
bergamot, bergamot oil, 20, **20**
bergamot orange, 20
berries, 134, **134–135**
bible leaf (costmary), 118
bilberry, 134, **134**
bird chilies, **30, 31**
bitter aloe. *See* aloe vera
bitter orange, **160**
blackberry, 134, **135**
black cardamom, 49
black cohosh, 158, 208, 209
black haw. *See* viburnum
black horehound, 130, 175
black pepper, 132, **132**, 169
black psyllium, 88
black walnut, 136, **137**
bladder infections, 172, 206. *See also* urinary tract infections
bladder seed. *See* lovage
bleeding control, 108, 110, 136, 196. *See also* wound treatments
bloating remedies, 180
angelica, 9
anise, star anise, 10, 178
caraway, 25
coriander, 36
dill, 39
fennel, 46
perilla, 87
thyme, 124
white horehound, 130
blond psyllium, 88
blood clot prevention, 52, 54
blood lipids, 8
blood sugar control, 56, 93, 132
blood vessel problems, 136
bloodwort. *See* yarrow
blue cohosh, 209
blue flag, 63
blue ginger, 49
blue vervain, 127
bog myrtle (sweet gale), 114
boils, 195
borage, 21, **21**, 155
Borago officinalis, 21, **21**, 155
bore tree. *See* elder
boswellia (*Boswellia serrata*), 198, 199
botanical (Latin) names, 162
bottle-brush (field horsetail or shave grass), 61
bouquet garni, **19**, 83, **150**
Bowle's (woolly) mint, 79
boxthorn, **160**
BPH (benign prostatic hyperplasia), 134, 212, 213
brahmi, 22, **22**, **161**, 187
brain function, 22, 55. *See also* memory, concentration aids
breast cancer, 116
breastfeeding aids, 39, 46, 172

breech births, 211
bridewort. *See* meadowsweet
broadleafed peppermint, 42
broad-leafed thyme, 123
broad-leaf sorrell, 112
bronchitis remedies
heartease, 58
hyssop, 62
licorice, 72
marsh mallow, 75
primrose, 91
red clover, 93
scented geranium, 111
white horehound, 130
bruises, 12, 21, 35, 88, 194, 196
buckeye. *See* horse chestnut
buckler-leaf (French) sorrel, 112, **112**
burdock, 23, **23**
burnet bloodwort, 108
burn treatments, 8, 24, 48, 57, 108, 194
'Bush BBQ' thyme, **123**

C

cabbage loopers, 41
cabbage moths, 107
cabbage white butterfly, 62
cajeput oil, 122
calendula (*Calendula officinalis*), 24, **24**, 153, 169, 194, 201, 210
Californian poppy, 89, **89**
Camellia sinensis, 120, **120, 121**
camphor plant, 118
Canada onion, 50
Canary Island jasmine, 64
Canary Island lavender, 67
cancer prevention and treatment
cat's claws for, 172
garlic for, 52
green tea for, 120
pau d'arco for, 173
saffron for, 132
sorrel for, 112
sweet violet for, 116
turmeric and, 125
cancer treatment support, 172
cape aloe, 8
Caprese salad, *16*, **16**
Capsicum annuum, 30, **30**
Capsicum baccatum, 30
Capsicum chinense, 30, **31**
Capsicum frutescens, 30
Capsicum pubescens, 30
Capsicum sp., 30–33, **30, 31, 32,** *33,* **33**
caput monachi. *See* dandelion
caraway, 25, *25,* **25**, 180, **180**
caraway crackers, *25,* **25**
caraway (seedcake) thyme, 123
cardiovascular problems, 48, 120, 136, 172, 202–203
cardiovascular system, 200–203. *See also specific ailments*

carpenter's herb. *See* yarrow
carpet beetles, 63
Carthusian pink, 34
Carum carvi, 25, *25,* **25**, 180, **180**
Carum roxburghianum, 25
cassia, 132
cassumar ginger, 54
catarrh. *See* decongestant herbs
caterpillar food sources, 81, 84
catmint, 146
catnip, 26, **26**
catnip cat toy, 26, **26**
cat's claw, 172, **172**
Caulophyllum thalictroides, 209
cayenne, 33, 169
celeriac, 27
céleri bâtard, 74
celery, celery seed, 27, **27**, 199, **199**
centaury (flower essence), 170
Centella asiatica, 22, 57, **57,** **161**, 201
centifolia rose, 96, **96**
Centranthus ruber, 126
cerato (flower essence), 170
Ceylon citronella, 70
Chamaemelum nobile, 28, **28**
chamomile, 28, **28**, 146, **148**
chapped skin, 98
chaste tree, 134, **135**, 190, **190**, 204, **204**, 205
chermoula, 125
Cherokee people, **173**
cherry laurel, 17
cherry plum (flower essence), 170
chervil, 29, **29**, 155
chestnut bud (flower essence), 170
Chewing John, 49
chi (qi), 160, 212
chia, 105
chickweed, 191, 194
chicory (flower essence), 170
childbirth. *See* pregnancy and childbirth
child safety, 162, **162**
chili, 30–33, **30, 31, 32,** *33,* **33**
chili and lime sauce, *33*
chiliblains remedy, 48
chimichurri sauce, *83*
Chinese basil. *See* perilla
Chinese celery (kin tsai), 27
Chinese chives, 50
Chinese date, **160**
Chinese decoctions, 165, **165**
Chinese (Korean) ginseng, 56, **56, 160**, 184, 212, **212**, 213
Chinese haw, **160**
Chinese herbalism, 160–161
Chinese keys (fingerroot), 49, **49**
Chinese (Mongolian) licorice, 72
Chinese onion (rakkyo), 50

Chinese parsley. *See* coriander
Chinese peony, 86. *See also* peony
Chinese rhubarb, 181
Chinese star anise, 10, **10**, 180
Chinese wormwood (qing hao), 13, **160**
chipotle chili, **33**
chives, 50, 53, **53**, **146**, 155
cholesterol-lowering herbs, 202–203
fenugreek, 93, 132
flaxseed oil, 48
garlic, 52
ginger, 54
milk thistle, 173
plantain, 88
turmeric, 125, 182
chronic venous insufficiency, 200, 201
cilantro (Mexican coriander), 36, **36**
Cinnamomum cassia, 132
Cinnamomum verum, 132, **133**
cinnamon, 132, **133**
cinnamon myrtle, 114
circulation problems, 101, 136, 200
Citrus aurantium, 20, **160**
Citrus bergamia, 20
clary (muscatel) sage, 105, 205
cleaning sprays, 68
cleavers (goosegrass), 117, 183, 190
clematis (flower essence), 170, **170**
Clematis vitalba, **170**
Cleopatra, 8
Cleveland sage, 106
clocks and watches. *See* dandelion
clove pinks, 34, **34**
clover, 45
cloves, clove oil, 132, **133**, 193
Cochin (East Indian) lemon grass, 70
cockroach repellents, 26, 80
codeine, 89, 90
Codonopsis pilosula, 172
coffee substitute, 182, **183**
cold and flu remedies, 174–175
andrographis, 172
Chinese wormwood, 13
echinacea, 40, 176
elder, 41
eyebright, 177
garlic, 52
ginger, 54
horseradish, 60
hyssop, 62
lime, 73
meadowsweet, 78
nasturtium, 129
oregano, 77
perilla, 87
scented geranium, 111

thyme, 124
white horehound, 130
Wilde als, 13
cold hands and feet, 54. *See also* Raynaud's syndrome
cold sores, 62, 69, 104, <u>193</u>
colic remedies
anise, star anise, 10
bergamot, 20
caraway, 25
catnip, 26
chamomile, 28
cumin, 132
dill, 39, 180
ginger, 54
lemon verbena, 71
marjoram, 77
parsley, 83
star anise caution, 180
yarrow, 131
colitis, 75, 88, 125
Colorado beetles, **118**
colorectal cancer, 52
comfrey, 35, **35**, 196, **196**
Commiphora myrrha, 193
common anise. *See* anise.
common balm. *See* lemon balm
common jasmine, 64, **64**
common oregano, 76
common peony, 86. *See also* peony
common plantain, 88
common (garden) sage, 105, **105**
common (garden) thyme, 123, **123**, **124**
compass plant. *See* rosemary
compresses, 168, **168**
coneflower. *See* echinacea
conehead thyme, 123
Confucius, 54
congestion. *See* decongestant herbs
Conium maculatum, 113, 163, **163**
conjunctivitis, 45, 98
constipation, 48, 88, <u>181</u>, 182. *See also* laxative herbs
container gardens, 146–149, **146**, **147**, **148**, **149**
Cook, James, 122
cooking with herbs, 111, 150–151. *See also* recipes; *specific herbs*
coriander, 36, **36**, 146, **150**
Coriandrum sativum, 36, **36**, 146, **150**
Cornish lovage. *See* lovage
Cornish yarg cheese, 81, **81**
Corsican mint, 79
Corymbia citriodora, 42
costmary (alecost or bible leaf), 118
cotton lavender, 67, **67**
cough remedies
garlic, 52

hyssop, 62
lemon grass, 70
licorice, 72
marsh mallow, 75
oregano, 77
perilla, 87
poppy, 90
primrose, 91
red clover, 93
scented geranium, 111
schisandra, 134
thyme, 175
cowslip (paigle), 91, **91**
crab apple (flower essence), 170
crafts, 26, **26**
cramp bark (viburnum), 128, **128**, 152, 197, 205
cranberry, 134, 206, **206**
Crataegus laevigata, 202
Crataegus monogyna, 202
Crataegus pinnatifida, **160**, 202
Crataegus sp., 136, **136**
creeping savory, 109
crimson clover, 93
crisp-leafed (fern-leafed or curly) tansy, 118
Crocus sativus, 132, **133**
Crohn's disease, 125
crown flax, 48
Cryptotaenia japonica, 82, 83
culinary herbs, 150–151, **150**, **151**
cumin, 132, **132**
Cuminum cyminum, 132, **132**
Curacao aloe. *See* aloe vera
Curcuma longa, 125, **125**, **161**, 182, 191, 202–203
curcumin, 125
curly parsley, 82, **82**, 83
curly spearmint, 79
curly (crisp-leafed or fern-leafed) tansy, 118
curry plant, 37, **37**
curry tree, 37, **37**
cuts and scrapes. *See* wound treatments
cutting leaf celery. *See* celery.
Cymbopogon citratus, 70, **70**
Cymbopogon flexuosus, 70
Cymbopogon martinii, 70
Cymbopogon nardus, 70
Cymbopogon winterianus, 70
cystitis, 58, 129, 134, <u>206–207</u>

D

Damask rose, 96
dame's violet (sweet rocket), 94
dandelion, 35, 38, **38**, 182, 183, **183**, 206, 207
dang shen, 172
dan shen, 107, **160**
Daoism, 160
Daphne, 17
deadly nightshade (belladonna), 163

decoctions, 165, **165**
decongestant herbs
eucalyptus oil, 42
eyebright, 45, 177
fennel, 46
horseradish, 60, 177
licorice, 72
marjoram, 77
peppermint, 80
plantain, 88
poppy, 90
primrose, 91
sweet violet, 116
Wilde als, 13
dehydration, 179
dementia and Alzheimer's, 55, 57, 107, 187, 213
De Mestral, George, 23
deodorizers, 68, 74, 107, 122
depression, and hops, 59, 188
depression remedies, <u>185</u>
jasmine essential oil, 64
lavender, 68
lemon balm, 69
rosemary, 101
St. John's wort, 104, 204–205, 208
dermatitis, 44, 87, 110, 191
detoxifying herbs, <u>183</u>
blue flag, 63
burdock, 23
cleavers, 190
dandelion, 38
horsetail, 61
milk thistle, 173
nettle, 81
sorrel, 112
sweet woodruff, 117
devils' bane, 127
devil's claw, 172, 196–197, 198, 199
devil's wood. *See* elder
dew of the sea. *See* rosemary
diabetes aids
aloe vera, 8
fenugreek, 93, 132
ginseng, 56
green tea, 120
'Holy Basil,' 15
psyllium, 203
sorrel, 112
tarragon, 119
diabetic neuropathy, 44
Dianthus carthusianorum, 34
Dianthus caryophyllus, 34, **34**
Dianthus plumarius, 34
diarrhea, 25, 134, 136
digestive aids and tonics
andrographis, 172
angelica, 9
dang shen, 172
devil's claw, 172
golden seal, 173
licorice, 72
magnolia, 136
meadowsweet, 78

milk thistle, 173
New Zealand flax, 48
nigella, 132
oregano, 77
parsley, 83
passionflower, 84
rocket, 95
rosemary, 101
scented geranium, 111
wilde als, 13
wormwood, 13
digestive system, 158, <u>178–183</u>. *See also specific ailments*
Digitalis sp., 128
dill, dill seed, 39, **39**, 155, 180, **180**
Diplotaxis tenuifolia, 94, **94**
disinfectant herbs
basil, 16
clove, 132
golden seal, 173
lavender, 68
nasturtium, 129
New Zealand tea tree oil, 195
rosemary, 103
sage, 107
tea tree oil, 122
thyme, 124
Dittany of Crete, 77
diuretic herbs, <u>206–207</u>
bachu, 172
celery seed, 27
dandelion, 38, 183
parsley, 83
sorrel, 112
sweet woodruff, 117
diviner's sage, 106
Di Yu, 108
Doctrine of Signatures, 45
dolomite, 141
dong quai, **160**, 204, **204**, 205
Doronicum orientale, 12
doshas, 161
douglasii, 109
drawing agent, 195
dried herbs
buying, 151, 155
making, **18**, 152–155, **152**, **153**
tinctures from, 167, **167**
dropwort, 78
drug interactions, 163
dry skin remedy, 21
Dutch rush (rough horsetail), 61
dwarf curry plant, 37
dwarf orange marigold, 52
dyer's chamomile, 28
dyes, plant-based, 35
dyspepsia, 9

E

ear infections, 41, 45
East Indian basil, 15

East Indian (Cochin) lemon grass, 70
eau d'anges, 114
echinacea (*echinacea* sp.), 40, **40**, 158, **158**, 176, **176**
Echinacea angustifolia, 40, 176, **176**
Echinacea pallida, 40, 176, **176**
Echinacea paradoxa, 40
Echinacea purpurea, 40, 176, **176**
ecology, 154
eczema remedies, 191
   aloe vera, 8
   blue flag, 63
   borage seed oil, 21
   calendula, 169
   cleavers, 183
   evening primrose oil, 44
   flax, 48
   heartease, 58
   marsh mallow, 75
   nettle, 81
   red clover, 93
   scented geranium oil, 110
   sweet violet, 116
   sweet woodruff, 117
edible flowers, 58, 98, 116
Edward I (King of England), 72
Egyptian (walking or tree) onion, 50
Egyptians, ancient, 8, 50, 68, 193
elder, 41, **41**, 153, **154**, 174, **174**, 175
elements, in TCM, 161
elephant garlic, 52, **52**
Eleutherococcus senticosus, 56, 186
Elizabeth I (Queen of England), 78
elm (flower essence), 170
emerald risotto, *83*
emotional problems, 12, 170–171. *See also* anxiety remedies; depression remedies
enchanter's plant, 127
English (true) lavender, 66, **66**, 68
English myrrh, 113
EPO (evening primrose oil), 44, **44**
Equisetum arvense, 61, **61**
Equisetum hyemale, 61
erigeron, **148**
Eruca sativa, 94–95, **94**, **95**
Eryngium foetidum, 36, **36**
eschallots (shallots or scallions), 50
Eschscholzia californica, 89, **89**
Essiac Tea, 112
eucalyptus (*Eucalyptus* sp.), 42, **42**, *43*
Eucalyptus dives, 42
eucalyptus essential oil, 42

Eucalyptus globulus, 42
Eucalyptus gummifera, 42
Eucalyptus haemostoma, 42
Eucalyptus radiata, 42
Eucalyptus smithii, 42
Eucalyptus staigeriana, 42
Eugenia polyantha, 17
Euphrasia brevipila, 45
Euphrasia officinalis, 45, **45**, 177
Euphrasia rostkoviana, 45
European annual red (field) poppy, 89–90, **89**, **90**
European cranberry bush. *See* viburnum
European red elder, 41
evening primrose, 44, **44**
evening primrose oil (EPO), 44, **44**
exhaustion. *See* tiredness and fatigue
eyebright, 45, **45**, 177
eye health, 134
eye infections, 45, 98

F

fairy clocks. *See* dandelion
false celery, 74
fatigue. *See* tiredness and fatigue
fennel, 46, **46**, 146, 155, **180**
fenugreek, 93, 132, **133**, **161**
fern-leafed (curly or crisp-leafed) tansy, 118
fernleaf lavender, 67
fern-leaf yarrow, 131
fertilizers, 143, 148
Ferula asafetida, 132, **132**
feverfew, 47, **47**, 189
fever remedies, 174
   bergamot, 20
   catnip, 26
   devil's claw, 172
   hyssop, 62
   lemon grass, 70
   lemon verbena, 71
   oregano, 77
   sorrell, 112
   vervain, 127
   wormwood, 13
   yarrow, 131
fibroids, 86
field horsetail (bottle-brush or shave grass), 61
field (red) poppy, 89–90, **89**, **90**
fig cakes, 36
Filipendula rubra, 78
Filipendula ulmaria (meadowsweet), 78, **78**, 153, **159**, 178, **178**
Filipendula vulgaris, 78
fine herbs, 29, **29**, 53
fingerroot (Chinese keys), 49, **49**
first aid, 194–195
Five Hundred Good Points of Husbandry (Tusser), 91

flat-leaf parsley, **82**, 83
flatulence remedies, 180
   angelica, 9
   anise, star anise, 10, 178
   asafetida, 132
   bergamot, 20
   caraway, 25
   catnip, 26
   coriander, 36
   cumin, 132
   dill, 39
   fennel, 46
   galangal, 49
   gentian, 178
   ginger, 54
   lemon balm, 69
   lemon verbena, 71
   marjoram, 77
   oregano, 77
   parsley, 83
   peppermint, 80
   thyme, 124
   white horehound, 130
   wormwood, 13
flax, flaxseed oil, 48, **48**, 191, **191**
flea repellents, 46, 70, 80, 103, 118
fleur de lis, 63
Florence fennel, 46, **46**
Florida anise, 10
flower essences, 170–171
flowers
   edible, 58, 98, 116
   harvesting and drying, 153–154, **153**
flu. *See* cold and flu remedies
fluid retention, 206–207
fly repellents, 118
Foeniculum vulgare (fennel), 46, **46**, 146, 155, **180**
Four Thieves Vinegar, *106*
foxgloves, 128
fractures, 35, 196
Fragaria vesca, 134, **135**
Frau Holle. *See* elder
freezing herbs, 155, **155**
French marigold, 24
French (Italian) parsley, 82
French (buckler-leaf) sorrel, 112, **112**
French tarragon, 119, **119**
fresh herbs, buying, 150–151
fringed lavender, 67
fruit salad (peach) sage, 106
fungal diseases, in plants, 15, 25, 28, 30, 37
fungal infections (skin), 24, 122, 192
fusarium wilt, 15

G

galangal, 49, **49**
galilica roses, 96, 97, **97**
Galium aparine, 117, 183, 190
Galium odoratum, 117, **117**

Galium verum, 117, **117**
gallbladder support, 38, 173, 182
gamma-linolenic acid (GLA), 21, 44
garbage cans, cleaning, 122
garden chervil. *See* chervil
garden cress, 129
gardening. *See also specific herbs*
   buying plants, 142–143, **142**
   container gardens, 146–149, **146**, **147**, **148**, **149**
   planting, 142–145, **143**, **145**
   plant labels, 145, 152
   soils and soil testing, 140–141, **140**, **141**
   sowing seed, 144, **144**
   stem cuttings, 144
   stratifying seed, 40
garden lovage. *See* lovage
garden (common) sage, 105, **105**
garden (common) thyme, 123, **123**, **124**
gari (Japanese or myoga ginger), 54
garlic, 50–53, **51**, 174–175, **175**, 202, 203
garlic chives, 50
garlic leek (sweet leek or Levant garlic), 50
gas. *See* flatulence remedies
gastritis, 78, 88
gastrointestinal remedies
   garlic, 52
   hops, 59
   lemon grass, 70
   marsh mallow, 75
   poppy, 89
   thyme, 124
   valerian, 126
   vervain, 127
genital herpes, 104
gentian, 178
gentian (flower essence), 170, **170**
Gentiana asclepiadea, **170**
Gentiana lutea, 178
George III (King of Great Britain), 56
geranium (palmarosa or rosha) grass, 70
Gerard, John, 91, 108
German chamomile, 28, **28**, 179, **179**
giant blue hyssop, 11
giant garlic (Russian garlic or sand leek), 50
gillyflower, 34
ginger, 54, **54**, 169, 179, 198–199, **198**, 199, 210, 211
ginkgo (*Ginkgo biloba*), 55, **55**, 160, 187, **187**, 200, 213, **213**
ginseng, 56, **56**, 160

GLA (gamma-linolenic acid), 21, 44
Glycyrrhiza glabra, 72, **72**
Glycyrrhiza pallidiflora, 72
Glycyrrhiza uralensis, 72
gobo (Japanese burdock), 23
golden buttons, 118
golden chia, 105
golden psyllium, 88
golden seal, 154, 158, 173, **173**
golden variegated sage, **107**
golds. *See* calendula
goosegrass (cleavers), 117, 183, 190
gorse (flower essence), 171
gotu kola, 22, 57, **57**, **161**, 201
gout, 27, 83, 134, 198–199
grapeseed, 200, 206–207
grape vine, **207**
gratiola, 62
great burdock, 23
greater burnet (pimpernel), 108
greater plantain. *See* plantain
Grecian bay. *See* bay
Greek basil, **15**
Greek myrtle, 114
Greek oregano, 76
green lavender, 67
green tea, 120
guajillo chili, **33**
guelder rose. *See* viburnum
gully gum, 42
gum nuts, **42**
gums and teeth. *See* oral health remedies
gum tree, 42
Gymnema sylvestre, **161**

H
habañero chili, **31**, **33**
hairbrushes, cleaning, 103
hair care, 103, 110
hair growth, 129
Hamamelis virginiana, 136, **137**, 181, **181**, 196, 210
Hamburg (turnip-rooted) parsley, 82, 83
hanging gardens, 148
hardening of the arteries, 52, 73, 125
Harpagophytum procumbens, 172, 196–197, 198, 199
Harry Potter and the Chamber of Secrets (Rowling), 163
harvest of herbs, 153–155, **153**
hawthorn, 136, **136**, 202, **202**, 203, **203**
hay fever, 15, 41, 81, 87, 177
headache remedies, 189
   feverfew, 47
   lavender, 68
   lemon grass, 70
   marjoram, 77
   passionflower, 84
   peppermint, 80
   poppy, 89

valerian, 126
white willow, 136
heartburn. *See* indigestion remedies
heart disease. *See* cardiovascular problems
heartease, 58, **58**, 148
heather (flower essence), 171
Hecate (goddess), 128
Helichrysum angustifolium, 37
Helichrysum italicum, 37, **37**
Helichrysum stoechas, 37
hemlock, 113, 163, **163**
hemorrhoids, 88, 108, 181, 210
herbal aperitifs, 178
herbal creams, 167
herbal medicine. *See also* specific ailment or body system
   Bach flower essences, 170–171
   berries used in, 134, **134–135**
   Eastern philosophy, 160–161
   medicinal herb list, 172–173, **172**, **173**
   medicinal preparations, 164–169, **164–169**
   professional practitioners, 162, 163
   safe use of herbs, 162–163
   spices used in, 132, **132–133**
   trees used in, 136, **136–137**
   Western philosophy, 158–159
herbal vinegar spray, 107
herb cocktail, *108*
herbes de Provence, 68, *109*
herb Louisa, 71
herb of grace, 127
herb of the cross, 127
herbs. *See also specific herbs*
   buying, 150–151, 155
   container gardens, 146–149, **146**, **147**, **148**, **149**
   cooking with, 150–151
   deadly, 163, **163**
   freezing, 155, **155**
   growing in garden, 140–145, **140**, **143**, **145**
   harvesting and drying, **18**, 152–155, **152**, **153**
   medicinal use (*See* herbal medicine)
   safety concerns, 152, 154, 162–163
   storing, 150–155, **152**
herb Venus, 127
Hesperis matronalis, 94
hiccup remedy, 39
high blood pressure aids, 202–203
   evening primrose oil, 44
   garlic, 52
   lemon grass, 70
   lime, 73

olive, 136
sage, 107
high blood pressure caution, 163
high cholesterol. *See* cholesterol-lowering herbs
Hippocratic tradition, 158
HIV, 112
holly (flower essence), 171
hollyhock, 75, **75**
'Holy Basil,' 14, 15
holy herb, 127
honeysuckle (flower essence), 171
hops, 59, **59**, 188
horehound, 130, **130**
hormone balancing herbs, 190, **190**. *See also* women's health
hornbeam (flower essence), 171
horse chestnut, 136, **136**, 200, 201, **201**
horseradish, 60, **60**, 177
horsetail, 61, **61**
hot flashes, 208, 209
huacatay, 24
Huang Di Nei Jing, 160
hummingbird mint, 11
humors, in TCM, 161
Humulus lupulus, 59, **59**, 188
Hungary water, 103
Hydrastis canadensis, 173, **173**
Hypericum perforatum (St. John's wort), 104, **104**, 163, 169, 185, 197, **197**, 204–205, 208
hyssop, 62, **62**
Hyssopus officinalis, 62, **62**

I
Illicium anisatum, 10, 180
Illicium floridanum, 10
Illicium verum, 10, **10**, 180
immune support, 40, 56, 111, 172, 176, 186
impatiens (flower essence), 171
incensier. *See* rosemary
incontinence, 61
Indian cress (nasturtium), 129, **129**
Indian ginseng (withania), 56, **161**, 186
indigestion remedies, 178
   coriander, 36
   cramp bark, 128
   dandelion root, 182
   dill, 39
   galangal, 49
   ginger, 54
   meadowsweet, 78
   peppermint, 80
   thyme, 124
   turmeric, 125
   white horehound, 130
   yarrow, 131

Indonesian bay, 17
infused oils, 169, **169**
infused vinegar, 111
infusions, 164, **164**
Insalata Caprese, 16, **16**
insect bites and stings, 68, 110, 194
insect repellents. *See also* specific insects
   apple geranium, 110
   bog myrtle, 114
   Four Thieves Vinegar, *106*
   lavender, 68
   lemon grass, 70
   pennyroyal, 80
   peppermint, 80
   sage, 107
insomnia remedies, 188. *See also* sleep aids
   dill, 39
   hops, 59
   lemon balm, 209
   lemon verbena, 71
   passionflower, 84
   poppy, 89
   primrose, 91
   schisandra, 134
   valerian, 126
   withania, 56
Intermedia lavenders, 66, 68
intermittent claudication, 55, 200
intestinal infections, 77
intestinal parasites, 136
iris (*Iris* sp.), 63, **63**
Iris pallida, 63
Iris pseudacorus, 63
Iris versicolor, 63
Iroquois people, 127
irritable bowel syndrome, 80, 88, 180
Isabella (Queen of Hungary), 103
Isatis tinctoria, 35
Italian cress, 94–95
Italian (pepper) fennel, 46
Italian lavender, 67
Italian (Spanish) licorice, 72
Italian lovage. *See* lovage
Italian (French) parsley, 82

J
jagged lavender, 67
Jamaican mint bush, 109
Japanese beetles, 21
Japanese burdock (gobo), 23
Japanese ginger (myoga ginger or gari), 54
Japanese ginseng, 56
Japanese medicine (Kampo), 87
Japanese parsley (mitsuba), 82, 83
Japanese peppermint (North American cornmint), 79
Japanese star anise, 10, 180
jasmine, 64, **64**, **65**

jasmine essential oil, 64
Jasminum azoricum, 64
Jasminum floribundum, 64
Jasminum multiflorum, 64
Jasminum nitidum, 64, **64**
Jasminum odoratissimum, 64
Jasminum officinale, 64, **64**
Jasminum polyanthemum, 64
Jasminum sambac, 64
Jasminum sp., 64, **64**, **65**
Java citronella, 70
Jell-O, 111, **111**
jessamine, 64, **64**, **65**
Jesus Christ, 68, 84, 127
Johnny-jump-up. *See* heartease
joint problem aids
    arnica, 12
    burdock, 23
    devil's claw, 196–197
    lemon grass, 70
    meadowsweet, 78
    New Zealand flax, 48
    peppermint, 80
Judaism, 130
Judas tree. *See* elder
Juglans nigra, 136, **137**
juniper, 134, **135**
Juniperus communis, 134, **135**

K

Kaempferia galanga, 49
Kaempferia pandurata, 49, **49**
Kalmia latifolia, 17
Kampo (Japanese medicine), 87
kapha, 161
kidney problems, 172, 206
kin tsai (Chinese celery), 27
kiss-me-quick (red valerian),
    126
knitbone. *See* comfrey
knot (sweet) marjoram, 76,
    76, 77
Korean (Chinese) ginseng, 56,
    56, **160**, 184, 212, **212**, 213
Korean mint, 11, **11**

L

labels for herbs, 145, 152, 153
Lacnunga (medical texts), 88
ladies' (Our Lady's or yellow)
    bedstraw, 117, **117**
lad's love, 13
lady of the meadow. *See*
    meadowsweet
lady's leek (nodding onion), 50
larch (flower essence), 171
laryngitis, 175
Latin (botanical) names, 162
Laurus azorica, 17–18
Laurus nobilis (bay), 17–18, **17**,
    18, **18**, **19**, **150**
Lavandula angustifolia, 66, **66**,
    68, 185, **185**, 194
Lavandula buchii, 67
Lavandula canariensis, 67
Lavandula dentata, 67, **67**

Lavandula lanata, 67
Lavandula latifolia, 66
Lavandula maroccana, 67
Lavandula multifida, 67
Lavandula pinnata, 67
Lavandula sp., 66–68, **66**, **67**, **68**
Lavandula stoechas, 67
Lavandula viridis, 67
lavender, **66**, **67**, **68**, **102**, **185**
    for anxiety, 185
    fertilizing, 143
    harvesting, 153
    infused oil, 169
    profile of, 66–68
    use caution, 195
lavender essential oil, 66, 68,
    185, 194, **194**
lavender (Spanish) sage, 105
laxative herbs, 88, 132, 173, <u>181</u>
leafhoppers, 41
Lebanese cress, 129
Lebanese oregano, 76
leeks, 50
leg ulcers, 136, <u>201</u>. *See also*
    ulcers (skin)
lemon balm, 69, **69**, 184, 193,
    193, 209, **209**
lemon basil, 14, **14**
lemon beebrush, 71
lemon bergamot, 20
lemon grass, 70, **70**
lemon ironbark, 42
lemon myrtle, 114
lemon poppy-seed cake, *90*, **90**
lemon (African) savory, 109
lemon-scented gum, 42
lemon thyme, 123, **124**
lemon verbena, 71, **71**
leopard's bane. *See* arnica
Lepidium sativum, 129
leprosy, 62
Leptospermum scoparium, 195
Leptospermum sp., 122
Levant garlic (garlic leek or
    sweet leek), 50
Levisticum officinale (lovage),
    74, **74**, **148**
lice repellents, 70, 110
Li Chung Yon, 57
licorice, 72, **72**, 163
'Licorice Basil', 14
licorice mint, 11
lime (herb), 73, **73**, 203
lime (soil amendment), 141
lime basil, 14
linden tree. *See* lime (herb)
linseed oil, 48
Linum usitatissimum, 48, **48**,
    191, **191**
Little John, 49
liver support, <u>182</u>
    astragulus for, 172
    dandelion for, 38
    magnolia for, 136
    milk thistle for, 173
    sage for, 107

schisandra for, 134
turmeric for, 125
vervain for, 127
white horehound for, 130
yarrow for, 131
London rocket, 94
long-stalked flax, 48
lovage, 74, **74**, **148**
love ache, 74
love-lies-bleeding. *See*
    heartease
love parsley. *See* lovage
Low John, 49
lucerne (alfalfa), 93
lung cancer, 116
Lycium barbarum, **160**
lymphatic system, 183

M

madder, 117
Maggi plant, 74
magnolia, 136, **136**
Magnolia officinalis, 136, **136**
maidenhair tree. *See* ginkgo
maiden's ruin, 13
mail-order plants, 143
mallow, 75. *See also* marsh
    mallow
Malva moschata, 75
Malva sylvestris, 75
Manchuian licorice, 72
Mandragora officinarum, 163,
    163
mandrake, 163, **163**
manuka (New Zealand tea
    tree), 195
manzanilla (Roman
    chamomile), 28, **28**
marathon (fennel), 46
marigold. *See* calendula; dwarf
    orange marigold; Mexican
    mint marigold
marjoram, 76–77, **76**, 146
marjoram and sausage pasta,
    77, **77**
Marrubium vulgare, 130, **130**,
    175
marsh mallow, 75, **75**, 175,
    206, 207
Mary Magdalene, 68
Mary's mantle. *See* rosemary
Matricaria matricarioides, 28
Matricaria recutita, 28, **28**, 179,
    179
maypops. *See* passionflower
meadow honeysuckle. *See* red
    clover
meadow queen. *See*
    meadowsweet
meadowsweet, 78, **78**, 153,
    159, 178, **178**
meadow trefoil. *See* red clover
mealybugs, 8
Medicago sativa, 93
medicinal herbs. *See* herbal
    medicine

Mediterranean rocket (smooth
    mustard), 94
Melaleuca alternifolia, 122, **122**,
    190, 192, 195
Melaleuca iridiflora, 122
Melaleuca leucadendron, 122
Melaleuca quinquenervia, 122
Melaleuca sp., 122
Melaleuca viridiflora, 122
melissa (*Melissa officinalis*), 69,
    69, 184, 193, **193**, 209, **209**
memory, concentration aids,
    <u>187</u>
    brahmi, 22
    ginkgo, 55
    gotu kola, 57
    green tea, 120
    'Holy Basil', 15
    lemon balm, 209
    peony, 86
    rosemary, 101
    sage, 107
menopause support, <u>208–209</u>
    cramp bark for, 128
    hops for, 59
    parsley for, 83
    red clover for, 93
    sage for, 107
    St. John's wort for, 104
men's health, <u>212–213</u>. *See
    also specific issues*
menstrual problem aids,
    <u>204–205</u>
    chamomile, 28
    chaste tree, 134
    cramp bark, 128
    evening primrose oil, 44
    ginger, 54
    ginkgo, 55
    hops, 59
    hyssop, 62
    magnolia, 136
    marjoram, 77
    peony, 86
    St. John's wort, 104
    valerian, 126
    vervain, 127
    witch hazel, 136
    wormwood, 13
    yarrow, 131
Mentha aquatica, 79
Mentha canadensis, 79
Mentha pulegium, 79, 80, **80**
Mentha requinii, 79
Mentha sp., 79–80, 146, 148, 155
Mentha spicata, 79, **79**, 80
Mentha suaveolens, 79, **79**
Mentha x gentilis, 79
Mentha x piperita, 79, **79**, 80,
    179, 180, 189
Mentha x villosa, 79
Mexican coriander (cilantro),
    36, **36**
Mexican marigold, 24, **24**
Mexican mint marigold, 119,
    119

Mexican tarragon, 119, **119**
migraine headaches, 47, 189
milfoil. *See* yarrow
milk thistle (St. Mary's thistle), 173, **173**, 182, **182**
milk vetch. *See* astragalus
mimulus (flower essence), 171
mint, 79–80, **79**, 146, 148, 155
mint jelly, *80*
mites, 41
mitsuba (Japanese parsley), 82, 83
mold, in showers, 122
mole poblano, 33
Monarda (*Monarda* sp.), 20
Monarda citriodora, 20
Monarda didyma, 20, **20**
Monarda fistulosa, 20, **20**
Monarda menthifolia, 20
Monarda punctata, 20
Mongolian (Chinese) licorice, 72
monkshood, 128
monk's pepper. *See* chaste tree
morning sickness. *See* pregnancy and childbirth
morphine, 89, 90
mosquito repellents, 26, 70, 110, 118, 193
mother of thyme, 124
moth repellents
  camphor plant, 118
  iris, 63
  lavender, 67, 68
  rosemary, 103
  sage, 107
  tansy, 118
motion sickness. *See* nausea remedies
mountain laurel, 17
mountain tobacco. *See* arnica
mouth health. *See* oral health remedies
moxibustion, 211
mugwort, 13, 211
Murraya koenigii, 37, **37**
muscatel (clary) sage, 105, 205
muscle cramps, 86, 101, 197
muscle pain remedies
  arnica, 12
  cramp bark, 197
  infused oils, 169
  lemon grass, 70
  marjoram, 77
  meadowsweet, 78
  peppermint, 80
musculoskeletal system, 198–199. *See also specific ailments*
mushroom poisoning, 173
musk mallow, 75
mustard (flower essence), 171
myoga ginger (Japanese ginger or gari), 54
Myrica gale, 114
Myrica pensylvanica, 17
myrrh, 193

Myrrhis odorata, 113, **113**
Myrtus communis, 114, **114**

N
Napoléon Bonaparte, 72, 115
Nardus italica, 66
narrowleaf echinacea, 40
narrow-leafed peppermint, 42
Nashia inaguensis, 127
nasturtium (Indian cress), 129, **129**
Nasturtium officinale (watercress), 129, **129**, 146
Native American herbalism, 127, 158, **173**. *See also specific herbs*
native wormwood (white sage), 13
nausea remedies, 179
  angelica, 9
  chamomile, 28
  galangal, 49
  gentian, 178
  ginger, 54
  lemon balm, 69
  peppermint, 80
  perilla, 87
Nepeta cataria, 26, **26**
Nepeta mussinii, 26
Nepeta x faassenii, 26
nerve pain, 70, 89, 104, 169, 197
nerve tonics, 13, 22
nervous irritability, 15
nervous system, 184–189. *See also specific ailments*
nettle, 81, **81**, 212, 213
neuralgia, 70, 84, 104
New Zealand flax, 48, **48**
New Zealand tea tree (manuka), 195
niaouli oil, 122
nigella, 132, **133**, **161**
Nigella sativa, 132, **133**, **161**
nightshade (belladonna), 163
night sweats, 86, 107
nipples, cracked, 210
nodding onion (lady's leek), 50
North American cornmint (Japanese peppermint), 79
northern bayberry, 17
nosebleeds, 13
notoginseng, 56
nurseries, 142–143, **142**

O
oak (flower essence), 171
oak bark, 136, **137**
oats (oat straw), 184, **184**
obsessive compulsive disorder, 104
Ocimum americanum, 14, **14**
Ocimum basilicum, 14, **15**, 16
Ocimum campechianum, 14
Ocimum gratissimum, 15
Ocimum minimum 'Greek', **15**

Ocimum sp. (basil), 14–16, **14**, **15**, *16*, **16**, 143, 150, 155
Ocimum tenuiflorum, 14, 15
Oenothera biennis, 44, **44**
Oenothera lamarckiana, 44
Oenothera parviflora, 44
Oenothera sp., 44
oil of aspic, 66
oils, infused, 169, **169**
old man, 13
old man banksia, 171
old warrior, 13
old woman, 13
Olea europaea, 136, **137**
oleum origani, 77
oleum spicae, 66
olive (flower essence), 171
olive chili, **31**
olive tree, 136, **137**
omega-3 fatty acids, 48, 105, 191
omega-6 fatty acids, 21, 44, 191
onchomycosis, 192
onions, 50–53, **51**
opium poppy, 89, 90
Oracle of Delphi, 17
oral health remedies, 193
  calendula, 24, 210
  catnip, 26
  green tea, 120
  marsh mallow, 75
  plantain, 88
  sage, 106–107
  tea tree oil, 122
orange peel (Azores) thyme, 123
oregano, 76–77, **76**, **102**
oregano de la Sierra, 20
oregano essential oil, 77
organic matter, in soil, 140, **140**
Origanum creticum, 77
Origanum dictamnus, 77
Origanum marjorana, 76, **76**, 77, 146
Origanum maru, 76
Origanum minutiflorum, 76
Origanum onites, 76
Origanum pulchellum, 76
Origanum sp., 76–77
Origanum syriacum, 76
Origanum vulgare, 76, 77
orris root, 63, **63**
Osmorhiza longistylis, 113
Oswego tea, 20, **20**
Our Lady's (ladies' or yellow) bedstraw, 117, **117**
overuse injuries, 196–197

P
Paeonia lactiflora, 86, **86**, 204, 205, **205**
Paeonia officinalis, 86
Paeonia suffruticosa, 86
paigle (cowslip), 91, **91**
pain relief, 196, 199. *See also specific pains*

pale purple echinacea, 40
palmarosa (geranium grass or rosha grass), 70
Panax ginseng, 56, **56**, **160**, 184, 212, **212**, 213
Panax japonicus, 56
Panax pseudoginseng, 56
Panax quinquefolius, 56
Panax sp., 56, 56
Papaver rhoeas, 89–90, **89**, **90**
Papaver somniferum, 89, 90
paprika, 33
parasitic infections, 13
Parma violets, 115
parsley, **19**, 82–83, **82**, 146, **150**, 155
pasilla chili, **33**
Passiflora edulis, 84
Passiflora incarnata, 84, **85**, 188, **188**
passionflower, 84, **85**, 188, **188**
passionfruit, 84
passionfruit cordial, *84*
Passion of Christ, 84
Passover plate, 130, **130**
pau d'arco, 173, 192, **192**
peach (fruit salad) sage, 106
pelargonium, 148
Pelargonium capitatum, 110
Pelargonium citrosum, 111
Pelargonium graveolens, 110, **110**
Pelargonium nervosum, 110
Pelargonium odoratissimum, 110
Pelargonium quercifolium, 111
Pelargonium quercifolium 'Fair Ellen,' **110**
Pelargonium radens, 110
Pelargonium reniforme, 111
Pelargonium sidoides, 111
Pelargonium sp., 110–111
Pelargonium x asperum, 110, 111
Pelargonium x capitatum, 111
Pelargonium x citronellum, 110
Pelargonium x concolor, 111
Pelargonium x graveolens, 111
Pelargonium x scabrum, 111
Pelargonium x scarboroviae, 111
pennyroyal, 79, 80, **80**
peony, 86, **86**, 204, 205, **205**
peppercorns, **19**
pepper (Italian) fennel, 46
peppermint, 79. **79**, 80, 179, 180, 189
perennial basils, 15
perfumery, 34, 96, 114
perilla, 87, **87**, 177
Perilla frutescens, 87, **87**, 177
peri peri, 33
peripheral circulation issues, 200
Persian cumin. *See* caraway
Persicaria odorata, 79, **80**
persillade, 83

'Peruvian Basil,' 14
Peruvian black mint, 24
pesticides, 154
Peter Rabbit, 83
Petroselinum crispum, 82, **82**, 83
Petroselinum sp. (parsley), **19**, 82–83, 146, **150**, 155
petunias, **148**
pewterwort, 61
Phormium tenax, 48, **48**
Phyla scaberrima, 71
pidgeonweed, 127
Pimenta racemosa, 17
pimentos, **33**
pimpernel (greater burnet), 108
Pimpinella anisum, 10, **10**, 178
pine (flower essence), 171
pineapple (apple) mint, 79, **79**, **146**
pineapple sage, 106, **106**
pineapple verbena, 127
pineapple weed, 28
pink savory, 109
Piper nigrum, 132, **132**
pipe tree. *See* elder
piss-en-lit. *See* dandelion
pitta, 161
pizza topping, 103
plague, 9, 17
Plantago arenaria, 88
Plantago asiatica, 88
Plantago indica, 88
Plantago lanceolata, 88
Plantago major, 88
Plantago major 'Rosularis', 88, **88**
Plantago ovata, 88, 181, 183, 203
Plantago psyllium, 88, 181, 183, 203
plantain (*Plantago* sp.), 45, 88, **88**
plant identification, 154, 162
plants. *See* gardening
Pliny, 59
PMS remedies, 204–205
    chaste tree, 134, 190
    evening primrose oil, 44
    ginkgo, 55
    peony, 86
    St. John's wort, 104
pollution, and herb harvest, 154
polycystic ovarian syndrome, 86
Polygonum odoratum, 36
Pontefract (pomfret) cakes, 72
poor man's leek (Welsh onion), 52
poppy, 89–90, **89**, **90**
Portuguese lavender, 67
Portulaca oleracea, 92, **92**
postnasal drip, 45
post-traumatic stress disorder (PTSD), 126
potato onion, 50

pot marigold, 24
pot (Turkish) marjoram, 76
Potter, Beatrix, 83
potting mixes, 147–148, 149
poultices, 168, **168**
pregnancy and childbirth, 132, 134, 162, 172, 210–211. *See also specific herbs*
premenstrual syndrome. *See* PMS remedies
prickly ash, 136, **137**
primrose, 91, **91**
Primula officinalis, 91
Primula veris, 91, **91**
Primula vulgaris, 91
professional herbalists, 162, 163
propagation of herbs, 144
prostate health, 61, 81, 134, 212–213
Prunus laurocerasus, 17
psoriasis remedies, 191
    aloe vera, 8
    borage seed oil, 21
    flax, 48
    red clover, 93
    sweet violet, 116
    sweet woodruff, 117
    turmeric, 125
psyllium, 88, 181, 183, 203
pterostachys lavenders, 67
PTSD (post-traumatic stress disorder), 126
purple clover. *See* red clover
purple passionflower. *See* passionflower
purslane, 92, **92**
purslane soup, 92

Q

qi (chi), 160, 212
qing hao (Chinese wormwood), 13, **160**
queen of the meadow. *See* meadowsweet
Quercus robur, 136, **137**

R

rakkyo (Chinese onion), 50
ramps (wood leeks), 52
ramsons (bear's garlic), 50
ras el hanout, 49, 68, 98
rashes, 13, 81, 194
raspberry, 134, **134**, 210–211, **211**
rat-tail plantain. *See* plantain
rau ram (Vietnamese coriander), 36
rau ram (Vietnamese mint), 79, **80**
Raynaud's syndrome, 55, 136, 200
recipes
    basil oil, *16*, **16**
    caraway crackers, *25*, **25**
    chili and lime sauce, *33*

chimichurri sauce, *83*
emerald risotto, *83*
fig cakes, *36*
Four Thieves Vinegar, *106*
herb cocktail, *108*
herbes de Provence, *109*
Insalata Caprese, *16*, **16**
lemon poppy-seed cake, *90*, **90**
marjoram and sausage pasta, *77*, **77**
mint jelly, *80*
passionfruit cordial, *84*
purslane soup, *92*
Roman salad, *95*, **95**
rose petal jelly, *98*, **98**
sage and thyme stuffing, *107*, **107**
salad greens, *95*, **95**
vanilla bay custard, *18*, **18**
red blood-wood, 42
red chestnut (flower essence), 171
red clover, 93, **93**, 208, **208**, 209
red (field) poppy, 89–90, **89**, **90**
red spider mite, 115
red valerian (kiss-me-quick), 126
Remembrance Day, 89
repotting herbs, 148
Rescue Remedy, 170
respiratory system, 174–179. *See also specific ailments*
resurrection lily, 49
rheumatic pain, 70, 77, 89, 104
rheumatism. *See* arthritis remedies
rheumatoid arthritis. *See* arthritis remedies
Rheum palmatum, 181
rhizomes, harvesting and storing, 154–155
Ribwort plantain, 88
ringworm treatments, 48
risotto, emerald, *83*
rocket (arugula), 94–95, **94**, **95**
rock hyssop, 62
rock rose (flower essence), 171
rock water (flower essence), 171
rocoto pepper, 30
rodent deterrents, 80
Roman chamomile, 28, **28**
Roman (sweet) fennel, 46
Roman nettle, 81
Roman rocket, 94–95
Romans, ancient, 18, 68, 95, 116, 127
Roman salad, 95
Roman wormwood, 13
rooibos tea, 120
roots, harvesting and storing, 154–155
roquette sauvage, 94, **94**
Rosa canina, 97, 98, **99**, 210
Rosa gallica, 98

Rosa gallica 'Officinalis', 96
Rosa gallica 'Rosa mundi', 97, **97**
Rosa sp., 96–98
Rosa x damascena, 96, 98
rose, 96–98, **96**, **97**, **99**, 153
rose geranium, 110, **110**
rosehips, rosehip oil, 97, **97**, 210
rosemary, 100–103, **100**, **101**, **102**, **103**, 150, 169, 187
rose oil, 98
rose petal jelly, 98, **98**
rose plantain, 88, **88**
rosewater, 98
rosha (palmarosa or geranium) grass, 70
Rosmarinus eriocalys, 100
Rosmarinus officinalis, 100–103, **100**, 187
Rosmarinus tomentosus, 100
rough horsetail (Dutch rush), 61
Rowling, J. K., 163
Rubia tinctorium, 117
Rubus fruticosus, 134, **135**
Rubus idaeus, 134, **134**, 210–211, **211**
Ruchetta selvatica, 94
rucola, 94–95
ruddles. *See* calendula
rugosa roses, 97
rugula, 94–95
Rumex acetosa, 112, **112**
Rumex acetosella, 112
Rumex crispus, 112, 181
Rumex scutatus, 112, **112**
Russian garlic (giant garlic or sand leek), 50
Russian licorice, 72
Russian oregano, 76
Russian tarragon, 119

S

SAD (seasonal affective disorder), 104
safety concerns, 152, 154, 162–163. *See also specific herbs*
saffron, 132, **133**
sage, 102, 105–107, **105**, **106**, **146**, 150, 174, **208**, 209
sage and thyme stuffing, *107*, **107**
Saibokuto, 87
salad burnet, 108, **108**
salad greens, 95, **95**
Salix alba, 136, **137**, 189, **189**, 196, 197, 199, **199**
Salvia apiana, 105
Salvia clevelandii, 106
Salvia columbariae, 105
Salvia divinorum, 106
Salvia dorisiana, 106
Salvia elegans, 106, **106**
Salvia fruticosa, 105
Salvia hispanica, 105

Salvia lavandulifolia, 105
Salvia miltiorrhiza, 107, **160**
Salvia officinalis, 105, **105**, 106–107, 174, **208**, 209
Salvia officinalis 'Icterina', **107**
Salvia officinalis 'Tricolor', **105**
Salvia polystachya, 105
Salvia pomifera, 106
Salvia sclarea, 105, 205
Salvia sp., 105–107, **105**
Sambucus nigra (elder), 41, **41**, 153, **154**, 174, **174**, 175
Sambucus racemosa, 41
sand leek (Russian garlic or giant garlic), 50
Sanguisorba minor, 108, **108**
santolina, 67, **67**
Santolina chamaecyparissus, 67, **67**
Satureja biflora, 109
Satureja hortensis, 109, **109**
Satureja montana, 109, **109**
Satureja sp., 109
Satureja thymbra, 109
Satureja viminea, 109
savory, 109, **109**
savory of Crete, 109
saw palmetto, 134, **135**, 212, **212**, 213
scale insects, 18
scallions (shallots or eschallots), 50
scar treatments, 8, 201
scented geranium, 110–111, **110**
schisandra, 134, **135**, **160**, 182
Schisandra chinensis, 134, **135**, **160**, 182
sciatica, 104, 197
science, and Western herbalism, 159
scleranthus (flower essence), 171
scouring rush, 61, **61**
Scoville Heat Units, 31
scribbly gum (white gum kino), 42
seasickness. *See* nausea remedies
seasonal affective disorder (SAD), 104
seder (Passover plate), 130, **130**
seedcake (caraway) thyme, 123
seeds
  harvesting and storing, 154
  sowing, 144, **144**
  stratifying, 40
senna, 173
Senna alexandrina, 173
Serenoa repens, 134, **135**, 212, **212**, 213
Seville orange, 20
shallots (eschallots or scallions), 50
shamrock, 93

sharp-leaf galangal, 49
shave grass (field horsetail or bottle-brush), 61
sheep's sorrel, 112
shell shock, 126
shingles, 104
shiso. *See* perilla
shock, from injuries, 12
shower cleaning spray, 122
Siamese ginger, 49
Siberian ginseng, 56, 186
side effects of herbs, 162–163
silverfish repellents, 67
Silybum marianum, 173, **173**, 182, **182**
simpler's joy, 127
sinusitis, 41, <u>177</u>
Sisymbrium altissimum, 94
Sisymbrium erysimoides, 94
Sisymbrium irio, 94
skin conditions, <u>190–195</u>. *See also specific skin conditions*
  bog myrtle for, 114
  burdock for, 23
  calendula for, 169, 194
  cat's claws for, 172
  chamomile for, 28
  chickweed for, 194
  lavender for, 68
  oak for, 136
  salad burnet for, 108
  scented geranium for, 110
  sorrell for, 112
sleep aids, 68, 69, 73, 126. *See also* insomnia remedies
slippery elm, 178, 195
smallage. *See* celery, celery seed
smooth mustard (Mediterranean rocket), 94
sneezewort, 131
society garlic, 50
Socrates, 163
soft tissue injuries, 197
soil and soil testing, 140–141, **141**, 143, 147–148, 149
sore throat, 13, 75, 106, 111, 124, <u>174–175</u>
sorrell, 112, **112**
sour grass, 112
southernwood, 13
soy foods, 209
Spanish lavender, 67
Spanish (Italians) licorice, 72
Spanish (lavender) sage, 105
Spanish thyme, 123
spartan oregano, 76
spearmint, 79, **79**, 80
sphagnum moss, 148
spices, 132, **132**, **133**, 151. *See also specific spices*
spike lavender, 66
splinter remedy, 195
sports injuries, <u>196–197</u>
spotted bergamot, 20

sprains and strains, 12, 21, <u>196–197</u>
stagbush. *See* viburnum
stain removal, 42
star anise, 10, **10**, 180
starflower. *See* borage
Star of Bethlehem (flower essence), 171
Stellaria media, 191, 194
stem cuttings, 144
stinging nettle, 81, **81**
St. John's wort, **104**, **197**
  for depression, 185
  infused oil, 169
  for nerve pain, 197
  profile of, 104
  side effects, 163
  for women's health, 204–205, 208
St. Mary's thistle (milk thistle), 173, **173**, 182, **182**
stoechas lavenders, 67, **67**
stomach cancer, 52
stomach cramps, 9, 70, 128
stomach upsets, 68
storage of herbs, 150–155, **152**. *See also specific herbs*
St. Patrick, 93
St. Peter, 91
stratifying seed, 40
strawberry pots, 149, **149**
strawflower Italian everlasting, 37
stress remedies, <u>184</u>
  ginseng, 56
  'Holy Basil,' 15
  licorice, 72
  poppy, 89
  primrose, 91
  valerian, 126
  withania, 56
stretch marks, 210
strewing herbs, 78, 91, 117
Sturt Desert pea, 171, **171**
styes, 45
sulphur, 141
summer savory, 109, **109**
sunburn protection, 120
suncups, 44
sundrops, 44
sunshine wattle, 171
Swainsona formosa, **171**
sweet balm. *See* lemon balm
sweet basil, 14, 143
sweet bay. *See* bay
sweet chestnut (flower essence), 171
sweet cicely, 113, **113**
sweet (Roman) fennel, 46
sweet gale (bog myrtle), 114
sweet leek (Levant garlic or garlic leek), 50
sweet mace, 119, **119**
sweet (knot) marjoram, 76, **76**, 77

sweet myrtle, 114, **114**
sweet rocket (dame's violet), 94
sweet violet, 115–116, **115**, **116**
sweet woodruff, 117, **117**
Symphytum asperum, 35
Symphytum grandiflorum, 35
Symphytum officinale, 35, **35**, 196, **196**
synergy, 159
Syrian hyssop (white oregano), 76
syrups, 167, **167**
Syzygium aromaticum, 132, **133**, 193

T

tabasco, 33
Tabebuia impetiginosa, 173, 192, **192**
Tagetes lucida, 119, **119**
Tagetes minuta, 24
Tagetes patula, 52
Tagetes sp., 24, **24**
Tagetes terniflora, 24
taijitu, 160
Tale of Peter Rabbit, The (Potter), 83
tall rocket (tumbling mustard), 94
tamarind, 132, **133**, **161**
Tamarindus indica, 132, **133**, **161**
Tanacetum balsamita, 118
Tanacetum cinerariifolium, 118
Tanacetum coccineum, 118
Tanacetum parthenium, 47, **47**, 189
Tanacetum vulgare, 118, **118**
tansy, 118, **118**
Taoism, 160
Taraxacum officinale, 35, 38, **38**, 182, 183, **183**, 206, 207
tarragon, 119, **119**, 145, **145**, 155
TCM (traditional Chinese medicine), 160–161
tea, 120, **120**, 121
tears of Isis, 127
tea tree, 122, **122**, 190, 192, 195
teething pain remedy, 26
tension. *See* stress remedies
'Thai Basil,' 14, **15**
Thai chilies, **33**
Thai ginger, 49
Theophrastus, 44
three-leafed sage, 105
thujone, 118
thyme, **19**, **102**, *107*, 123–124, **123**, **124**, 146, 148, **148**, **150**, 175
thyme-leafed gratiola, 22
thyme-leafed savory, 109
Thymus caespititius, 123
Thymus capitatus, 123

Thymus herba-barona, 123
Thymus hyemalis, 123
Thymus mastichina, 123
Thymus micans, 123
Thymus nummularium, 123
Thymus pseudolanuginosis, 124
Thymus quinquecostatus, 124
Thymus serpyllum, 124
Thymus sp., 123–124
Thymus vulgaris, 123, **123**, 124, **124**, 175
Thymus vulgaris 'Silver Posie,' **123**
Thymus x citrodorus, 123, **124**
Tiberius, 18
tick repellents, 70, 110, 193
tilia. *See* lime (herb)
Tilia cordata, 73, **73**, 203
Tilia platyphyllos, 73, 203
Tilia x europaea, 73, 203
tilleul, 73
tinctures, 166–167, **166**, **167**
tinnitus, 55
tiredness and fatigue, 56, 70, 72, 101, 172, 186
toenail fungus, 192
tomatoes, for prostate, 213
tomato hornworms, 21
tonsillitis, 106, 111, 117, 124, 174, 175
toothaches, 193. *See also* oral health remedies
toute bonne. *See* sage
toxins. *See* detoxifying herbs; pollution
traditional Chinese medicine (TCM), 160–161
transplant shock, 143, 148
trauma, emotional, 12, 56
tree basil, 15
tree (Egyptian or walking) onion, 50
tree peony, 86. *See also* peony
trees, 136, **136–137**
tree wormwood, 13, **13**
Trifolium incarnatum, 93
Trifolium pratense, 93, **93**, 208, **208**, 209
Trifolium repens, 93, **93**
Trifolium sp., 45
Trigonella foenum-graecum, 93, 132, **133**, **161**
Tropaeolum majus, 129, **129**
true (English) lavender, 66, **66**, 68
Tulbaghia violacea, 50
tumbling mustard (tall rocket), 94
turberculosis, 111
Turkish delight, 98, **98**
Turkish (pot) marjoram, 76
turmeric, 125, **125**, **161**, 182, 191, 202–203
turnip-rooted (Hamburg) parsley, 82, 83
Tusser, Thomas, 91

U

ulcers (skin), 8, 48, 136, 172, 201
ulcers (stomach or intestinal), 24, 72, 75, 78, 88, 125
Ulmus rubra, 178, 195
umckaloabo, 111
Uncaria guaianensis, 172
Uncaria tomentosa, 172
upland (winter cress), 129
upper respiratory infections, 40, 42, 56, 60, 172. *See also* bronchitis remedies; cold and flu remedies
urinary tract infections, 206–207
 bachu for, 172
 celery for, 27
 horseradish for, 60
 horsetail for, 61
 nasturtium for, 129
 parsley for, 83
 uva-ursi for, 173
Urtica dioica, 81, **81**, 212, 213
Urtica pilulifera, 81
uva-ursi, 173

V

Vaccinium macrocarpon, 134, **134**, 206, **206**
Vaccinium myrtillus, 134, **134**
valerian, 126, **126**, 163, 188
Valeriana officinalis, 126, **126**, 163, 188
vampires, 127
vanilla bay custard, 18, **18**
varicose veins, 48, 57, 136, 200, 210
variegated sage, **105**
vata, 161
Velcro, 23, **23**
Venus (goddess), 114
Verbena hastate, 127, **127**
Verbena officinalis, 127, **127**
verticillium wilt, 30
vertigo remedy, 55
vervain (flower essence), 171
vervain (herb), 127. **127**
viburnum (cramp bark), 128, **128**, 152, 197, 205
Viburnum opulus, 128, **128**, 152, 197, 205
Viburnum prunifolium, 128
Viburnum trilobum, 128
Vietnamese coriander (rau ram), 36
Vietnamese mint (rau ram), 79, **80**
vine (flower essence), 171
Vinegar of the Four Thieves, 106
Viola odorata, 115–116, **115**, **116**
Viola tricolor (heartease), 58, **58**, 148

Virgin Mary, 68, 73, 101
vision. *See* eye health; eye infections
vitamin C, 97
Vitex agnus-castus, 134, **135**, 190, **190**, 204, **204**, 205
Vitis vinifera, 200, 206–207

W

walking (Egyptian or tree) onion, 50
walnut (flower essence), 171
walnut hulls, 136, **137**
wasabi, *Wasabia japonica*, 60, **60**, **177**
watercress, 129, **129**, 146
water hyssop, 22
watering herbs, 148
water mint, 79
water violet (flower essence), 171
weevils, in pantry, 18
weigh-loss aid, 120
Welsh onion (poor man's leek), 52
white chestnut (flower essence), 171
white clover, 93, **93**
whitefly repellent, 41
white gum kino (scribbly gum), 42
white horehound, 130, **130**, 175
white oregano (Syrian hyssop), 76
white peony, 86, 204, 205, **205**
white sage (*Artemisia* sp.), 13
white sage (*Salvia* sp.), 105
white willow bark, 136, **137**, 189, **189**, 196, 197, 199, **199**
wild apricot. *See* passionflower
wild arugula, 94, **94**
wild bergamot, 20, **20**
wild clover. *See* red clover
wilde als, 13
wild garlic, 50, **50**
wild harvest, 154
wild marjoram, 76
wild oat (flower essence), 171
wild pansy. *See* heartease
wild passionflower. *See* passionflower
wild rocket, 94, **94**
wild rose (flower essence), 171
wild strawberry, 134, **135**
willow (flower essence), 171
wind. *See* flatulence remedies
winter cherry (withania), 56, **161**, 186
winter cress (upland), 129
winter-flowering thyme, 123
winter savory, 109, **109**
winter tarragon, 119, **119**
witch hazel, 136, **137**, 181, **181**, 196, 210
withania (*Withania somnifera*), 56, **161**, 186

woad, 35
women's health, 204–211. *See also* specific issues
wood leeks (ramps), 52
woolly lavender, 67
woolly (Bowle's) mint, 79
woolly thyme, 124
woolly yarrow, 131
World War I, 50, 89, 126
World War II, 97, 100, 122
worms, intestinal, 136
wormwood, 13
wound treatments
 aloe vera, 8
 calendula, 24, 194
 chamomile, 28
 comfrey, 35
 devil's claw, 172
 gotu kola, 57, 201
 horsetail, 61
 lavender, 68
 nasturtium, 129
 New Zealand flax, 48, **48**
 plantain, 88
 salad burnet, 108
 scented geranium, 110
 tea-tree oil, 195
 yarrow, 131
wrinkle treatments, 8, 98

Y

yarrow, 131, **131**, 174, 175
yellow (ladies' or Our Lady's) bedstraw, 117, **117**
yellow coneflower, 40
yellow dock, 112, 181
yellow echinacea, 40
Yellow Emperor's Inner Classic, The, 160
yellow flag, 63
yerba buena, 109
yin and yang, 160–161
yi zhi, 49

Z

za'atar, 76, **76**
za'atar rumi, 109
Zanthoxylum americanum, 136, **137**
Zeus, 69
Zingiber cassumar, 54
Zingiber mioga, 54
Zingiber officinale (ginger), 54, **54**, 169, 179, 198–199, **198**, 199, 210, 211
Ziziphus jujuba, **160**

Acknowledgments

The publishers wish to thank the following individuals, companies and organizations for their help during the preparation of *The Essential Book of Herbs*.

Alex Jordan. Ambiance Interiors. Australia Post. Australia's Open Garden Scheme. Baytree. Beclau.
Blooms the Chemist. British Sweets & Treats. Buds and Bowers Florist. Bulb. Bunnings. Chee Soon and Fitzgerald.
Chinese Ginseng & Herb Co. Coles Supermarkets Australia. Darling Street Health Centre. Domayne.
Dong Nam A & Co. Doug Up on Bourke. Dulux.
Feed Ya Face. Flower Power Nursery. Freedom Furniture. Fruitique. Funkis Swedish Forms.
Gardens R Us. Glebe Newsagency. Glenmore House. Gold's World of Judaica. Gundabluey.
Herb Herbert. House of Herbs and Roses.
Julie Pilcher Flowers. Mint Condition. Moss River. Mr Copy. Mrs Red and Sons. New Directions Australia. No Chintz. Oishi. Oxford Art Supplies.

Paper Couture. Paper2. Pet City. Price War. Reln Plastics. Rococo Flowers.
Ros Andrews. Royal Botanic Gardens, Sydney. Sally Stobo. Spotlight Australia.
St. Vincent de Paul Society. Stark's Kosher Supermarket. Summers Floral Woollahra.
Swadlings Timber and Hardware. The Barn Café and Grocery.
The Floral Decorator. The Nut Shop. The Tegal Garden. Urban Balcony. Vicino.
Wholefoods House. Yarrow's Pharmacy.

Special thanks to Fratelli Fresh for the supply of fresh herbs
for photography.
Herbie's Spices. Ici et La.

Photography Credits

Adobe Stock: 22 *bl* vaivirga; 64 *r* kazmulka; 72 *tr* LianeM; 79 *bl* Manfred Ruckszio; 96 *tr* jbphotographylt; 97 *tl* Josie Elias; 119 *tr* amy_lv; 127 *bl* Golden Shark; 132 *br* ub-foto; 133 *tr* Sergey; 133 *tl* Jivko Nakev; 133 *cl* Peter Flindell; 133 *bl* wiha3; 133 *cr* viperagp; 135 *cr* hjschneider; 135 *cl* Alferova Evgeniya (Geshas); 137 *cl* paolofusacchia; 137 *bl* MarinoDenisenko; 137 *tr* Maria Brzostowska; 154 *bc* Branimir; 163 *tc* Estelle R; 163 *tr* espy3008; 171 *br* Rafael Ben-Ari; 172 *tr* Alexander Ruiz; 195 *tr* lovelyday12; 205 *c* Madeleine Steinbach; 213 *cr* espy3008

Carole Orbell: 63 *tr*; 90 *bl*; 91 *tr*

ChrisLJones Photo: 11 *tr*; 52 *br*; 56 *tr*; 80 *bl*; 88 *t*; 110 *bl*; 112 *bl*; 141 *ct*; 141 *cb*; 141 *tr*; 141 *br*; 144 *tc*; 144 *c*; 144 *bc*; 144 *br*; 149 *all*

Dreamstime: 134 *br* Jonathan Wilson; 135 *tl* Elena Ray

Forest & Kim Starr: 92 *tr*; 192 *tr*; 133 *br*

istock photos*: 32 *full pg.* jclegg; 38 *bl* lelepado; 55 *tr* mahroch; 68 *tr* BonyChan; 69 *bl* JCOLL/(C) Caplio R2 User; 89 *tr* meltonmedia; 89 *bl*; 93 *bl* esemelwe; 135 *br* Diana Lundin; 136 *cr* Roger Whiteway; 137 *tl* istera; 137 *cr* benoitrousseau; 163 *tl* pjclark; 170 *tr* briannolan; 173 *tr* Douglas Atmore; 175 *t* Floortje; 178 *tr* Anna Milkova/adel66; 183 *tr* Hanis; 185 *br* Andreas G. Karelias/ akarelias; 187 *tr* mahroch; 189 *t* gardendata; 203 *tr*; 212 *tl* LindaCharlton

Photolibrary: 42 *bl* Bob Gibbons

Premaphotos / Alamy Stock Photo: 127 *tr*

Shutterstock: 3 *tc* angelakatharina; 6 *full pg.* Robyn Mackenzie; 9 *tr* Pavel_D; 10 *tr* Alexandr Kanōkin; 12 *tr* indykb; 14 *tr* Volosina; 16 *tr* B.G. Photography; 18 *r* Madlen; 20 *bl* Maslov Dmitry; 21 *bc* Savo Ilic; 23 *tl* Sergey Yasenev; 24 *tr* Kardash; 26 *tr* bonchan; 28 *tr* almgren; 34 *bl* Sergey Ryzhov; 34 *tr* Gala_Kan; 35 *tr* Florin Capilnean; 37 *tr* attem; 41 *bl* trabachar; 43 *full pg.* LianeM; 44 *tr* Le Do; 46 *bl* Franco Deriu; 46 *tr* DeSerg; 48 *tr* Dionisvera; 48 *bl* Ant Clausen; 55 *bl* diyanski; 59 *br* NinaM; 60 *bl* matin; 61 *tr* dabjola; 61 *br* Scisetti Alfio; 66 *tr* blueeyes; 69 *tr* Kuttelvaserova Stuchelova; 72 *bl* urbanbuzz; 72 *br* Madlen; 73 *tr* Elena Schweitzer; 75 *tr* Sue Smith; 78 *t* dabjola; 81 *br* Monkey Business Images; 83 *c* Chirtsova Natalia; 85 *full pg.* Kenneth Keifer; 92 *br* Peter Zijlstra; 94 *bl* bonchan; 97 *br* Vaide Seskauskiene; 99 *full pg.* Douglas Freer; 104 *bl* LianeM; 114 *br* s74; 115 *tr* miltonia; 116 *tl* Marek Mierzejewski; 117 *bl* Artem and Olga Sapegin; 117 *tr* Simone Voigt; 118 *bl* Seroff; 119 *br* eye-blink; 120 *tr* Scorpp; 121 *full pg.* Worldpics; 122 *tr* Tamara Kulikova; 128 *tr* Irina Burakova; 128 *bc* kredo; 129 *bl* Larisa Lofitskaya; 129 *tr* Happy Stock Photo; 129 *br* Joerg Unfried; 131 *br* Volosina; 132 *tr* Gumirov; 132 *c* Ivan Tihelka; 134 *tr* Nata Naumovec; 134 *cr* Matauw; 136 *br* Arnold John Labrentz; 177 *br* matin; 186 *bc* Lim Yong Hian; 188 *br* Katinkah; 197 *tr* LianeM; 208 *tr* Bertold Werkmann

Tafel: 174 *c*; 179 *tr*; 180 *tr*; 182 *tr*; 184 *tr*; 191 *tr*; 193 *tr*; 201 *tl*

Any images not listed above are RD owned.